HANDBOOK OF

Critical Care Drug Therapy

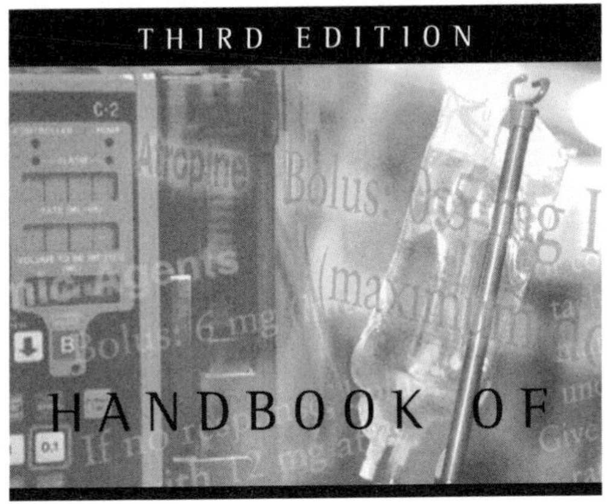

Critical Care Drug Therapy

Gregory M. Susla
Anthony F. Suffredini
Dorothea McAreavey
Michael A. Solomon
William D. Hoffman
Paul Nyquist
Frederick P. Ognibene
James H. Shelhamer
Henry Masur

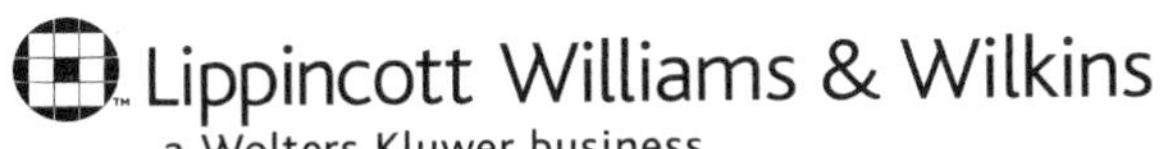
Lippincott Williams & Wilkins
a Wolters Kluwer business
Philadelphia • Baltimore • New York • London
Buenos Aires • Hong Kong • Sydney • Tokyo

Acquisitions Editor: Brian Brown
Developmental Editor: Louise Bierig
Project Manager: Jennifer Harper
Manufacturing Coordinator: Kathleen Brown
Marketing Manager: Angela Panetta
Designer: Stephen Druding
Production Services: TechBooks
Printer: R.R. Donnelley, Crawfordsville

530 Walnut Street
Philadelphia, PA 19106 USA
LWW.com

Printed in the USA

Library of Congress Cataloging-in-Publication Data

Handbook of critical care drug therapy / editors, Gregory M. Susla . . . [et al.]– 3rd ed.
p. ; cm.
Includes index.
ISBN 0-7817-9763-2 (soft : alk. paper)
ISBN 978-0-7817-9763-4
1. Drugs—Handbooks, manuals, etc. 2. Chemotherapy—Handbooks, manuals, etc.
3. Critical care medicine—Handbooks, manuals, etc. I. Susla, Gregory M. II. Title.
[DNLM: 1. Drug Therapy—Handbooks. 2. Critical Care—Handbooks. 3. Pharmaceutical Preparations—administration & dosage—Handbooks. WB 39 H23567 2006]
RM301.12.H37 2006
615.5′8—dc22 2006002920

Care has been taken to confirm the accuracy of the information presented and to describe generally accepted practices. However, the authors, editors, and publisher are not responsible for errors or omissions or for any consequences from application of the information in this book and make no warranty, expressed or implied, with respect to the currency, completeness, or accuracy of the contents of the publication. Application of this information in a particular situation remains the professional responsibility of the practitioner.

The authors, editors, and publisher have exerted every effort to ensure that drug selection and dosage set forth in this text are in accordance with current recommendations and practice at the time of publication. However, in view of ongoing research, changes in government regulations, and the constant flow of information relating to drug therapy and drug reactions, the reader is urged to check the package insert for each drug for any change in indications and dosage and for added warnings and precautions. This is particularly important when the recommended agent is a new or infrequently employed drug.

Some drugs and medical devices presented in this publication have Food and Drug Administration (FDA) clearance for limited use in restricted research settings. It is the responsibility of the health care provider to ascertain the FDA status of each drug or device planned for use in their clinical practice.

To purchase additional copies of this book, call our customer service department at (800) 638-3030 or fax orders to (301) 223-2320. International customers should call (301) 223-2300. Visit Lippincott Williams & Wilkins on the Internet: http://www.lww.com. Lippincott Williams & Wilkins customer service representatives are available from 8:30 am to 6 pm, EST, Monday through Friday, for telephone access.

10 9 8 7 6 5 4 3 2

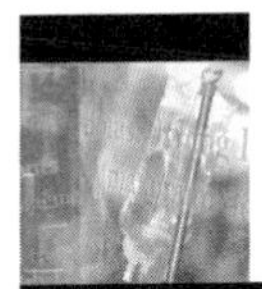

Preface

The Handbook of Critical Care Drug Therapy was originally developed because of the complexity of critical care medicine. Remembering the drugs of choice for arrhythmias, infections, electrolyte emergencies, sedation, poisonings, and a host of other problems has always been daunting. With new drugs and increasingly complex patients, the tasks of choosing the proper drug and selecting the proper dose and dilution are even more challenging.

The third edition of *The Handbook of Critical Care Drug Therapy* continues to be a quick reference for drug therapy and ideally should be used when rapid decisions need to be made, before more extensive information can be obtained. It is not a textbook and should not substitute for more detailed descriptions regarding how to manage specific syndromes. Also, it should not be used in the absence of clinical judgment: its recommendations are general and must be considered in light of a patient's specific circumstances.

In this era of computer access, we continue to find a hard copy book to be an essential element in the deep pockets of our white coats, along with our stethoscopes. This handbook can be accessed from a handheld device, but when quickly writing orders, scanning a hard copy can still be quick and useful.

There are three basic types of tables in this book: (a) tables that list disease entities and indicate therapies of choice; (b) tables that list drugs and highlight their indications, advantages, and disadvantages; and (c) three appendices that provide information on how to mix and administer parenteral drugs, how to convert intravenous medications to equivalent oral doses, and guidelines for dosing oral drugs commonly prescribed for critically ill patients.

Generic drug names are used throughout the book. However, every drug is listed in the index both by generic and brand names so that reference to the appropriate tables and pages can be made regardless of which drug name the clinician is familiar with.

This work represents the clinical experience of the authors in the Critical Care Medicine Department at the National Institutes of Health, in critical care units at other hospitals in the Washington–Baltimore area, and at institutions where staff members have been recruited for leadership positions. The authors of this book are physicians with board certification in critical care medicine, pulmonary medicine, cardiology, infectious diseases, anesthesiology, and allergy/immunology, supplemented by an extraordinarily knowledgeable and versatile critical care pharmacist.

We hope that the content and organization of this book prove useful for care providers from a wide variety of specialties and backgrounds who care for hospitalized patients, especially those in medical, surgical, and neurological critical care units.

Greg Susla
Anthony F. Suffredini
Henry Masur

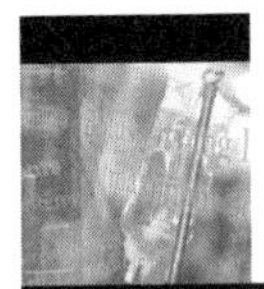

Contributors

William D. Hoffman, MD
Director, Cardiac Surgical Intensive Care Unit
Massachusetts General Hospital
Boston, Massachusetts

Henry Masur, MD, FCCM, FACP
Chief, Critical Care Medicine Department
National Institutes of Health
Bethesda, MD

Dorothea McAreavey, MD, FACC
Staff Clinician
Director, Critical Care Medicine Fellowship Program
Critical Care Medicine Department
National Institutes of Health
Bethesda, Maryland

Paul Nyquist, MD
Assistant Professor of Neurology and Anesthesia and Critical Care
John Hopkins University Medical School
Baltimore, Maryland

Frederick P. Ognibene, MD, FCCM, FACP
Director, Office of Clinical Research Training Program and Medical Education
Director, Clinical Research Training Program
Attending Physician, Critical Care Medicine Department
National Institutes of Health
Bethesda, Maryland

James H. Shelhamer, MD
Deputy Chief, Critical Care Medicine Department
National Institutes of Health
Bethesda, Maryland

Michael A. Solomon, MD, FACC
Staff Clinician
Critical Care Medicine Department
National Institutes of Health
Bethesda, Maryland

Anthony F. Suffredini, MD, FCCM
Senior Investigator, Critical Care Medicine Department
National Institutes of Health
Bethesda, MD

Gregory M. Susla, PharmD, FCCM
Pharmacy Manager
VHA, Inc.
Frederick, Maryland

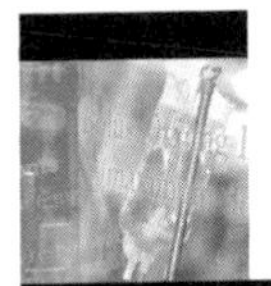

Contents

CHAPTER 1

Acute Resuscitation

CHAPTER 2

Anesthesia: Analgesia, Sedation, and Neuromuscular Blockade

CHAPTER 3

Cardiovascular Therapies

CHAPTER 4

Pulmonary Therapies

CHAPTER 5

Renal, Electrolyte, and Acid Base Disturbances

CHAPTER 6

Endocrine Therapies

CHAPTER 7

Gastroenterology, Liver, and Nutrition Therapies

CHAPTER 8

Hematologic Therapies

CHAPTER 9

Neurologic and Psychiatric Therapeutics

CHAPTER 10

Infectious Diseases

CHAPTER 11

Allergy

CHAPTER 12

Poisonings

CHAPTER 13

Drug Monitoring

APPENDIX 1

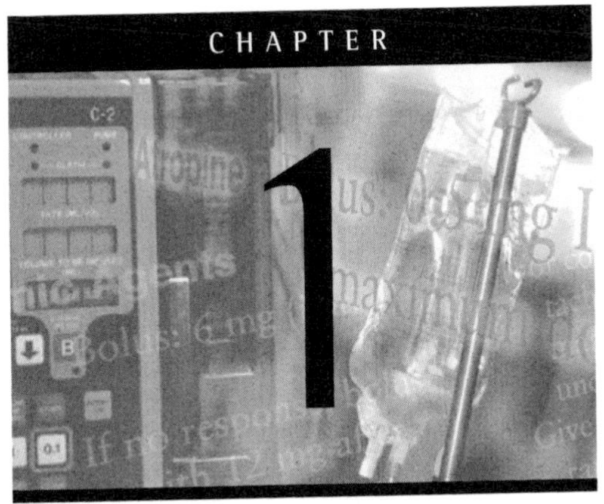

Acute Resuscitation

TABLE 1.1. Advanced Cardiac Life Support (ACLS) Drugs

Drug	Dosage	Indications/Comments
Antiarrhythmic Agents		
Adenosine	Bolus: 6 mg (initial) If no response, bolus with 12 mg after 1–2 min	For conversion of PSVT unresponsive to vagal maneuvers
	May repeat 12 mg once	Give as rapid IV bolus over 1–3 s followed by rapid 10 ml fluid bolus May use lower bolus dose of 3 mg if central line available Be cautious of interactions with theophylline (inhibits adenosine), dipyridamole (potentiates adenosine), other drugs that prolong QT interval
Amiodarone	300 mg bolus IV	For VF or pulseless VT refractory to shock; may repeat 150 mg bolus IV in 3–5 min
	150 mg bolus IV followed by 1 mg/min for 6 h and then 0.5 mg/min for 18 h	For stable wide-complex tachycardia up to a total dose 2.2 g IV per 24 h May use for narrow complex atrial arrhythmias, as adjunct to cardioversion Monitor for bradycardia and hypotension
Atropine	Bolus: 0.5 mg IV (maximum dose 3 mg)	For either absolute (<60 beats/min) or "relative" symptomatic bradycardia
	Bolus: 1 mg IV	For bradycardia manifesting with lack of pulse, PEA or for asystole unresponsive to epinephrine May repeat dose every 3–5 min up to maximum dose 0.04 mg/kg or 3 mg
	ETT bolus: 2–3 mg	Dilute up to 10 ml in NS or sterile water (IV preferred)
Diltiazem	0.25 mg/kg IV bolus over 2 min (typically 15–20 mg) May repeat once 0.35 mg/kg IV bolus over 2 min (typically 25 mg) Maintenance infusion 5–15 mg/h	For control of ventricular response rate in A fib or A flutter, or other narrow complex tachycardia Do not use in wide-complex tachycardia Negative inotrope, so use cautiously if reduced LV function
Epinephrine	Bolus: 1 mg IV (10 ml of 1:10,000 solution)	Therapy for refractory VF or pulseless VT; dose should be followed by CPR and defibrillation; may be repeated every 3–5 min Initial therapy for PEA; may repeat every 3–5 min Initial therapy for asystole; may repeat every 3–5 min
	ETT bolus: 2–2.5 mg	Dilute up to 10 ml NS or sterile water (IV preferred)
	Infusion: 2–10 μg/min	For treatment of symptomatic bradycardia unresponsive to atropine and transcutaneous pacing; alternative to dopamine
Ibutilide	1 mg IV infused over 10 min; may be repeated after 10 min Use 0.01 mg/kg if <60 kg	For treatment of atrial arrhythmias Monitor electrolytes and EKG Increased risk for torsade de pointes if elderly, abnormal LV function (EF <35%), or electrolyte abnormalities Monitor for 4–24 h

(continued)

TABLE 1.1. *(continued)* **Advanced Cardiac Life Support (ACLS) Drugs**

Drug	Dosage	Indications/Comments
Isoproterenol	Infusion: 2–10 μg/min	May be used in torsade de pointes unresponsive to magnesium Use with extreme caution; at higher doses is considered harmful *Not indicated* for cardiac arrest, hypotension, or bradycardia
Lidocaine	Bolus: 1–1.5 mg/kg	For wide-complex tachycardia of uncertain type, stable VT, and control of PVCs May be followed by boluses of 0.5–0.75 mg/kg every 5–10 min up to a total of 3 mg/kg Only bolus therapy should be used in cardiac arrest
	Bolus: 1.5 mg/kg	Initial bolus dose suggested when VF is present and defibrillation and epinephrine have failed
	ETT bolus: 2–4 mg/kg	Diluted in 5–10 ml NS or sterile water (IV preferred)
	Infusion: 2–4 mg/min	Continuous infusion used after bolus dosing and following return of perfusion to prevent recurrent ventricular arrhythmias Because half-life of lidocaine increases after 24–48 h, the dose should be reduced after 24 h, or levels should be monitored Therapeutic levels 1–4 mg/L Full-loading dose but reduced infusion rate in patients with low cardiac output, hepatic dysfunction, or age over 70 years
Magnesium sulfate	Bolus: 1–2 g (8–16 mEq)	Drug of choice in patients with torsade de pointes For recurrent/refractory VT or VF For hypomagnesemia For ventricular dysrhythmias, administer over 1–2 min For magnesium deficiency, administer over 60 min
	Infusion: 0.5–1 g/h (4–8 mEq/h)	Rate and duration of infusion determine clinically or by magnitude of magnesium deficiency
Naloxone	0.4 mg IV is typical	Onset of action 2 min IV and <5 min IM/SC
	May give 0.4–2 mg IV every 2–3 min (maximum dose is 10 mg) 0.8 mg IM/SC	Duration of action ~45 min Give 0.4 mg diluted in 10 ml NS or sterile water slowly to avoid abrupt narcotic withdrawal Hypertension/hypotension, cardiac arrhythmias, pulmonary edema may occur Monitor for reoccurring respiratory depression because narcotics typically last longer than naloxone
	ETT: 2 mg diluted in 5–10 ml NS or sterile water	(IV preferred)

(continued)

TABLE 1.1. *(continued)* **Advanced Cardiac Life Support (ACLS) Drugs**

Drug	Dosage	Indications/Comments
Procainamide	12–17 mg/kg; administer at rate of 20–30 mg/min (maximum 50 mg/min)	Infrequently used Recommended when lidocaine is contraindicated or has failed to suppress ventricular ectopy Use higher dose for more urgent situations (VF or pulseless VT) Maximum total dose of 17 mg/kg Continue bolus dosing until arrhythmia suppressed, hypotension, QRS complex widens by 50% of original width, or maximum total dose given Rapid infusion may cause precipitous hypotension Avoid in patients with QT prolongation (>30% above baseline) or torsade de pointes
	Infusion: 1–4 mg/min	Continuous maintenance infusion, after return of perfusion, to prevent recurrent arrhythmias Reduce dosage in renal failure Monitor blood levels in patients with renal failure or with >24-h infusion Therapeutic levels: procainamide 4–10 mg/L, N-acetyl-procainamide (NAPA) 10–20 mg/L
Vasopressin	40 U IV push, one dose only	As an alternative to 1st or 2nd dose epinephrine in refractory VF, asystole, or PEA resume epinephrine after 3–5 min
Verapamil	Bolus: 2.5–10 mg over 2–3 min May repeat in 15–30 min prn Max. cumulative = 20 mg	Only give to patients with narrow complex PSVT unresponsive to adenosine Diltiazem (0.25 mg/kg) is an alternative to verapamil because it has less negative inotropy
Vasopressor Agents		
Dopamine (For other vasopressors, Table 3.8)	Infusion: 2–20 μg/kg/min	For treatment of symptomatic bradycardia unresponsive to atropine and transcutaneous pacing For treatment of hypotension that is unresponsive to volume
Electrolyte Agents		
Sodium bicarbonate	Bolus: 1 mEq/kg	Helpful in limited clinical conditions: hyperkalemia, bicarbonate responsive acidosis, tricyclic antidepressant overdose Not recommended in the majority of arrest cases (hypoxic lactic acidosis) Guide therapy by blood gas analyses and calculated base deficit to minimize iatrogenic alkalosis

A fib, atrial fibrillation; A flutter, atrial flutter; CPR, cardiopulmonary resuscitation; EF, ejection fraction; EKG, electrocardiogram; ETT, endotracheal tube; IM, intramuscular; IV, intravenous; LV, left ventricular; MI, myocardial infarction; NS, normal saline; PEA, pulseless electrical activity; PSVT, paroxysmal supraventricular tachycardia; PVC, premature ventricular contraction; SC, subcutaneous; VF, ventricular fibrillation; VT, ventricular tachycardia

TABLE 1.2. Shock—General Management

Type of Shock	Initial Therapy	Subsequent Therapy
Cardiogenic Shock		
Massive myocardial infarction	Supplemental oxygen, aspirin, pain relief, venous access Therapy for ACS (see Table 3.1) Optimize volume status and ensure adequate preload Treat arrhythmias Consider RHC Determine need for inotropic agents; diuretics; vasodilators; vasopressors (see Tables 3.3 and 3.8) Consider mechanical ventilation	Early IAB, coronary arteriography, and revascularization by PCI or bypass grafting Consider thrombolytic agent if cardiac catheterization not possible
Nonischemic cardiomyopathy	Therapy as above, but omit therapy for ACS	Consider IAB or assist devices as bridge to transplantation Consider reversible causes (e.g., acute valvular regurgitation requiring emergent valve replacement, thyrotoxicosis)
Oligemic Shock		
Massive hemorrhage, severe dehydration, etc.	For hemorrhage, large bore peripheral or central venous access Volume resuscitation with packed RBCs and 0.9% NaCl Consider use of blood warmer If large bleed, consider platelets, fresh frozen plasma, and supplemental calcium For dehydration, volume resuscitation with 0.9% NaCl or Ringer's lactate Monitor electrolytes and coagulation	If hypotension persists despite volume resuscitation, consider: possibility of coexisting sepsis, tamponade, or ACS; RHC; inotropic and/or vasopressor agents Consult GI and surgery for massive gastrointestinal hemorrhage (see Table 7.1)
Extracardiac Obstructive Shock		
Tamponade	Confirm suspected diagnosis with echocardiography and/or RHC, temporize by increasing filling pressures with bolus 0.9% NaCl IV; support BP	Urgent percutaneous pericardiocentesis, surgical pericardiotomy, or pericardial window
Massive pulmonary embolism	Correct hypoxemia; administer heparin or LMWH; thrombolytic therapy (alteplase 100 mg IV over 2 h); give inotropic support such as dobutamine for right heart strain and failure	Consider percutaneous catheter suction thrombectomy or thoracotomy with embolectomy Consider IVC filter long term See Table 4.11
Tension pneumothorax	Emergent needle or tube thoracostomy	Tube thoracostomy

(continued)

TABLE 1.2. *(continued)* **Shock-General Management**

Type of Shock	Initial Therapy	Subsequent Therapy
Distributive Shock		
Septic shock	Emergent broad-spectrum antibiotics IV after blood cultures; IV crystalloid; if shock persists, consider RHC If shock persists despite adequate preload, add dopamine 2–20 μg/kg/min; or norepinephrine 2 μg/min	Consider vasopressin in refractory shock Stress dose steroids hydrocortisone 100 mg IV q8h; optional fludrocortisone 50 μg po qd Consider baseline cortisol level prior to glucocorticosteroid therapy and corticotropin stimulation test Role of drotrecogin alfa is not established[a]
Anaphylaxis	Epinephrine 0.3–0.5 mg for severe symptoms of hypotension, bronchospasm, or laryngeal edema; given as 0.3–0.5 ml of 1:1,000 SC or 0.5–1.0 ml of 1:10,000 solution IV; also give diphenhydramine 50 mg IV; repeat 25–50 mg IV q4h prn; abnormal permeability causes intravascular depletion, which should be corrected with volume	Cautious administration prn of additional epinephrine; give corticosteroids (Methylprednisolone 60 mg IV or equivalent) and cimetidine 300 mg IV q12; these will have delayed rather than immediate effect For persistent symptoms and patient on β-blockers, give glucagon 1 mg IV
Hypoadren-alism	Administer dexamethasone 4 mg IV q6h together with fluids	To confirm diagnosis, perform corticotropin stimulation test (dexamethasone will not interfere); draw baseline cortisol level, give 250 μg IV cosyntropin, and repeat cortisol level 30 min later
Neurogenic	Trendelenburg position; fluids	If hypotension persists, consider vasopressors (e.g., phenylephrine or metaraminol)

ACS, acute coronary syndrome; BP, blood pressure; GI, gastroenterology; IAB, intra-aortic balloon; IV, intravenous; IVC, inferior vena cava; LMWH, low molecular weight heparin; PCI, percutaneous coronary intervention; RBCs, red blood cells; RHC, right heart catheterization

[a]While some authors recommend drotrecogin alfa (recombinant activated protein C) in highly selected patients with a high risk of death (Apache score of ≥25) and a low risk of bleeding, the role of drotrecogin alfa in septic patients has not been clearly established. It has no effect or is harmful in septic patients with Apache score of <25, in surgical patients with single organ dysfunction, and in pediatric sepsis. The risk of serious bleeding including intracerebral hemorrhage is increased in patients receiving drotrecogin alfa.

TABLE 1.3. Hypovolemic Shock

	Mild	Moderate	Severe	Life-threatening
% loss of intravascular volume	≤10–15%	15–30%	30–40%	>40%
Loss of intravascular volume (cc)	<700–800	800–1500	1500–2000	>2000
Mean arterial pressure	WNL	WNL	Reduced	Reduced
Heart rate	80–100	101–119	120–140	>140
Pulse pressure	WNL/ increased	101–119 Reduced	120–140 Reduced	>140 Reduced
Respirations (breaths/min)	15–20	21–29	30–35	>35
Capillary refill test[a]	≤2 s	>3 s	>3 s	>3 s
Urine output (cc/h)	≥30	20–30	5–15	Oliguria
Mental status	Uneasy	Mild anxiety	Anxiety or confusion	Confusion or lethargy
Volume replacement	Crystalloid	Crystalloid	Crystalloid or blood if indicated	Crystalloid or blood if indicated

[a]The capillary refill test is performed by pressing on the fingernail or the hypothenar eminence. The test is not valid in hypothermic patients.
WNL = within normal limits.

TABLE 1.4. Crystalloids and Colloids

Fluid	Dosage	Comments
0.9% NaCl	≥500 ml[a]	Hyperchloremic metabolic acidosis secondary to vigorous NaCl replacement may occur
Lactated Ringer's	≥500 ml[a]	Balanced electrolyte composition (mEq/L): Na^+ 130, K^+ 4, Ca^{++} 3, Cl^- 110, lactate 28 Not compatible with blood products
5% albumin	0.25–1 g/kg[b]	Each 250 ml contains 12.5 g albumin
25% albumin	0.25–1 g/kg[b]	Each 100 ml contains 25 g albumin
6% hetastarch	≥500 ml[a]	Chemically modified glucose polymer Large doses, especially >1500 ml, can lead to coagulopathies (factor VIII deficiency) and platelet abnormalities Can cause artifactual hyperamylasemia Anaphylactoid reactions have occurred Total amount should not exceed 1,500 ml/d (20 ml/kg) Cautious use in cardiac bypass and septic patients
6% hetastarch in lactated electrolyte injection	500–1,000 ml	Chemically modified glucose polymer Balanced electrolyte composition (mEq/L): Na^+ 143, K^+ 3, Ca^{++} 5, Cl^- 124, Mg^{++} 0.9, lactate 28, dextrose 0.99 g/L A volume expander used to support oncotic pressure and provide electrolytes Doses >1,500 ml are rarely required Can cause artifactual hyperamylasemia Use with caution in anticoagulated patients

[a]Most crystalloids are given in 500 ml aliquots as quickly as possible (i.e., over 10–15 minutes) to increase blood pressure or perfusion. If initial aliquot is not successful in increasing blood pressure, then repeat until hemodynamic stability or the addition of a vasopressor agent occur.
[b]Colloid has no proven outcome benefit in general ICU patients; it may have a role in hypotensive patients. Dextrans and gelatins are rarely used plasma expanders.

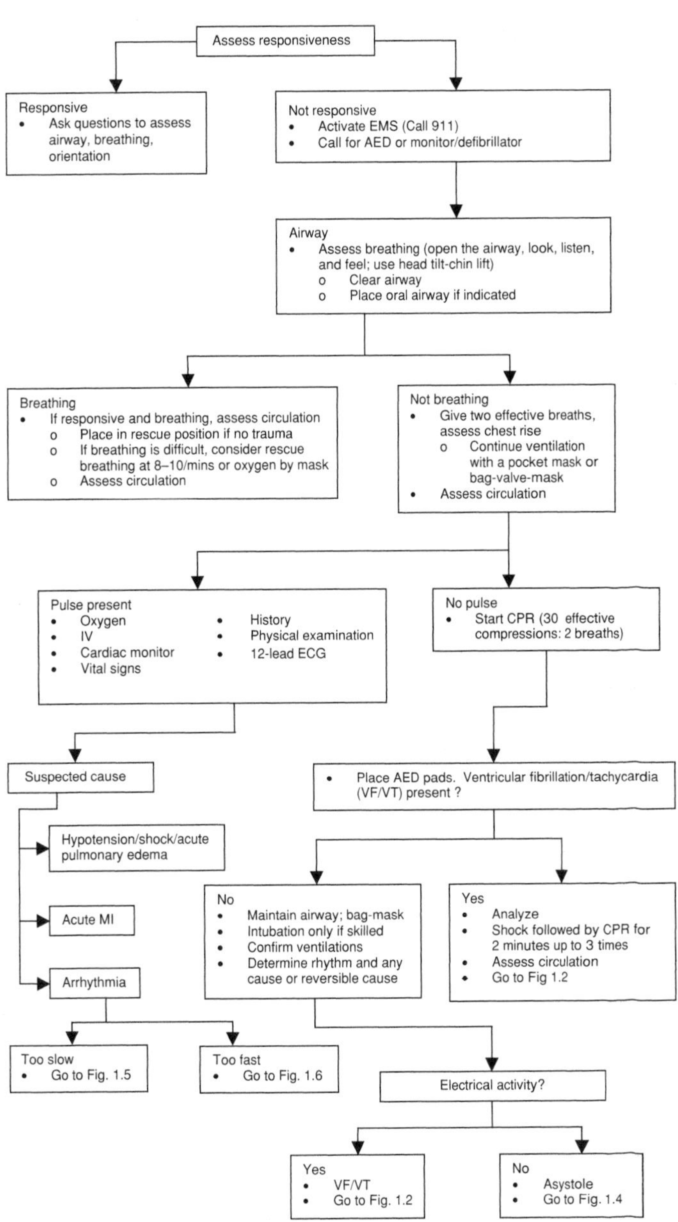

FIGURE 1.1. Universal Algorithm for Adult Emergency Cardiac Care

AED, automatic external defibrillator; CPR, cardiopulmonary resuscitation; ECG, electrocardiogram; EMS Emergency Management Service; IV, intravenous; MI, myocardial infarction (The American Heart Association in collaboration with the International Liaison Committee on Resuscitation: Guidelines 2000 for Cardiopulmonary Resuscitation and Emergency Cardiovascular Care Circulation 2000; 102: 8 Suppl I with permission; also adapted from Circulation 2005;Suppl III:1–130.)

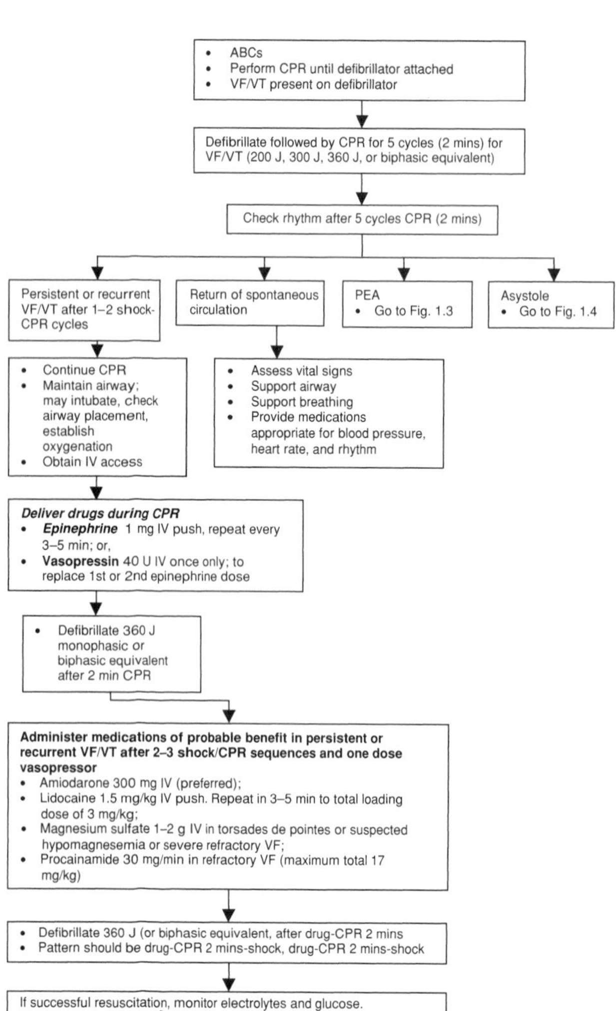

FIGURE 1.2. Algorithm for Ventricular Fibrillation (VF) and Pulseless Ventricular Tachycardia (VT)

ABC, airway breathing circulation; CPR, cardiopulmonary resuscitation; IV, intravenous; PEA, pulseless electrical activity

Give drugs typically at 3–5 minute intervals: Vasopressin 40 U IV single dose (wait 10 minutes before giving epinephrine)

(The American Heart Association in collaboration with the International Liaison Committee on Resuscitation: Guidelines 2000 for Cardiopulmonary Resuscitation and Emergency Cardiovascular Care. Circulation 2000; 102: 8 Suppl I, with permission; also adapted from Circulation 2005;Suppl III:1–130.)

PEA includes

- Electromechanical dissociation (EMD)
- Pseudo-EMD
- Idioventricular rhythms
- Ventricular escape rhythms
- Bradyasystolic rhythms
- Postdefibrillation idioventricular rhythms

- Effective CPR
- IV access
- Maintain airway; may intubate
- Assess blood flow using Doppler ultrasound

↓

Consider and treat possible causes
(Parentheses, possible therapies and treatments)

- Hypovolemia (volume infusion)
- Hypoxia (ventilation)
- Cardiac tamponade (pericardiocentesis)
- Tension pneumothorax (needle decompression)
- Hypothermia
- Massive pulmonary embolism (surgery, thrombolytics)
- Drug overdoses such as tricyclics, digitalis, β-blockers, calcium channel blockers
- Hyperkalemia/hypokalemia*
- Acidosis†
- Massive acute myocardial infarction

↓

- ***Epinephrine*** 1 mg IV push, repeat every 3–5 min
- ***Vasopressin 40 IU IV*** *once only, instead of 1st or 2nd epinephrine dose*

↓

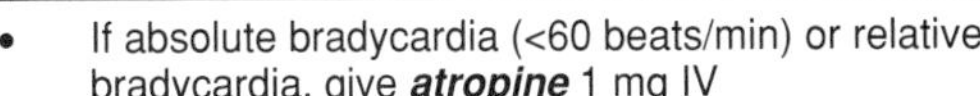

- If absolute bradycardia (<60 beats/min) or relative bradycardia, give ***atropine*** 1 mg IV
- Repeat every 3–5 min up to a total of 0.04 mg/kg

FIGURE 1.3. Algorithm for Pulseless Electrical Activity (PEA)

CPR, cardiopulmonary resuscitation; EMD, electromechanical dissociation; IV, intravenous
Class I: definitely helpful. Class IIa: acceptable, probably helpful. Class IIb: acceptable, possibly helpful. Class III: not indicated, may be harmful.
*Sodium bicarbonate 1 mEq/kg: is Class I: if patient has known pre-existing hyperkalemia.
†Sodium bicarbonate 1 mEq/kg: Class IIa: if known pre-existing bicarbonate-responsive acidosis; if overdose with tricyclic antidepressants; to alkalinize the urine in drug overdoses. Class IIb: if intubated and long arrest interval; upon return to spontaneous circulation after long arrest interval. Class III: hypoxic lactic acidosis.
(The American Heart Association in collaboration with the International Liaison Committee on Resuscitation: Guidelines 2000 for Cardiopulmonary Resuscitation and Emergency Cardiovascular Care. Circulation 2000; 102: 8 Suppl I with permission; also adapted from Circulation 2005;Suppl III:1–130.)

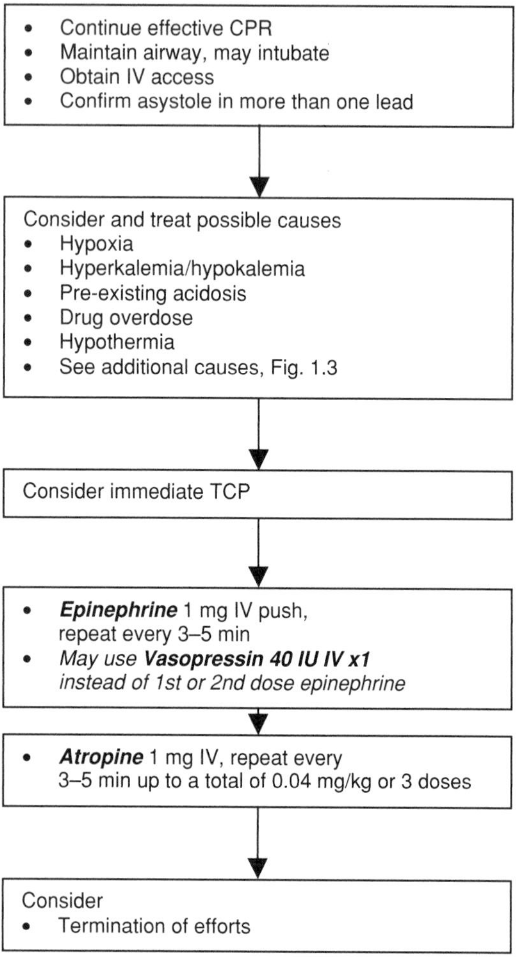

- Continue effective CPR
- Maintain airway, may intubate
- Obtain IV access
- Confirm asystole in more than one lead

↓

Consider and treat possible causes

- Hypoxia
- Hyperkalemia/hypokalemia
- Pre-existing acidosis
- Drug overdose
- Hypothermia
- See additional causes, Fig. 1.3

↓

Consider immediate TCP

↓

- ***Epinephrine*** 1 mg IV push, repeat every 3–5 min
- *May use **Vasopressin 40 IU IV x1** instead of 1st or 2nd dose epinephrine*

↓

- ***Atropine*** 1 mg IV, repeat every 3–5 min up to a total of 0.04 mg/kg or 3 doses

↓

Consider

- Termination of efforts

FIGURE 1.4. Asystole Treatment Algorithm

CPR, cardiopulmonary resuscitation; IV, intravenous; TCP, transcutaneous pacing

(The American Heart Association in collaboration with the International Liaison Committee on Resuscitation: Guidelines 2000 for Cardiopulmonary Resuscitation and Emergency Cardiovascular Care. Circulation 2000; 102: 8 Suppl I, with permission; also adapted from Circulation 2005;Suppl III:1–130.)

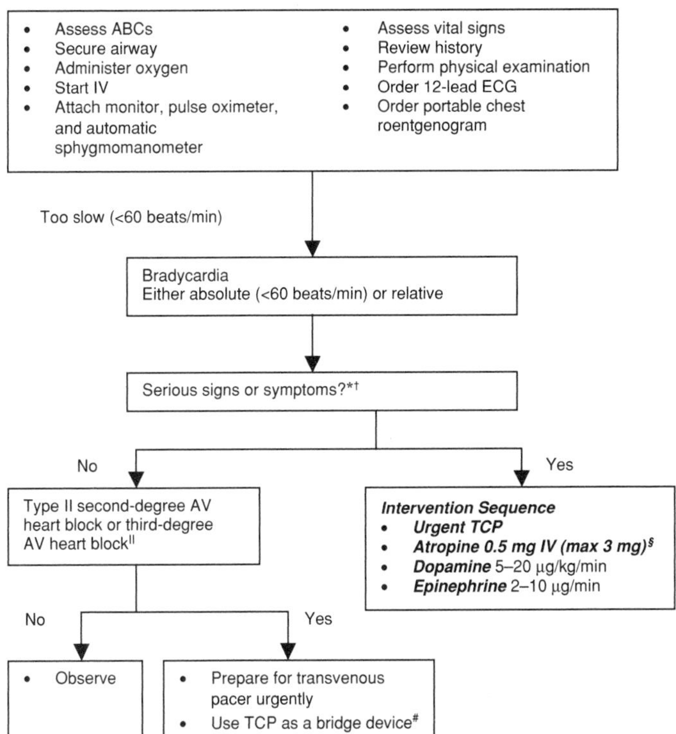

FIGURE 1.5. Bradycardia Algorithm (Patient not in Cardiac Arrest)

ABC, airway breathing circulation; AV, atrioventricular; BP, blood pressure; ECG, electrocardiogram; HF, heart failure; IV, intravenous; MI, myocardial infarction; TCP, transcutaneous pacemaker

*Serious signs or symptoms must be related to the slow rate. Clinical manifestations include: symptoms (chest pain, shortness of breath, decreased level of consciousness) and signs (low BP, shock, pulmonary congestion, HF, acute MI).

†Do not delay TCP while awaiting IV access or for atropine to take effect if patient is symptomatic.

§Atropine should be given in repeat doses in 3–5 minutes up to total of 0.04 mg/kg.

‖Never treat third-degree heart block plus ventricular escape beats with lidocaine.

#Verify patient tolerance and mechanical capture. Use analgesia and sedation as needed.

(The American Heart Association in Collaboration with the International Liaison Committee on Resuscitation: Guidelines 2000 for Cardiopulmonary Resuscitation and Emergency Cardiovascular Care. Circulation 2000; 102: 8 Suppl I, with permission; also adapted from Circulation 2005;Suppl III:1–130.)

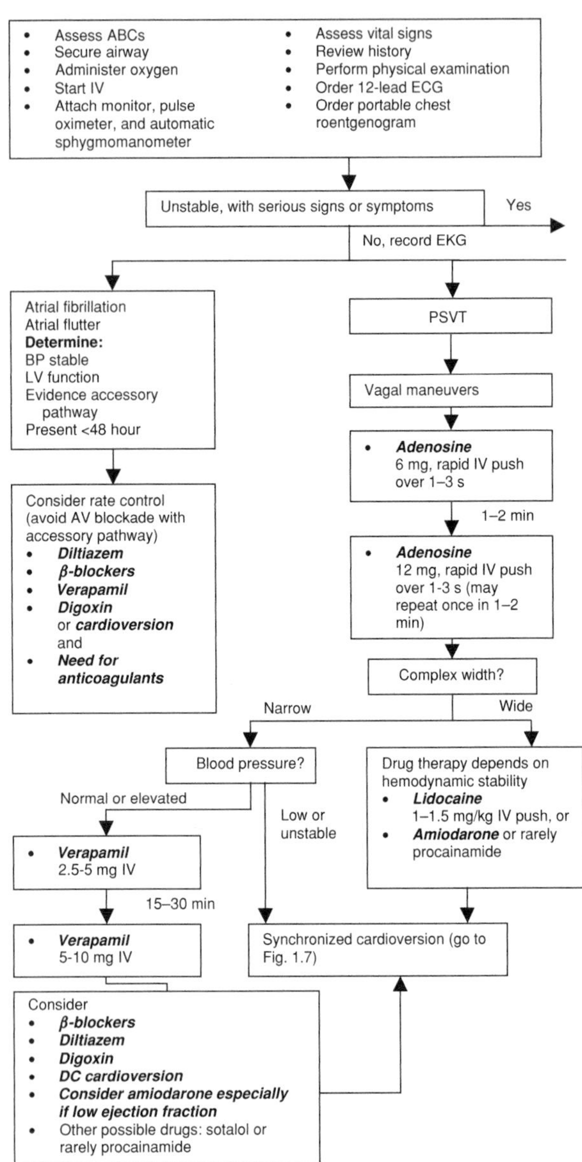

FIGURE 1.6. Tachycardia Algorithm

ABC, airway breathing circulation; AV, atrioventricular; BP, blood pressure; DC, direct current; ECG, electrocardiogram; LV, left ventricular; PSVT, paroxysmal supraventricular tachycardia; VT, ventricular tachycardia
(The American Heart Association in collaboration with the International Liaison Committee on Resuscitation: Guidelines 2000 for Cardiopulmonary Resuscitation and Emergency Cardiovascular Care. Circulation 2000; 102: 8 Suppl I, with permission; also adapted from Circulation 2005;Suppl III:1–130.)

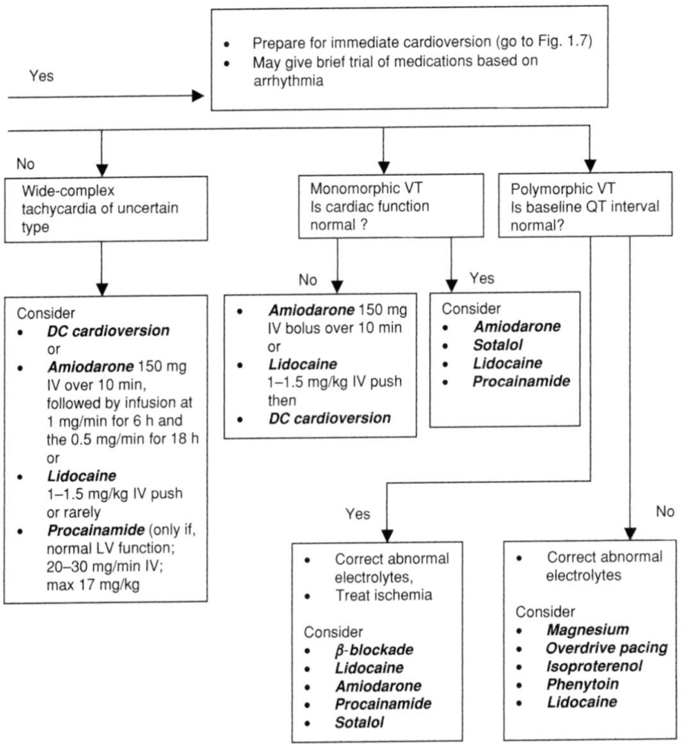

FIGURE 1.6. Tachycardia Algorithm (continued)

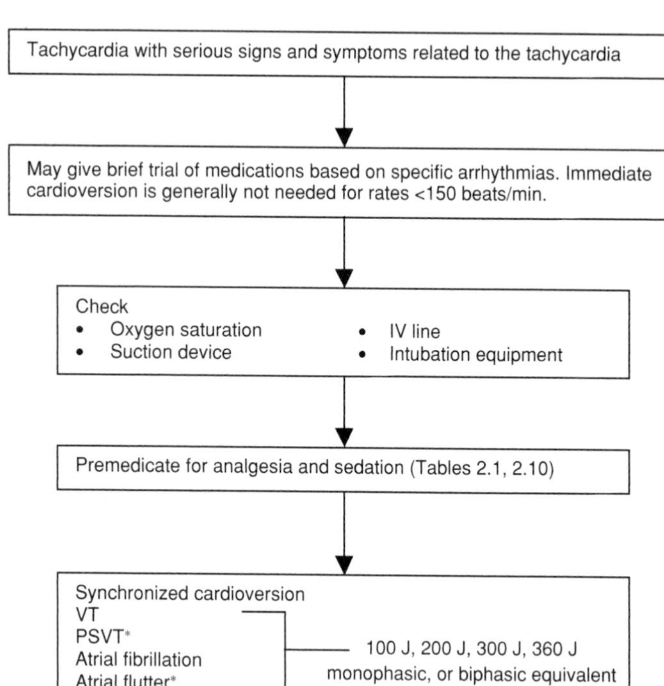

FIGURE 1.7. Electrical Cardioversion Algorithm (Patient not in Cardiac Arrest)

IV, intravenous; VT, ventricular tachycardia
*PSVT (paroxysmal supraventricular tachycardia) and atrial flutter often respond to lower energy levels (start with 50 J)
(The American Heart Association in collaboration with the International Liaison Committee on Resuscitation: Guidelines 2000 for Cardiopulmonary Resuscitation and Emergency Cardiovascular Care. Circulation 2000; 102: 8 Suppl I, with permission; also adapted from Circulation 2005;Suppl III:1–130.)

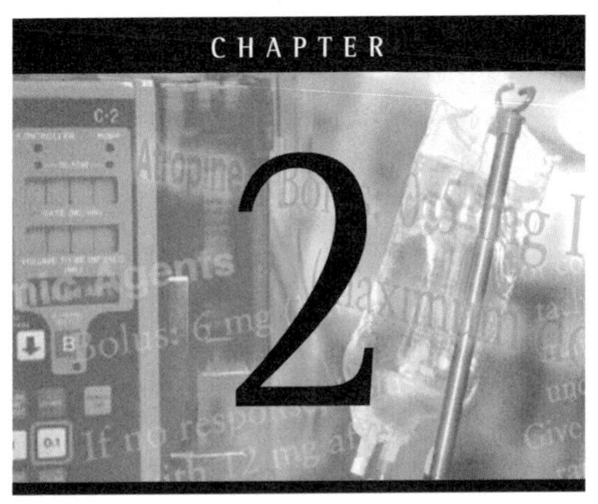

CHAPTER 2

Anesthesia: Analgesia, Sedation, and Neuromuscular Blockade

TABLE 2.1. Commonly Used Agents for Intravenous Sedation/Anesthesia

Drug	Initial IV Dosage[a]	Maintenance Infusion[a]	Comments
Barbiturates			
Pentobarbital	5–20 mg/kg Onset: <1 min Duration: 15 min	1–4 mg/kg/h	Infuse loading dose over 2 h Rapid administration produces hypotension and hemodynamic instability
Thiopental	3–4 mg/kg Onset: 10–20 s Duration: 5–15 min	Not applicable	Alkaline solution; decreases cardiac index
Benzodiazepines			
Diazepam	0.1–0.2 mg/kg Onset: 1–3 min Duration: 1–2 h	Not applicable	Active metabolite with long half-life (desmethyldiazepam) contributes to activity
Lorazepam	0.04 mg/kg Onset: 5–15 min Duration: 1–6 h	0.02–0.1 mg/kg/h	No active metabolites Approximately 5 times more potent than diazepam
Midazolam	0.025–0.035 mg/kg Onset: 1–3 min Duration: 30 min–3 h	0.05–5 μg/kg/min	Elderly patients may develop apnea when midazolam is administered with narcotics Approximately 3–4 times more potent than diazepam Active metabolites accumulate in renal failure Unpredictable elimination in critically ill patients (e.g., shock, liver failure) Initial dose: 0.5–1 mg and titrate to effect in 0.5–2 mg increments
Other			
Propofol	1–2 mg/kg Onset: <1 min Duration: 5–10 min	5–75 μg/kg/min	Generally a rapid recovery Pain on injection is common with peripheral administration Hypotension may occur especially with rapid bolus in hypovolemic or elderly patients Propofol may increase serum triglyceride levels when used at high infusion rates; take caution when using in patients with pancreatitis Doses of propofol of 5 mg/kg/h have been associated with cardiac failure and death Safety of propofol has not been established for ICU sedation of children Propofol contains 1.4 mmol of $PO_4^{=}$ /100 ml

(continued)

TABLE 2.1. *(continued)* **Commonly Used Agents for Intravenous Sedation/Anesthesia**

Drug	Initial IV Dosage[a]	Maintenance Infusion[a]	Comments
Dexmedetomidine	1 μg/kg IV over 10 min	0.2–0.7 μg/kg/h for up to 24 h	Alpha-2 adrenergic agonist with analgesic and sedative properties Numerous cardiovascular effects including brady- and tachyarrhythmias, hyper- and hypotension, and atrioventricular block Does not produce respiratory depression
Ketamine	1–2 mg/kg (or 5–10 mg/kg IM) Onset: <1 min Duration: 5–10 min	9–45 μg/kg/min	Usually preserves airway reflexes Central sympathetic stimulation; hypertension; tachycardia; advantageous in hypovolemic patients Tachyphylaxis is rare
Etomidate	0.3–0.4 mg/kg Onset: <1 min Duration: 3–5 min	Not recommended Produces adrenal suppression in continuous infusion	Minimal cardiovascular effects Myoclonic muscle movements Pain on IV injection
Remifentanil	0.05 μg/kg Onset: <1 min Duration: <4 min	0.05–0.2 μg/kg/min	Ultrashort acting narcotic analgesic; used primarily as an intraoperative analgesic; elimination not dependent on liver or kidney function

CNS, central nervous system; ICU, intensive care unit; IM, intramuscular; IV, intravenous
[a]Bolus doses and rates of infusion should be individualized to provide the desired level of sedation with consideration of potential hemodynamic compromise. Doses should generally be reduced for elderly and hypovolemic patients. It may be beneficial to wake patients daily and assess their CNS function during maintenance infusions to determine the minimal dose required for sedation.

TABLE 2.2. Tracheal Intubation Techniques

Technique	Clinical Setting	Procedural Features	Cautions
All listed below	Indications: Upper airway obstruction Airway protection Tracheal toilet	Minimum required monitoring ECG, BP, pulse oximetry Prepare patient for 100% O_2 Establish IV access for rapid administration of resuscitative drugs and fluids if necessary Equipment and drugs: Oxygen bag-mask ventilation equipment, monitors, suction laryngoscopes, ETT, stylettes, cuff, syringes, "Code Blue" cart Anesthetics: Neuromuscular blocking agents, Sedative/hypnotic agents	Aspiration Loss of airway Dental damage Trauma to airway Hemodynamic compromise
Awake	Anticipated difficult laryngoscopy Full stomach Minimize risk of airway loss as a result of sedation or neuromuscular blockade Assessment and protection of neurologic function in cervical spine instability Can be performed without depression of airway reflexes Requires patient cooperation	Patient maintains airway and ventilation	Vomiting from pharyngeal stimulation Hypertension and tachycardic response to intubation is undesirable in certain clinical settings (e.g., myocardial ischemia, cerebral or aortic aneurysm) Topical anesthesia of larynx or nerve blocks of larynx obtunds protective airway reflexes
Conscious: Oral	Allows largest diameter ETT	Topical anesthesia of pharynx or pharyngeal nerve blocks Intubation with direct vision	

(continued)

TABLE 2.2. *(continued)* **Tracheal Intubation Techniques**

Technique	Clinical Setting	Procedural Features	Cautions
Conscious: Blind nasal		Apply vasoconstrictor and topical anesthetic to nasal mucosa Gently dilate nasal passage with soft nasal airways Gently advance ETT from nose to trachea during inhalation	Nasal bleeding, avoid in coagulopathic patients Sinusitis Avoid in craniofacial trauma
Fiberoptic (oral or nasal)		Consider administering an antisialagogue (glycopyrrolate 0.2 mg IV) Topical anesthetic and vasoconstrictor (for nasal) Insert bronchoscope through ETT and directly into trachea Advance ETT over bronchoscope and remove bronchoscope	
Not Awake	Uncooperative patients Preexisting loss of consciousness (e.g., cardiac arrest, heavy sedation) Blunts tachycardic and hypertensive response Minimizes unpleasantness of procedure		Risk of apnea, aspiration, airway loss
Unsedated uncon-scious	Cardiac arrest	Bag-mask ventilation until intubation equipment available Immediate oral laryngoscopy and intubation	
Rapid-sequence: oral (see Table 2.3)	Full stomach or risk of aspiration in a patient without an anatomically difficult airway for laryngoscopy	Administration of sedative and neuromuscular blocking agents Cricoid pressure Rapid intubation after onset of neuromuscular blockade Check ETT placement Remove cricoid pressure	Risk of airway loss Hemodynamic compromise may result from sedation or positive pressure ventilation

(continued)

TABLE 2.2. *(continued)* **Tracheal Intubation Techniques**

Technique	Clinical Setting	Procedural Features	Cautions
Reintubation	Nonfunctioning ETT (e.g., cuff leak) Placement of an ETT with different features (e.g., larger diameter)	Sedate and administer neuromuscular blockade	Chronically intubated patients may have swelling or traumatic changes of larynx making reintubation difficult Patients who are dependent on high oxygen concentrations or PEEP may become hypoxemic
Direct vision extubation and reintubation	Laryngoscopy possible	Perform laryngoscopy with existing ETT in place If glottis is visualized, remove existing ETT and replace with new one	Loss of airway
Styletted reintubation[a]	Difficult laryngoscopy anticipated	Insert stylette into existing ETT Remove ETT without removing stylette Insert new ETT over stylette	

BP, blood pressure; ETT, endotracheal tube; ECG, electrocardiogram; IV, intravenous; PEEP, positive end-expiratory pressure

[a]Refers to specific intubating stylettes and not to those routinely used to stiffen ETT during routine intubation.

TABLE 2.3. Suggested Drugs for Rapid Sequence Intubation

Drug	Dosage	Comment
Sedatives/Anesthetics		
Thiopental	3–4 mg/kg IV	Reduce dose in elderly and hemodynamically unstable patients (0.25–1 mg/kg) May produce hypotension and hemodynamic instability Blunts intracranial hypertensive response to intubation and is useful in hemodynamically stable patients with elevated ICP
Ketamine	1–2 mg/kg IV 4–10 mg/kg IM	Useful in hypovolemic patients as this drug tends to support the circulation; may rarely produce myocardial depression Produces hypertension, tachycardia, and elevates ICP; therefore, avoid in patients with myocardial ischemia, severe hypertension, or intracranial mass lesions
Etomidate	0.3–0.4 mg/kg IV	Hemodynamic stability Patients often have benign nonpurposeful muscle movements during induction which may be blunted by low doses of fentanyl (50–100 μg)
Propofol	1–2.5 mg/kg IV	Reduce dose in elderly and hemodynamically unstable patients (0.25–0.5 mg/kg) May produce hypotension and hemodynamic instability
Muscle Relaxants[a]		
Cisatracurium	0.15–0.2 mg/kg IV	Slower in onset than succinylcholine Less histamine release than atracurium Hemodynamic stability Duration of action is dose-dependent (30 min–1 h)
Rocuronium	0.6–1.2 mg/kg IV	Reported as most rapid onset of nondepolarizing neuromuscular blocking drugs (60–90 s) Not recommended in Caesarean section patients Hemodynamic stability Duration of action is dose dependent (30 min–1 h)
Succinylcholine	1 mg/kg IV	Depolarizing agent Because of rapidity of onset, drug of choice unless specifically contraindicated (see Table 2.4) Duration of action ≅10 min for patients with normal pseudocholinesterase activity
Vecuronium	0.1–0.28 mg/kg	Slower onset than succinylcholine Hemodynamic stability Duration of action is dose dependent (30 min–1 h)

ICP, intracranial pressure; IM, intramuscular; IV, intravenous
[a] For most clinical situations, cost may be the overriding consideration when choosing among the available nondepolarizing muscle relaxants.

TABLE 2.4. Neuromuscular Blockade—Bolus Dosing

Agent	Dosage	Onset/Duration	Comments
Depolarizing Relaxant			
Succinylcholine[a]	Bolus: 1–2 mg/kg	Onset: 1 min Duration: 10 min	Prolonged effect in pseudocholinesterase deficiencies Contraindications: family history of malignant hyperthermia, neuromuscular disease, hyperkalemia, open eye injury, major tissue injury (burns, trauma, crush); increased intracranial pressure; not indicated for routine use in children or adolescents Side effects: bradycardia (especially in children), tachycardia, increased serum potassium
Nondepolarizing Relaxants			
Atracurium	Bolus: 0.5 mg/kg	Onset: 2 min Duration: 30–40 min	Rapid injection of atracurium bolus doses >0.6 mg/kg releases histamine and may precipitate asthma or hypotension Metabolized in the plasma by Hofmann elimination and ester hydrolysis Duration not prolonged by renal or liver failure; otherwise, see comments with vecuronium
Cisatracurium	Bolus: 0.15 mg/kg	Onset: 2 min Duration: 30–40 min	Less histamine release than racemic atracurium (see above) Metabolism and duration of action similar to atracurium
Mivacurium	Bolus: 0.15 mg/kg followed in 30 s by 0.10 mg/kg	Onset: 1.5 min Duration: 25 min	Inject over 30 s May cause histamine release Metabolized by pseudocholinesterase
Rocuronium	Bolus: 0.6 mg/kg	Onset: 1 min Duration: 30–40 min	Metabolized by liver, prolonged duration in hepatic failure Duration not prolonged by renal failure Used when succinylcholine is contraindicated or not preferred

(continued)

TABLE 2.4. *(continued)* **Neuromuscular Blockade—Bolus Dosing**

Agent	Dosage	Onset/Duration	Comments
Vecuronium	Bolus: 0.1 mg/kg	Onset: 2 min Duration: >30–40 min	Metabolized by liver; duration not significantly prolonged by renal failure
	Bolus: 0.28 mg/kg	Onset: 60 s Duration: 100 min	Used when succinylcholine is contraindicated or not preferred No cardiovascular effects

[a]The pharmaceutical companies that manufacture succinylcholine have changed the package insert to indicate that the drug should not be used routinely in children, except for airway emergencies, risk of aspiration, and special situations. This practice is a response to reported complications including malignant hyperthermia, masseter muscle rigidity, rhabdomyolysis, and sudden cardiac arrest in children with undiagnosed myopathies.

TABLE 2.5. Neuromuscular Blockade—Maintenance Dosing

Agent	Maintenance Dosage	Duration	Comments
Short Acting			
Mivacurium	0.01–0.1 mg/kg Infusion: 9–10 μg/kg/min	15 min	Metabolized by pseudocholinesterase
Intermediate Acting			
Atracurium[a]	0.08–0.10 mg/kg Infusion: 5–9 μg/kg/min	15–25 min	Elimination independent of renal or hepatic function
Cisatracurium[a]	0.01–0.02 mg/kg Infusion: 1–2 μg/kg/min	15–25 min	Elimination independent of renal or hepatic function
Rocuronium[a]	0.1–0.2 mg/kg Infusion: 10–12 μg/kg/min	10–25 min	Metabolized primarily by the liver Active metabolite significantly less potent than parent compound
Vecuronium[a]	0.01–0.15 mg/kg Infusion: 1 μg/kg/min	15–25 min	Bile is main route of elimination Minimal dependence on renal function, although active metabolite accumulates in renal failure
Long Acting			
Doxacurium[a]	0.005–0.01 mg/kg Infusion: 0.25 μg/kg/min (not generally recommended)	35–45 min	Cardiovascular stability Predominantly renal elimination significant accumulation in renal failure
Pancuronium[a]	0.01–0.015 mg/kg Infusion: 1 μg/kg/min (not generally recommended)	25–60 min	Tachycardia (vagolytic effect) Active metabolite accumulates in renal failure

[a] Prolonged infusions of neuromuscular blocking drugs have been associated with undesirable prolongation of neuromuscular blockade and myopathy. When indicated, general guidelines for use of infusions include: (a) periodic monitoring of neuromuscular function (train-of-four stimulation) during administration of infusions, and (b) infusions should be stopped every 24–28 hours to allow recovery of function. Concurrent steroid administration may increase likelihood of this complication.

TABLE 2.6. Reversal of Nondepolarizing Neuromuscular Blocking Drugs

Drug	Dosage	Onset/Duration	Comments
Neostigmine-Glycopyrrolate	25–75 μg/kg 5–15 μg/kg	Onset: 3–8 min Duration: 40–60 min	
Pyridostigmine-Glycopyrrolate	100–300 μg/kg 5–15 μg/kg	Onset: 2–5 min Duration: 90 min	Must be used to reverse long-acting neuromuscular blocking agents (i.e., doxacurium, pancuronium)
Edrophonium-Atropine	500–1000 μg/kg 10 μg/kg	Onset: 30–60 s Duration: 10 min	Rapid onset; not useful for deep blockade

Use lower doses to reverse minimal blockade, maximum doses for deep blockade. The anticholinergic agent must be given to block undesired muscarinic effects of anticholinesterase drug; this applies even when the patient has a baseline tachycardia. Reversal of neuromuscular blockade is associated with a high incidence of transient arrhythmias.

TABLE 2.7. Topical Anesthetics

Agent	Concentration	Use	Comments
Cocaine	4%	Topical to nares and nasopharynx prior to nasal intubation	Vasoconstriction Controlled substance
Lidocaine	1–4%	Solution: oropharynx, tracheobronchial tree Viscous: nasal and oral pharynx	Vasodilating, therefore must be used in conjunction with a vasoconstrictor during nasal intubation Dilute solutions (1–2%) may be nebulized and inhaled to provide anesthesia for bronchoscopy Total dose should be less than 400 mg Large doses have been associated with methemoglobinemia
Eutectic Mixture Lidocaine and Prilocaine (EMLA)		Apply to skin for 1 h prior to procedures involving skin puncture	Application to inflamed skin may increase absorption Ineffective when rubbed into skin

TABLE 2.8. Local Anesthetics for Infiltration and Nerve Blocks

Drug	Concentration (Maximum Dose)	Use	Features
Lidocaine	0.5% (400 mg without epinephrine; 500 mg with epinephrine)	Local infiltration	Relatively short duration Epinephrine prolongs block and decreases peak levels
Lidocaine	1–2% (400 mg without epinephrine; 500 mg with epinephrine)	Nerve blocks	Short duration Epinephrine prolongs block and decreases peak levels
Bupivicaine	0.25–0.75% (2.5–3 mg/kg)	Nerve blocks Epidural	Long duration, slow onset Addition of epinephrine may not prolong block but may decrease systemic absorption

Avoid epinephrine-containing solutions in areas supplied by end-arteries (e.g., fingers, toes, penis). Nerve blocks should be performed by personnel trained in the procedures and in treatment of local anesthetic toxicity.

TABLE 2.9. Comparison of Narcotic Analgesics

Drug	Route/Equivalence[a]	Onset of Action (min)	Peak Analgesic Effect (min)	Duration of Action (h)
Alfentanil	IM: 1 mg	IV: 1–2	IV: 1–2	IV: 0.25
Codeine	PO: 200 mg IM: 120 mg	PO: 30–45 IM: 10–30	PO: 60–120 IM: 30–60	PO: 4–6 IM: 4
Fentanyl	IM: 0.1 mg	IV: <1 IM: 7–5	IV: 1–2 IM: N/A	IV: 0.5–1 IM: 1–2
Hydromorphone	PO: 7.5 mg IM: 1.5 mg	PO: 30 IM: 30–60 IV: 10–15	PO: 90–120 IM: 4–5 IV: <20	PO: 4 IV: 2–3
Levorphanol	PO: 4 mg IM: 2 mg	PO: 10–60 IM: N/A	PO: 90–120 IM: 30–60 IV: <20	PO: 4–5 IM: 4–5 IV: 4–5
Meperidine	PO: 300 mg IM: 75 mg	PO: 15 IM: 10–15 IV: 1	PO: 60–90 IM: 60–120 IV: 15–30	PO: 2–4 IM: 2–4 IV: 2–4
Methadone	PO: 20 mg IM: 10 mg	PO: 30–60 IM: 10–20 IV: N/A	PO: 90–120 IM: 60–120 IV: 15–30	PO: 4–6[b] IM: 4–5[b] IV: 3–4[b]
Morphine	PO: 60 mg IM: 10 mg	PO: 15–60 IM: 10–30 IV: <1	PO: 60–120 IM: 30–60 IV: 20	PO: 4–5 IM: 4–5 IV: 4–5
Oxycodone	PO: 30 mg	PO: 15–30	PO: 60	PO: 4–6
Propoxyphene	Toxic[c]	PO: 15–60	PO: 120	PO: 4–6
Remifentanil[d]	IV: 0.05–0.15 μg/kg	IV: <1	IV: <1	IV: 3–4 min
Sufentanil	IM: 0.01–0.02 mg	IV: <1	IV: 1–2	IV: 0.25–1

IM, intramuscular; IV, intravenous; PO, by mouth
[a] Dose in mg therapeutically equivalent to morphine 10 mg IM. IM doses are used to specify equivalent doses but are not recommended when IV access is available.
[b] Increases with repetitive dosing due to accumulation of drug and/or metabolites.
[c] Dose equivalent to 10 mg of morphine would be too toxic to administer.
[d] Remifentanil is suitable for IV infusion only.

TABLE 2.10. Parenteral Analgesic Agents

Drug	Bolus Dosage	Continuous Infusion	Comments
Alfentanil	10–25 μg/kg	0.5–3 μg/kg/min	Safe to use in renal failure because lack of active metabolites
Codeine	15–60 mg	N/A	Usually effective for mild to moderate pain Recommended in renal failure
Fentanyl	25–50 μg	50–100 μg/h	Slows heart rate Chest wall rigidity can occur Increased half-life with continuous infusions
Hydromorphone	1–4 mg	N/A	Reserved for patients who are tolerant to and are receiving high doses of opiates Recommended in renal failure
Ketorolac	15–60 mg IV followed by 15–30 mg IV q6h		Parenteral NSAID; lower doses in elderly patients; especially useful for orthopedic pain; reversible platelet dysfunction; associated with acute renal failure when given for more than 5 d Advantage over opioids: no hemodynamic effects, respiratory depression, or ileus Combined IV/IM/PO therapy limited to 5 d
Levorphanol	2 mg	N/A	Optimal IV dose has not been established Avoid in patients with increased intracranial pressure, asthma, acute alcoholism
Meperidine	25–100 mg	5–35 mg/h	Highly lipid soluble Accumulation of neurotoxic (convulsant) normeperidine metabolite in renal failure and in patients receiving large cumulative doses Avoid in patients receiving MAOI
Methadone	2.5–10 mg	N/A	Duration of action and half-life increases with repetitive dosing With repetitive doses, the dose should be lowered or the interval lengthened to avoid excessive narcosis
Morphine	2–10 mg	2–5 mg/h	Less lipid soluble versus fentanyl Histamine release with bolus doses may cause hypotension or, rarely, bronchospasm Active metabolite morphine-6-glucuronide accumulates in renal failure, producing enhanced narcosis
Remifentanil	0.05 μg/kg	0.0125–0.025 μg/kg/min	Ultrashort action may limit its use for pain Bolus doses are not recommended to treat postoperative pain IV tubing must be cleared after administration to avoid inadvertent bolus dose
Sufentanil	0.2–0.6 μg/kg	0.01–0.05 μg/kg/min	May allow for volume reduction in patients receiving large doses of continuous infusion narcotics

IV, intravenous; MAOI, monoamine oxidase inhibitor; NSAID, nonsteroidal anti-inflammatory drug

TABLE 2.11. Patient-Controlled Analgesia (PCA) Guidelines

	Morphine	Fentanyl	Hydromorphone
Standard dilution	2 mg/mL	20 μg/mL	0.5 mg/mL
Demand dose	1 mg	20 μg	0.2 mg
Initial lockout	6 min	6 min	6 min
Initial basal rate	0	0	0
Considerations	Generally, opioid of choice unless patient has renal insufficiency or is intolerant to morphine: nausea, vomiting, pruritus	Less accumulation may result in less confusion in elderly patients; preferred over morphine in patients with renal insufficiency to avoid accumulation of morphine metabolites	

For patients who report pain on PCA, first assess the frequency of self-dosing. If the patient is not self-dosing at least 3 times per hour, encourage him or her to dose more often. Failing that, give the patient a bolus dose (2–5 mg of morphine or equivalent) and increase the demand dose to 1.5 or 2 mg of morphine or equivalent. Finally, consider an adjuvant drug (ketorolac) or a low basal rate (0.5 mg/h of morphine or equivalent).

TABLE 2.12. Oral Analgesic Agents

Agent	Onset/Duration	Dosage	Comments
Narcotic			
Codeine	Onset: 15–30 min Duration: 4–6 h	30–60 mg q4h	
Codeine with acetaminophen 300 mg	Onset: 15–30 min Duration: 4–6 h	1–2 tablets q4h	Available with codeine 7.5 mg, 15 mg, 30 mg, or 60 mg
Oxycodone 5 mg	Onset: 15–30 min Duration: 4–6 h	5–10 mg q4h	Sustained release preparation, Oxycontin, has been associated with illegal abuse and diversion; deaths have resulted when the pills have been crushed and the powder inhaled
Oxycodone 5 mg with acetaminophen 325 mg	Onset: 15–30 min Duration: 4–6 h	1–2 tablets q4h	
Oxycodone HCl 4.5 mg plus oxycodone terephthalate 0.38 mg with aspirin 325 mg	Onset: 15–30 min Duration: 4–6 h	1–2 tablets q4h	
Propoxyphene napsylate 50 or 100 mg with acetaminophen 325 mg	Onset: 15–60 min Duration: 4–6 h	1–2 tablets q4h	
Propoxyphene 32 or 65 mg	Onset: 15–60 min Duration: 4–6 h	32–65 mg q4h	
Non-narcotic			
Acetaminophen	Onset: 0.5–1 h Duration: 3–6 h	325–650 mg q4h	
Aspirin	Onset: 0.5 h Duration: 3–6 h	325–650 mg q4h	
Choline magnesium salicylate	Onset: 30–60 min Duration: N/A	1000–2000 mg bid	500 mg = ASA 650 mg May monitor with salicylate levels Does not affect platelet aggregation Available as a liquid 500 mg/5 ml
Ibuprofen	Onset: 0.5 h Duration: 3–6 h	400–800 mg tid-qid	Reversible effect on platelet aggregation Available as a liquid 100 mg/5 ml
Ketorolac	Onset: 30–60 min Duration: 4–6 h	10 mg q4–6h	Reversible platelet effect Reduce dose in elderly patients Maximum oral dose 40 mg/day Indicated only as continuation therapy to parenteral ketorolac up to a maximum duration of 5 d of combined IV/IM/PO administration
Tramadol	Onset: 1 h Duration: 3–6 h	50–100 mg q4–6h	Reduce dose in patients with renal or liver failure

IV, intravenous; IM, intramuscular, PO, by mouth

TABLE 2.13. Oral Sedative-Hypnotic Agents

Agent	Onset	Usual Dosage	Half-Life	Comments
Benzodiazepines				
Alprazolam	Intermediate	Sedative: 0.25–0.5 mg PO tid	12–15 h	No active metabolites
Diazepam	Fast	Sedative: 2–10 mg PO bid-qid Pre-op medication: 5–10 mg PO 1 h before procedure	20–200 h	Active metabolites accumulate with chronic dosing and contribute to pharmacologic effect Available in a liquid dosage form (1 mg/ml and 5 mg/ml)
Lorazepam	Intermediate	Sedative: 0.5–3 mg PO bid-tid Hypnotic: 0.5–4 mg PO qhs Pre-op medication: 1–4 mg PO 1–2 h before procedure	10–20 h	No active metabolites Safe to use in liver disease Available in a liquid dosage form (2 mg/ml) Amnesia may be produced for as long as 4–6 h without excessive sedation when lorazepam is used as a pre-op medication
Midazolam	Fast	Pre-op medication: 0.5–0.75 mg/kg PO 1–2 h before procedure	3–6 h	Use high potency 5 mg/ml injectable form and dilute in 3–5 ml of fruit juice
Oxazepam	Slow	Sedative: 10–30 mg PO tid-qid Hypnotic: 10–30 mg PO qhs	5–20 h	No active metabolites
Temazepam	Intermediate	Sedative: N/A Hypnotic: 7.5–30 mg PO qhs	10–17 h	No active metabolites
Barbiturates				
Pentobarbital	Fast	Sedative: N/A Hypnotic: 100 mg PO qhs Pre-op medication: 100 mg PO 1–2 h before procedure	22 h	Geriatric or debilitated patients may react to usual doses with excitement, confusion, or mental depression; lower doses may be required in these patients
Secobarbital	Fast	Sedative: N/A Hypnotic: 100 mg PO qhs Pre-op medication: 200–300 mg PO 1–2 h before procedure	28 h	Geriatric or debilitated patients may react to usual doses with excitement, confusion, or mental depression; lower doses may be required in these patients
Other agents				
Chloralhydrate	Intermediate	Sedative: 250 mg PO tid after meals Hypnotic:500–1000 mg PO qhs Pre-op medication: 25–75 mg/kg up to 2 g PO 1 h before procedure	8 h TCE	Active metabolite TCE Available in liquid (10 mg/ml) and suppository (500 mg) dosage forms
Diphenhydramine	Slow	Hypnotic: 25–50 mg PO qhs	1–4 h	Available in a liquid dosage form (12.5 mg/5 ml) Half-life is prolonged in patients with liver disease

(continued)

TABLE 2.13. *(continued)* **Oral Sedative-Hypnotic Agents**

Agent	Onset	Usual Dosage	Half-Life	Comments
Eszopiclone	Fast	Sedative: N/A Hypnotic: 1–3 mg PO qhs		Reduce to 1 mg in elderly patients, patients receiving CYP3A4 inhibitors and patients with severe hepatic disease
Zaleplon	Fast	Sedative: N/A Hypnotic: 5–10 mg PO qhs	1 h	The initial dose should be reduced to 5 mg in elderly and in patients with liver disease
Zolpidem	Fast	Sedative: N/A Hypnotic: 5–10 mg PO qhs	2.5 h	No active metabolites An initial dose of 5 mg should be used in patients with liver disease
Amitriptyline	Slow	25–100 mg qhs		Sedating tricyclic antidepressant Contraindicated in acute recovery phase of myocardial infarction
Quetiapine	Intermediate	25–100 mg qhs		Sedating dibenzothiazepine antiphychotic May result in orthostatic hypotension or tachyarrhythmias Anticholinergic effects (dry mouth, constipation)

PO, by mouth; TCE, trichloroethanol

TABLE 2.14. Malignant Hyperthermia—Therapy

Typical Presentation

Setting: Intraoperative or early postoperative.
Clinical: Tachycardia, tachypnea, ventricular arrhythmias, muscle rigidity, fever
Laboratory: Combined respiratory and metabolic acidosis, hyperkalemia, hypercalcemia, myoglobinuria, elevation in creatine phosphokinase.

Protocol for treatment

Discontinue triggering drug (succinylcholine, inhalational anesthetic).
Hyperventilate with 100% oxygen.
Dantrolene 2.5 mg/kg IV repeated every 5–10 min as dictated by the clinical situation. Although 10 mg/kg is often reported as a maximum total dose, more dantrolene may be needed.
Follow usual guidelines for treatment of metabolic acidosis, hyperkalemia (calcium has not been investigated in this setting), hyperthermia (external ice, gastric lavage), disseminated intravascular coagulation, prevention and treatment of myoglobinuric renal failure.
Procainamide as needed for arrhythmias refractory to general measures. Avoid calcium channel blockers in conjunction with dantrolene.
For health care providers having questions on patient management, the Malignant Hyperthermia Association of the United States operates a hot line: 1-800-644-9737.

IV, intravenous

TABLE 2.15. Neuroleptic Malignant Syndrome

Typical Presentation
Setting: Most cases within 30 days of antipsychotic (neuroleptic) drug administration (incidence ~0.07–0.4%) or withdrawal of dopamine agonist (e.g., levodopa, amantadine). Viewed as extreme extrapyramidal adverse effect versus idiosyncratic drug reaction related to antidopaminergic effects in central nervous system. Increased risk in highly agitated restrained patient.
Clinical Presentation: Hyperthermia caused by muscle rigidity, vasoconstriction, and possibly central nervous system effect. Dehydration, mental status changes (obtundation), autonomic instability (tachycardia, oscillations in blood pressure).
Laboratory: Elevated serum creatine phosphokinase, leukocytosis, metabolic acidosis.
Protocol for treatment
Discontinue antipsychotics if muscle rigidity impairs breathing or swallowing.
Control temperature (cooling blankets, ice baths, antipyretics; avoid NSAID because of renal effects), correct fluid and electrolyte disturbances.
Anticholinergics (if temperature <38.9°C): benztropine (up to 8 mg/d, PO, IM, IV), may worsen hyperthermia.
Dopamine agonists (if temperature >38.9°C): amantadine 200–300 mg/d PO, bromocriptine 7.5–75 mg/day PO, carbidopa/levodopa 300–800 mg/d PO.
Dantrolene 4–8 mg/kg/d PO/IV.

IV, intravenous; IM, intramuscular, PO, by mouth

Cardiovascular Therapies

TABLE 3.1. Treatment of Acute Coronary Syndromes (Unstable Angina, Non-ST Segment Elevation, and ST Segment Elevation Myocardial Infarction)

- All patients with ACS are candidates for antiplatelet and antithrombin therapies.
- STEMI are candidates for reperfusion therapy (fibrinolytic or catheter-based).
- NSTEMI are not candidates for fibrinolytic reperfusion agents but should receive catheter-based therapy when applicable.
- In treating ACS attention should also be paid to exacerbating factors such as fever, anemia, hypoxemia, hypertension, hypotension, and arrhythmias.
- If chest pain or hypotension remains refractory, intra-aortic balloon counterpulsation should be considered.
- In general, patients with ACS should undergo diagnostic coronary arteriography to evaluate for left main disease, triple vessel disease, proximal LAD disease or lesions amenable to PCI.
- Cocaine-induced ACS should be treated with intravenous nitroglycerin and a calcium channel blocker (e.g., diltiazem, verapamil) and coronary arteriography should be considered. There is evidence that β-adrenergic blockade can enhance cocaine-induced coronary artery vasoconstriction.

Agent	Dosage	Indications	Comments
MONA (Morphine, O_2, NTG, ASA)	See below	All patients with ACS.	Bedrest, IV access, telemetry, obtain serial ECGs and cardiac enzymes
Morphine sulfate	Initially 2–4 mg IV then increments of 2–8 mg IV q5–15 min prn pain	If pain not relieved with NTG then give until pain and anxiety relief is obtained or hypotension occurs	Reduces sympathetic tone; reduces preload; reduces myocardial O_2 demand
Oxygen	Initially 4 L/min by nasal cannula or 28% by venti-mask (adjust to maintain SaO_2 >90%)	Maximize O_2 delivery to ischemic myocardium	SaO_2 should be maintained over 90% and preferably over 95%
Nitrates (Contraindicated in patients on sildenafil or other PDE 5 inhibitors and patients with RV infarctions)			
Nitroglycerin	SL: 0.4 mg q5min ×3 Spray: 1–2 metered sprays (0.4 mg NTG/spray) onto or under the tongue; may repeat in 3–5 min, ×3 IV: 20 μg/min then titrate to effect (pain relief and/or to lower BP 10% to 20% if not hypotensive) Topical: 1–2 inches of 2% ointment q6h or equivalent patches	Nitrate preparations for acute use; initial pain relief; coronary vasodilation; reduces preload (predominant) and afterload	Causes headache; may increase myocardial O_2 demand by causing unintended tachycardia or hypotension; rapid tachyphylaxis
Isosorbide dinitrate	10–60 mg PO q4–6h	Useful for chronic management	Daily nitrate-free interval may ameliorate tachyphylaxis to antianginal effects

(continued)

TABLE 3.1. *(continued)* **Treatment of Acute Coronary Syndromes (Unstable Angina, Non-ST Segment Elevation, and ST Segment Elevation Myocardial Infarction)**

Agent	Dosage	Indications	Comments
Antiplatelet, Antithrombin, and Fibrinolytic Agents			
Aspirin (ASA)	Immediate: 162–325 mg tablet (chewed or ground up) then 75–162 mg PO qd PCI: 75–325 mg prior to (300–325 mg at least 2 h and preferably 24 h before PCI if not on daily ASA) then 325 mg qd for at least 1 m if BMS, 3 m if sirolimus-eluting and 6 m if paclitaxel-eluting then 75–162 mg indefinitely	All patients with ACS without ASA allergy Effective for primary and secondary MI prevention	Irreversibly inhibits prostaglandin cyclo-oxygenase, preventing formation of platelet aggregating factor thromboxane A2 Immediate antiplatelet effect; reduces mortality
Clopidogrel	ACS: Initially 300 mg PO then 75 mg PO qd PCI: 300 mg PO before PCI (preferably 6 h prior), then 75 mg PO qd for at least 1 m if BMS, 3 m if sirolimus-eluting and 6 m if paclitaxel-eluting and ideally up to 12 m if bleeding risk not high	As a substitute for ASA in individuals with true ASA allergy May be beneficial when added to daily ASA in NSTEMI (CURE trial) In addition to ASA for planned PCI	Inhibitor of ADP-induced platelet aggregation May be associated with increased risk of bleeding in patients undergoing CABG within 5–7 d of receiving clopidogrel
Heparin (UFH)	If adjunct to fibrinolytic agents: 60 U/kg IV bolus (max 4,000 U) then 12 U/kg/h infusion (max 1,000 U/h) for at least 48 h (maintain aPTT 1.5–2.0 × control) *otherwise* 60–70 U/kg IV bolus (max, 5,000 U) then 12–15 U/kg/h infusion (max 1,000 U/h) for at least 48 h (maintain aPTT 1.5–2.0 × control)	For persistent or recurrent angina; for fibrin-specific lytics; for increased risk of systemic emboli (e.g., coexisting atrial fibrillation, LV thrombus, large or anterior MI)	Enhances the action of antithrombin III Should be avoided in cases of known HIT or whenever a pre-existing coagulopathy would increase risk over perceived benefit
Bivalirudin	PCI: 0.75 mg/kg IV bolus immediately before the procedure then 1.75 mg/kg/h infusion for the duration of the procedure. Five min after bolus, an ACT should be done, and if needed an additional bolus of 0.3 mg/kg may be given.	As an alternative to UFH in patients with ACS undergoing PCI With "provisional use" of GPI IIb/IIIa (given for complications) as an alternative to UFH + GPI IIb/IIIa in patients undergoing PCI	Direct thrombin inhibitor (synthetic analogue of recombinant hirudin) Except in the setting of PCI there are limited data on efficacy and safety Use in conjunction with ASA (325 mg PO); safety and

(continued)

TABLE 3.1. *(continued)* **Treatment of Acute Coronary Syndromes (Unstable Angina, Non-ST Segment Elevation, and ST Segment Elevation Myocardial Infarction)**

Agent	Dosage	Indications	Comments
Bivalirudin (continued)	Continuation of the infusion for up to 4 h postprocedure is optional (after 4 h, an additional infusion may be continued at 0.2 mg/kg/h for up to 20 h)	(REPLACE-2 Trial) As a substitute for UFH with known HIT in patients undergoing PCI	efficacy have not been established when used in conjunction with platelet inhibitors other than ASA
Enoxaparin (LMWH)	30 mg IV bolus, then 1 mg/kg sq bid for 2–8 d (use with ASA 325 mg PO); avoid if age ≥75, serum Cr > 2 mg/dl in women or >2.5 mg/dl in men	Adjunctive therapy in ACS (age <75, and without clinically significant renal insufficiency) as an alternative to UFH	Direct thrombin inhibitor through complex with antithrombin III Avoid if pre-existing coagulopathy would increase risk over perceived benefit

Fibrinolytic Agents (For contraindications refer to Table 3.2)

- *Only for* STEMI, including true posterior MI, or presumed new left bundle branch block and <12 hours from onset (ideally ≤3 h from symptom onset; goal: door to drug <30 minutes).
- Consider PCI as an alternative based on local resources. In general PCI preferred if door to balloon <90 minutes, or cardiogenic shock present or late presentation (>3 hours) or contraindication to fibrinolysis. If ≤3 hours from symptom onset and PCI without delay then no preference for either strategy.
- Reteplase and alteplase are not known to be antigenic nor hypotensive-inducing. Tenecteplase has shown infrequent development of antibody titer at 30 days and reuse should be undertaken with precaution. It is also not hypotensive-inducing.
- Tenecteplase, reteplase, and alteplase should be used in conjunction with ASA 162–325 mg PO and heparin bolus of 60 U/kg (max 4,000 U) then 12 U/kg/h infusion (max 1,000 U/h) for at least 48 hours (maintain aPTT of 1.5–2.0 times control).

Agent	Dosage	Comments
Tenecteplase	IV bolus over 5–15 s <60 kg: 30 mg 60–69 kg: 35 mg 70–79 kg: 40 mg 80–89 kg: 45 mg ≥90 kg: 50 mg	Greater fibrin specificity then rtPA Give with ASA and heparin (see above)
Reteplase	10 U IV over 2 min, then repeat, 30 min later, 10 U IV over 2 min	Low fibrinolysis (relatively clot-selective) Give with ASA and heparin (see above)
Alteplase (rtPA)	>67 kg: 15 mg IV bolus, then 50 mg over 30 min, then 35 mg over 60 min ≤67 kg: 15 mg IV bolus, then 0.75 mg/kg over 30 min, then 0.5 mg/kg over 60 min	Low fibrinolysis (relatively clot-selective) Give with ASA and heparin (see above)

(continued)

TABLE 3.1. *(continued)* **Treatment of Acute Coronary Syndromes (Unstable Angina, Non-ST Segment Elevation, and ST Segment Elevation Myocardial Infarction)**

Agent	Dosage	Indications	Comments
Glycoprotein IIb/IIIa Receptor Inhibitors (GPI IIb/IIIa)			
• Platelet aggregation inhibitor; inhibits the integrin GP IIb/IIIa receptor in the platelet membrane; contraindications include active bleeding, bleeding diathesis (past 30 days), intracranial tumor, hemorrhage arteriovenous malformation, aneurysm, recent stroke or major surgery or trauma (past month), severe hypertension, aortic dissection, pericarditis, platelets <100,000. • Major benefit in NSTEMI troponin positive group with signs of persistent or recurrent ischemia (used in addition to aspirin or heparin). • Can be used as adjunctive therapy with PCI strategy. • Eptifibatide and tirofiban preferred in patients with USA/NSTEMI managed medically and abciximab and eptifibatide preferred in patients with USA/NSTEMI undergoing PCI. For planned PCI start treatment prior to procedure as early as feasible.			
Abciximab	0.25 mg/kg IV bolus (over 5 min) then 0.125 μg/kg/min (max 10 μg/min) infusion for 12–24 h	Consider for USA/NSTEMI undergoing PCI	A murine monoclonal antibody; readministration may result in hypersensitivity, thrombocytopenia, or diminished benefit due to formation of human antichimeric antibodies
Eptifibatide	0.18 mg/kg IV bolus (max 22.6 mg) then 2 μg/kg/min (max 15 mg/h) infusion up to 72 h	Consider for USA/NSTEMI undergoing PCI Adjunct to ASA and heparin in high risk USA/NSTEMI managed medically	If CrCl <50 mL/min or Cr >2 mg/dL, decrease infusion to 1 μg/kg/min (maximum 7.5 mg/h), contraindicated in renal dialysis
Tirofiban	0.4 μg/kg/min IV for 30 min then 0.1 μg/kg/min for 12–48 h	Adjunct to ASA and heparin in high risk USA/NSTEMI managed medically	CrCl <30 mL/min, decrease dose by half (0.2 μg/kg/min IV for 30 min, then 0.05 μg/kg/min)
Angiotensin Converting Enzyme—Inhibitors (Refer to Table 3.4)			
• Beneficial in setting of MI regardless of ejection fraction or presence of HF (oral route preferred). • Avoid IV ACE-I within the first 24 hours of symptom onset due to risk of hypotension.			
β-Blocking Agents (Refer to Table 3.5)			
• Indicated as treatment in the setting of ACS.			
Statins (Refer to Table 3.6)			
• For all patients with ACS without contraindication in first 24 hours. May reduce ACS associated inflammation, and increase nitric oxide level and thus may be useful irrespective of LDL-C level.			
Antiarrhythmic Agents (Refer to Tables 3.9 and 3.10)			
• *Do not* give prophylactically and *avoid* Class IC agents.			
Magnesium sulfate	1–2 g IV over 30–60 min, then 0.5–1 g IV q1–2 h for up to 24 h	Prophylactic use in ICU patients with ACS not recommended Some studies suggest reduction in mortality while others do not	Can cause conduction disturbances; mild hypotension; flaccidity; optimal dose unknown

(continued)

TABLE 3.1. *(continued)* **Treatment of Acute Coronary Syndromes (Unstable Angina, Non-ST Segment Elevation, and ST Segment Elevation Myocardial Infarction)**

Treatment of Complications of ACS

Please see the following tables:

- Cardiogenic pulmonary edema and shock (Therapy; Table 3.3)
- Heart failure (Tables 3.3, 3.4, 3.5)
- Arrhythmia (antiarrhythmic agents Tables 3.9 and 3.10)

Secondary Prevention After Acute MI

- ASA 75–162 mg PO qd indefinitely
- ACE inhibitor indefinitely (Table 3.4)
- β-blocker indefinitely (Table 3.5)
- Statin indefinitely if LDL-C $\geq$100 mg/dl (Table 3.6)

ACS, acute coronary syndromes; ADP, adenosine diphosphate; aPTT, activated partial thromboplastin time; ASA, aspirin; BMS, bare metal stent; BP, blood pressure; CABG, coronary artery bypass graft; CURE, clopidogrel in unstable angina to prevent recurrent events; ECG, electrocardiogram; GPI IIb/IIIa, glycoprotein IIb/IIIa receptor inhibitor; HF, heart failure; HIT, heparin-induced thrombocytopenia; INR, international normalized ratio; IV, intravenous; LAD, left anterior descending coronary artery; LDL-C, low-density lipoprotein-cholesterol; LMWH, low molecular weight heparin; LV, left ventricle; NSTEMI, non-ST segment elevation myocardial infarction; NTG, nitroglycerin; O_2, oxygen; PCI, percutaneous coronary intervention; PDE, phosphodiesterase; PO, by mouth; REPLACE-2, Randomized Evaluation in PCI Linking Angiomax to Reduced Clinical Events-2; RV, right ventricle; SaO_2, arterial oxygen saturation; STEMI, ST segment elevation myocardial infarction; UFH, unfractionated heparin; USA, unstable angina

TABLE 3.2. Fibrinolytic Therapy for ST-Segment Elevation Acute Coronary Syndrome: Contraindications

Absolute Contraindications to Fibrinolytic Therapy

- Active bleeding or recent bleeding diathesis (excluding menses).
- Intracranial/cerebral vascular legion (e.g., malignant intracranial neoplasm, arteriovenous malformation, or aneurysm).
- Prior intracranial hemorrhage.
- Major closed head or facial trauma within 3 months.
- Ischemic stroke within 3 months (except acute ischemic stroke <3 hours).
- Suspicion of aortic dissection.

Relative Contraindications to Fibrinolytic Therapy

- Chronic hypertension—severe and poorly controlled.
- Presentation with severe uncontrolled hypertension (SBP >180 or DBP >110 mm Hg, consider absolute in "*low risk*" patients with STEMI).
- Prior ischemic stroke >3 months, dementia, or known intracranial pathology not covered under absolute.
- Recent internal bleeding (preceding 2–4 weeks) or active peptic ulcer disease.
- Noncompressible vascular punctures.
- Current anticoagulant use (bleeding risk proportional to INR).
- Pregnancy.
- Traumatic or prolonged cardiopulmonary resuscitation (>10 minutes) or major surgery (<3 weeks).

TABLE 3.3. Treatment of Hypervolemia, Pulmonary Edema, Cardiogenic Shock and Decompensated Heart Failure Associated with Systolic Dysfunction

- Assess BP, heart rhythm, adequacy of oxygenation, mentation, heart and lung sounds. Cardiovert for VT or rapid AF; initiate anti-ischemic (coronary arteriography referral in appropriate individuals), antihypertensive, or inotropic therapies as indicated.
- Consideration should be given to guiding management with continuous arterial monitoring and RHC determined hemodynamics, especially in patients not responding to initial therapies.
- Management of compensated chronic HF associated with systolic dysfunction should routinely include oral vasodilator therapy (Table 3.4), β-blockade (Table 3.5), and symptom relief with diuretics. In addition in selective patients with moderate to severe HF aldosterone antagonists (spironolactone [25–50 mg q24h for NYHA Class III–IV] or eplerenone [25–50 mg for HF post-MI]) and digoxin (adjusted to serum levels of 0.5–0.9 ng/ml) can be beneficial. Cardiac resynchronization therapy should be considered in appropriate candidates on optimal medical therapy with NYHA Class III–IV symptoms and LVEF ≤35%, QRS duration ≥0.12 s, and LV end diastolic dimension ≥30 mm (indexed to height). An implantable cardioverter defibrillator should be considered in selective HF patients per guidelines.

Agent	Dosage	Comments

3.3.1 Therapy of Pulmonary Edema or Significant Hypervolemia

- If patient not hypotensive then put head of bed at 60–90°. If patient is hypotensive then also refer to Table 3.8.
- For patients with hypoxemia, consider noninvasive ventilatory support with CPAP.
- For pulmonary edema associated with hypertensive crisis also see Table 3.11. If aortic dissection is a concern then β-blockade should be instituted prior to starting other antihypertensive agents.
- For patients with decompensated HF the goal would be to obtain PCWP <18 and preferably ≤15 mm Hg while avoiding symptomatic hypotension and organ hypoperfusion.

Agent	Dosage	Comments
Oxygen	Initially 4 L/min by nasal cannula or 28% by venti-mask (Adjust to maintain SaO_2 > 90%)	SaO_2 should be maintained over 90% and preferably over 95%
Morphine sulfate	Initially 2–4 mg IV then increments of 2–8 mg IV q5–15min prn pain and anxiety (avoid if hypotensive)	Reduces sympathetic tone; reduces preload; reduces myocardial oxygen demand
Nitroglycerin	IV: 20 μg/min then titrate to effect (pain relief and/or to lower BP 10% to 20% if not hypotensive) Topical: 1–2 inches of 2% ointment q6h or equivalent patches	Increase venous capacitance; reduces preload (predominant) and afterload, and can reduce myocardial O_2 demand; tachyphylaxis occurs Useful in patients with ischemia because of direct coronary vasodilation Causes headache and contraindicated in RV infarction or in patients on sildenafil or other PDE 5 inhibitors

Diuretics

- Reduce circulating blood volume; improve oxygenation; goal is to relieve symptoms without producing hypotension or azotemia.
- Initial therapy with IV loop diuretics is recommended for patients with pulmonary edema or anasarca or suspected GI edema, others may be tried on oral therapy.
- If GFR <30 cc/min then initial doses may need to be doubled.
- Poor response to traditional oral or IV bolus diuretic regimens may respond to IV infusions or sequential nephron blockade with a loop diuretic used in combination with either metolazone or hydrochlorothiazide or chlorothiazide.
- Diuretic refractory patients may be considered for ultrafiltration.

(continued)

TABLE 3.3. *(continued)* **Treatment of Hypervolemia, Pulmonary Edema, Cardiogenic Shock and Decompensated Heart Failure Associated with Systolic Dysfunction**

Agent	Dosage	Comments
Diuretics—Loop of Henle		
• Primary diuretic agents used intravenously for patients with pulmonary edema or anasarca. • Ototoxicity during therapy is most frequently associated with high doses and elevated blood concentrations. • Furosemide 40 mg ≈ torsemide 10–20 mg ≈ bumetanide 1 mg.		
Bumetanide	IV: Initial bolus: 0.5–1.0 mg Range: 0.5–6 mg titrate to effect q2–3 prn Infusion: 1 mg load then 0.5–2 mg/h Oral: Initial: 0.5–1.0 mg Range: 0.5–10 mg q24h, 12h, 8h, prn Max daily dose: 10 mg	Oral form duration of action 4–6 h; IV ≈4 h Maintenance doses should be given on an intermittent schedule, i.e., QOD or every 3–4 d alternating with a 1-2-d interval without drug
Furosemide	IV: Initial bolus: 20–40 mg Range: 20–250 mg titrate to effect q1–2 prn Infusion: 40–80 mg load then 5–20 mg/h Oral: Initial: 20–40 mg Range: 20–600 mg ÷ q12h, 8h, 6h, prn Max daily dose: 600 mg	Oral form duration of action 6–8 h; IV ≈2 h IV boluses are usually doubled until desired effect is obtained or maximal single dose range reached (250–400 mg)
Torsemide	IV: Initial bolus: 10–20 mg Range: 10–200 mg q24h titrate to effect Infusion: 20 mg load then 3–15 mg/h Oral: Initial: 10–20 mg q24h Range: 10–200 mg q24h Max daily dose: 200 mg	Oral and IV form duration of action ≈12 h Doses can be up-titrated by doubling until desired effect is obtained or maximal single dose reached (200 mg) IV dose = PO dose
Diuretics—Thiazide (Distal Tubule)		
• Primarily effects distal renal tubular mechanism of electrolyte reabsorption. • Adjunctive diuretic agents for treatment of pulmonary edema or anasarca. May be used with loop diuretics to provide sequential nephron blockade.		
Chlorothiazide	IV or oral: Initial: 250 mg q24h or q12h Range: 250–1,000 mg q24h, 12h Max daily dose: 1,000 mg	Oral or IV form duration of action 6–12 h
Hydrochlorothiazide	Initial: PO 25 mg q24h or q12h Range: PO 25–100 mg q24h, 12 h Max daily dose: 200 mg	Duration of action 6–12 h
Metolazone	Initial: PO 2.5 mg q24h Range: PO 2.5–20 mg q24h Max daily dose: 20 mg (If with loop diuretic for sequential nephron blockade then 2.5–10 mg 60 min before loop diuretic)	Duration of action 12–24 h Thiazide-like diuretic although primarily acts by inhibiting sodium reabsorption at the cortical diluting site

(continued)

TABLE 3.3. *(continued)* **Treatment of Hypervolemia, Pulmonary Edema, Cardiogenic Shock and Decompensated Heart Failure Associated with Systolic Dysfunction**

Agent	Dosage	Comments
Diuretics—Potassium Sparing (Aldosterone Antagonists)		
• Adjunctive diuretic agents for treatment of pulmonary edema or anasarca. May be used with loop diuretics in patients with refractory hypokalemia. • Beneficial in the treatment of chronic HF associated with systolic dysfunction. • These agents combined with ACE inhibitors may lead to hyperkalemia (monitor potassium levels). Risk increases progressively with serum Cr >1.6 mg/dl. If baseline K ≥5.0 mg/dl then avoid aldosterone antagonists.		
Eplerenone	Initial: PO 25 mg q24h Range: PO 25–100 mg q24h Max daily dose: 100 mg Max daily dose for chronic HF: 50 mg	For HF after MI, initially 25 mg q24h, increasing to 50 mg q24h within 4 wk if tolerated (EPHESUS). Selective aldosterone antagonist blocks mineralocorticoid but not glucocorticoid, androgen, or progesterone receptors
Spironolactone	Initial: PO 12.5–25 mg q24h Range: PO 12.5–200 mg q24h, 12h Max daily dose: 200 mg Max daily dose for chronic HF: 50 mg	Duration of action 48–72 h In severe HF, 25–50 mg q24h added to therapy with ACE-I and loop diuretics reduced risk of death or hospitalization (RALES).
Diuretics—Proximal Tubule		
Acetazolamide	IV or oral: Initial: 5 mg/kg (250–375 mg) Range: 250–500 mg ÷ q24h, 12h (Maintenance doses should be given on an intermittent schedule, i.e., qod or 2 out of every 3 d)	Oral form duration of action 6–12 h; IV ≈ 4–5 h Carbonic anhydrase inhibitor, causes bicarbonaturia Adjunctive diuretic agent for treatment of pulmonary edema or anasarca; may be used with loop diuretics in patients with metabolic alkalosis

3.3.2 Therapy of Hypoperfusion (characterized by low CI due to systolic dysfunction and abnormally high afterload [elevated SVR])

- For patients refractory to medical therapy consideration should be given to intra-aortic balloon counterpulsation (contraindications include severe aortic insufficiency, abdominal or aortic aneurysm, and severe calcific aortic-iliac disease or peripheral vascular disease).
- For patients with HF the goal would be to obtain SVR ≤1,200 while avoiding symptomatic hypotension and organ hypoperfusion.
- In appropriate medically refractory HF patients consideration should be given to referral for transplantation and/or evaluation for ventricular assist device placement.

(continued)

TABLE 3.3. *(continued)* **Treatment of Hypervolemia, Pulmonary Edema, Cardiogenic Shock and Decompensated Heart Failure Associated with Systolic Dysfunction**

Agent	Dosage	Comments
Inodilators (Inotropy and Afterload Reduction)		
• In chronic HF, scheduled intermittent (i.e., 48–72 hours once a week) or continuous prolonged inotrope infusions may palliate symptoms but do not improve survival and can have an adverse impact on survival.		
Dobutamine	Initial: 2.5 μg/kg/min IV Range: 2.5–20 μg/kg/min IV titrate to effect Usual: (in HF) 2.5–7.5 μg/kg/min Wean: taper slowly (i.e., 1 μg/kg/min q1h or slower)	Synthetic catecholamine with primarily β-1 adrenergic activity; 3+ inotropic effect; 2+ chronotropic effect; 1+ vasodilation In HF patients with CAD or associated secondary pulmonary HTN, consider using with NTG In HF, if hypoperfusion and elevated SVR persist then consider adding nitroprusside or milrinone May precipitate or worsen dysrhythmias
Milrinone	Load: 25–50 μg/kg IV over 10 min (Controversial—in HF several advocate no load, realizing initial effect will be delayed several h) then 0.25 or 0.375 μg/kg/min IV Range: 0.25 or 0.375 or 0.5 or 0.75 μg/kg/min IV Wean: taper slowly (i.e., adjust dose downward q2–3h or slower—elimination half-life is ≈2.3h)	Phosphodiesterase inhibitor; 2+ inotropic effect; 1+ chronotropic effect; 3+ vasodilation In refractory HF patients can be combined with dobutamine May precipitate or worsen dysrhythmias
Vasodilators		
Hydralazine	IV: 5–40 mg q2–4h	Predominantly reduces afterload and often combined with nitrates to achieve balanced arterial and venous effects Can cause a lupuslike syndrome For oral dosing in HF see Table 3.4
Nesiritide	Load: 2 μg/kg IV bolus over 60 s then Initial: 0.01 μg/kg/min IV Range: 0.01–0.03 μg/kg/min IV Titration: Increase by 0.005 μg/kg/min (after a bolus of 1 μg/kg IV) no more frequently than every 3 h up to a max dose of 0.03 μg/kg/min IV (limited experience with infusion durations >48 h)	Recombinant human B-type natriuretic peptide; natriuretic and vasodilatory (arterial and venous) effects Limit use to acutely decompensated HF with dyspnea at rest or with minimal activity (VMAC trial); sufficient evidence does not exist to recommend its use as an agent to replace diuretics or enhance diuresis Should not be used as primary therapy for cardiogenic shock or in patients with systolic BP <90 mm Hg May be associated with a dose-dependent increase in serum Cr

(continued)

TABLE 3.3. *(continued)* **Treatment of Hypervolemia, Pulmonary Edema, Cardiogenic Shock and Decompensated Heart Failure Associated with Systolic Dysfunction**

Agent	Dosage	Comments
Nitroglycerin	IV: 0.25–4 μg/kg/min (20–300 μg/min)	Useful with dobutamine in HF patients with CAD or associated secondary pulmonary HTN Useful in patients with ischemia because of direct coronary vasodilation Increase venous capacitance; reduces preload (predominant) and afterload Causes headache and contraindicated in RV infarction and in patients on sildenafil and other PDE 5 inhibitors For dosing of isosorbide dinitrate in CAD see Table 3.1 and in HF see Table 3.4
Nitroprusside	Initial: 0.2 μg/kg/min IV (10–15 μg/min) Usual: 1–4 μg/kg/min IV Titrate to effect in increments of 0.2–0.5 μg/kg/min IV q10–30min or slower Max: 10 μg/kg/min IV Wean: Taper slowly to prevent rebound increase in filling pressures and decrease in cardiac output	Onset of action <1 min; duration of action 1–10 min; usually used with invasive monitoring Preload and afterload reduction (balanced venous and arterial vasodilation); very effective for decreasing pulmonary congestion and increasing CI Methemoglobin levels should be monitored and elevated or rising levels are indications for discontinuing Be alert for thiocyanate toxicity (confusion, nausea, weakness, anion-gap acidosis, seizures), especially in renal insufficiency. Monitor thiocyanate levels if infusion >48 h Solution is light-sensitive

ACE-I, angiotensin converting enzyme-inhibitor; BP, blood pressure; CAD, coronary artery disease; CI, cardiac index; CPAP, continuous positive airway pressure; EPHESUS, Eplerenone Post MI Heart Failure Efficacy and Survival Study; GFR, glomerular filtration rate; HF, heart failure; HTN, hypertension; LVEF, left ventricle ejection fraction; MI, myocardial infarction; NTG, nitroglycerin; NYHA, New York Heart Association; O_2, oxygen; PCWP, pulmonary capillary wedge pressure; PDE, phosphodiesterase; PO, by mouth; RALES, Randomized Aldactone Evaluation Study; RHC, right heart catheterization; RV, right ventricle; SaO_2, arterial oxygen saturation; SVR, systemic vascular resistance; VMAC, Vasodilation in the Management of Acute Congestive HF

TABLE 3.4. Oral Vasodilator Therapy for the Treatment of Heart Failure Associated with Systolic Dysfunction or Postmyocardial Infarction

- ACE-I are considered first line therapy with ARB a suitable alternative in patients intolerant of ACE-I, particularly in those with ACE-I induced incessant cough.
- For HF associated with systolic dysfunction in patients intolerant of ACE-I and ARB, the combination of HYZ and ISDN is a reasonable alternative. In addition the combination of HYZ and ISDN when added to standard HF therapy that includes ACE-I (or ARB), β-blocker, and diuretic (many also received digoxin) has been shown to produce a further survival benefit in black patients with NYHA Class III–IV HF.

Agent	Dosage	Comments
Angiotensin Converting Enzyme Inhibitors		
• Survival benefit in NYHA Class II–IV HF patients and quality-of-life benefit in NYHA Class I patients (asymptomatic LV dysfunction). • Beneficial in setting of MI regardless of ejection fraction or presence of HF. • Cautiously begin low doses in setting of hypovolemia, hyper K, azotemia, or serum Na <130. • In patients with uni or bilateral renal artery stenosis, ACE-I can increase serum Cr or BUN. • Has been associated with angioedema, rash, hyperkalemia, and incessant cough.		
Captopril	Initial: PO 6.25 mg q6h Range: PO 12.5–50 mg q8h (advance over 24–72 h to max tolerated dose)	Reduction in HF or cardiac events following MI Beneficial in patients with LV dysfunction and prior or current HF symptoms
Enalapril	Initial: PO 2.5 mg q12h Range: PO 5–20 mg q12h	Beneficial in NYHA Class I–IV HF
Fosinopril	Initial: PO 5 mg qd Range: PO 10–40 mg qd	Beneficial in patients with LV dysfunction and prior or current HF symptoms
Lisinopril	Initial: PO 2.5 mg qd Range: PO 5–40 mg qd	Reduction in HF or cardiac events following MI Beneficial in patients with LV dysfunction and prior or current HF symptoms
Quinapril	Initial: PO 5 mq q12h Range: PO 10–20 mg q12h	Beneficial in patients with LV dysfunction and prior or current HF symptoms
Ramipril	Initial: PO 1.25 mg q12h Range: PO 2.5–5 mg q12h	Reduction in HF or cardiac events following MI
Trandolapril	Initial: PO 0.5 mg qd Range: PO 1–4 mg qd	Reduction in HF or cardiac events following MI
Angiotensin Receptor Blockers		
• Use cautiously and start in low doses in setting of hypovolemia, hyperkalemia, and azotemia.		
Candesartan	Initial: PO 4 mg qd Range: PO 8–32 mg qd	Beneficial in patients with LV dysfunction and prior or current HF symptoms
Losartan	Initial: PO 25 mg qd Range: PO 25–50 mg q12h	Beneficial in patients with LV dysfunction
Valsartan	Initial: PO 20 mg q12h Range: PO 40–160 mg q12h	Reduction in HF or cardiac events following MI Beneficial in patients with LV dysfunction and prior or current HF symptoms
Combined Arterial and Venous Vasodilatation		
Hydralazine (HYZ) and Isosorbide Dinitrate (ISDN)	Initial: HYZ 10–20 mg PO q6–8h ISDN 10–20 mg PO q6–8h Range: HYZ 25–75 mg PO q6–8h ISDN 20–40 mg PO q6–8h	For HF associated with systolic dysfunction in patients intolerant of ACE-I and ARB and in addition to ACE-I in black patients Use cautiously and start in low doses in setting of hypovolemia Also available in a fixed dosage form of HYZ 37.5 mg and ISDN 20 mg. Starting dose ½ to 1 tablet tid with max dose 2 tablets tid HYZ can cause a lupuslike syndrome; ISDN can cause headache and is contraindicated with sildenafil and other PDE 5 inhibitors

ACE-I, angiotensin converting enzyme-inhibitors; ARB, angiotensin receptor blocker; BUN, blood urea nitrogen; HF, heart failure; HYZ, hydralazine; ISDN, isosorbide dinitrate; K, potassium; LV, left ventricular; MI, myocardial infarction; Na, sodium; NYHA, New York Heart Association; PDE, phosphodiesterase

TABLE 3.5. β-Blockade Therapy for the Treatment of Heart Failure Associated with Systolic Dysfunction or Acute Coronary Syndrome

- β-blockade is indicated as treatment in the setting of ACS and for secondary prevention post-MI. It is beneficial in the setting of MI regardless of EF or presence of HF.
- β-blockade with either carvedilol or bisoprolol or metoprolol (CR/XL) is indicated for HF associated with systolic dysfunction. There is sufficient evidence from multiple randomized trials to recommend these agents in NYHA Class II–IV HF. Many experts would also advocate these agents in NYHA Class I HF. Appropriate candidates should be in a relatively compensated state with resting HR >60, and absence of 2nd- or 3rd-degree AV block or bronchospastic disease.
- β-blockers can cause bradycardia, hypotension, bronchospasm, worsened conduction disturbances, worsened HF in a decompensated HF patient, and rebound ischemia after discontinuation.
- There is evidence that β-adrenergic blockade augments cocaine-induced coronary artery vasoconstriction.

Agent	Dosage	Comments
Atenolol	IV (for ACS): 5 mg over 5 min, then 5 mg 10 min later then begin PO Range PO: 25–100 mg qd	Reduction in HF or cardiac events following MI β1 cardioselective at usual dose; long half-life allows qd dosing
Bisoprolol (HF indication)	HF therapy: Initial: PO 1.25 mg qd Range: PO 1.25–10 mg qd (Initial dose doubled after 1 wk then titrate over 1–4 wk intervals to max tolerated) Anti-ischemic range: PO 5–20 mg qd	Beneficial in patients with LV dysfunction and prior or current HF symptoms (NYHA Class III–IV HF) β1 cardioselective
Carvedilol (HF indication)	HF therapy: Initial: PO: 3.125 mg q12h Range: PO: 6.25–25 mg q12h (max dose 50 mg q12h if wt >85 kg) (Initial dose doubled after 1–2 wk then titrated as tolerated every 2 wk) Anti-ischemic range: PO 25–50 mg qd	Beneficial in patients with LV dysfunction and prior or current HF symptoms. (NYHA Class II–IV HF) Reduction in HF or cardiac events following MI Not cardioselective
Esmolol	IV: 250–500 μg/kg over 1 min then 50 μg/kg/min; rebolus and increase q5min by 50 μg/kg/min to max of 300 μg/kg/min	β1 cardioselective; its 7-min half-life allows effects to subside quickly Consider reducing loading dose in marginally or poorly compensated patients Use 100 mg vial for loading dose
Metoprolol (HF indication)	Succinate (HF therapy): Initial: (NYHA II) PO 25 mg qd Initial: (NYHA III–IV) PO 12.5 mg qd Range: PO 25–200 mg qd (Initial dose doubled after 1–2 wk then titrated as tolerated every 2 wk) Anti-ischemic range: PO 100–400 mg qd Tartrate (ACS therapy): IV: 5 mg q5min up to 15 mg then begin PO therapy 15 min after final IV dose Initial: PO 25–50 mg PO q6h for 48 h Range: PO 50–200 mg q12h	Succinate form beneficial in patients with LV dysfunction and prior or current HF symptoms (NYHA Class II–IV) Tartrate form associated with reduction in HF or cardiac events following MI β1 selective at daily doses totaling ≤200 mg

(continued)

TABLE 3.5. *(continued)* **β-Blockade Therapy for the Treatment of Heart Failure Associated with Systolic Dysfunction or Acute Coronary Syndrome**

Agent	Dosage	Comments
Nadolol	Range: PO 40–240 mg qd	Not cardioselective; long half-life allows qd dosing
Propranolol	Short acting: Range: PO: 10–80 mg q6h Long acting: Range: PO: 80–320 mg qd	Reduction in HF or cardiac events following MI Prototype β-blocker; not cardioselective
Timolol	Range: PO 5–20 mg bid	Reduction in HF or cardiac events following MI; not cardioselective

ACS, acute coronary syndrome; AV, atrioventricular; EF, ejection fraction; HF, heart failure; LV, left ventricular; MI, myocardial infarction; NYHA, New York Heart Association; O_2, oxygen

TABLE 3.6. Statins (HMG-CoA Reductase Inhibitors)

- For all patients with ACS without contraindication in first 24 hours. May reduce ACS associated inflammation, and increase nitric oxide level and thus may be useful irrespective of LDL-C level.
- For secondary prevention in patients with LDL-C >100 mg/dl.
- Reduction in LDL-C 18% to 55%, TG 7% to 30%, and increase in HDL-C 5% to 15%.
- Contraindicated in active or chronic liver disease.
- Side effects: Myopathy (monitor CK) or increased liver enzymes (monitor AST and ALT).
- Liver enzyme tests should be performed before and at 2–3 months following both the initiation of therapy and dose elevations, and periodically (e.g., semiannually) on chronic therapy.
- Reduce dose or discontinue if serum transaminase levels of 3 times the upper normal limit persist.
- Temporarily hold or discontinue if a condition suggestive of or predisposing to myopathy or renal failure develops.
- Concomitant therapy with cyclosporine, macrolides, protease inhibitors, azole antifungals, nefazodone, fibrates, or niacin may increase the risk of myopathy.

Agent	Equipotent Dosages (mg) (once-daily oral-dosing)				
Atorvastatin	5	10	20	40	80
Fluvastatin	40	80	N/A	N/A	N/A
Lovastatin	20	40	80	N/A	N/A
Pravastatin	20	40	80	N/A	N/A
Rosuvastatin	2.5	5	10	20	40
Simvastatin	10	20	40	80	N/A

ACS, acute coronary syndrome; ALT, alanine aminotransferase; AST, aspartate aminotransferase; CK, creatine kinase; HDL-C, high-density lipoprotein cholesterol; LDL-C, low-density lipoprotein-cholesterol; N/A, not applicable; TG, triglyceride

TABLE 3.7. Calcium Channel Antagonists

- In general, calcium channel antagonists are not used in the treatment of acute coronary syndromes.
- Used for treatment of hypertension.
- Nondihydropyridine forms are used for treatment of atrial arrhythmias.

Agent	Dosage	Comments
Nondihydropyridine		
Diltiazem	IV: 0.25 mg/kg over 2 min (typically 15–20 mg IV) (may repeat once in 15 min with 0.35 mg/kg, typically 25 mg IV) then 5–15 mg/h PO: 30–90 mg q6h	Compared to verapamil, slightly more vasodilator potency and less antiarrhythmic potency; relatively little negative inotropy
Verapamil	IV: 2.5–10 mg over 2–3 min (repeat in 15–30 min prn), Max cumulative = 20 mg PO: 40–160 mg q6h	Verapamil has the strongest antiarrhythmic potency, the most negative inotropy, and the weakest vasodilator potency; side effects include conduction disturbances, heart failure, hypotension, and constipation
Dihydropyridine		
Amlodipine	PO: 2.5–10 mg qd	Peripheral and coronary arterial vasodilator; acts directly on vascular smooth muscle; does not affect myocardial contractility or cardiac conduction; can cause dizziness and edema; once-daily dosing
Nicardipine	Initial: 5 mg/h IV Titrate: 2.5 mg/h every 5–15 min Range: 5–15 mg/h IV PO: 20–40 mg tid	Effects intermediate between amlodipine and nifedipine
Nifedipine	PO: 10–30 mg q8h	Minimal inotropic, antiarrhythmic, or conducting system effects; relative to verapamil or diltiazem, acts more as a pure vasodilator, including coronary vasodilatation; side effects include dizziness, headache, and flushing

TABLE 3.8. Intravenous Vasoactive Agents

- Vasoconstrictors usually are administered by central vein and should be used in conjunction with adequate volume repletion. All can precipitate myocardial ischemia. All except phenylephrine can cause tachyarrhythmias.
- Cautions should be used to avoid extravasation of vasoconstrictors. If extravasation occurs, 10–15 ml of 0.9% NaCl containing 5–10 mg of phentolamine should be infiltrated liberally throughout the affected area.

Agent and Dose	Systemic Vasoconstriction	Inotropy	Systemic Vasodilation	Comments
Vasoconstrictors				
Phenylephrine Start at 30 μg/min IV and titrate	++++ Alpha	0	0	Pure vasoconstrictor without direct cardiac effects; may cause reflex bradycardia. Doses up to 350 μg/min may be required in some settings
Vasopressin Start at 0.01 U/min and titrate; doses should be limited to 0.04 U/min	+++	0	0	May be beneficial in patients with refractory shock despite adequate fluid resuscitation and high dose conventional vasopressors. Exact mechanism of BP increase is unknown
Vasoconstrictors and Inotropes				
Dopamine 2–20 μg/kg/min Dopaminergic effects (++++)	+ Alpha	++++ Beta	0	Doses >20–30 μg/kg/min usually produce no added response. Increases in BP mainly due to increases in inotropy and HR
Epinephrine Start at 2 μg/min and titrate	+ Alpha	++++ Beta	0	Increases in BP mainly due to increases in inotropy and HR. Doses up to 0.5 μg/kg/min may be required in some settings
Norepinephrine Start at 2 μg/min and titrate	++++ Alpha	+ Beta	0	Increase in BP primarily due to increase in peripheral vasoconstriction. Doses up to 3 μg/kg/min may be required in some settings
Vasodilators and Inotropes				
Dobutamine 2.5–20 μg/kg/min	0	++++ Beta	++	Useful for acute management of low cardiac output states. Can be combined with nitroprusside, NTG, or milrinone

(continued)

TABLE 3.8. *(continued)* **Intravenous Vasoactive Agents**

Agent and Dose	Systemic Vasoconstriction	Inotropy	Systemic Vasodilation	Comments
Milrinone Loading dose 25–50 μg/kg over 10 min, then 0.25–0.75 μg/kg/min	0	++	+++	Useful for acute management of low cardiac output states Can be combined with dobutamine
Vasodilators				
Nesiritide Load 2 μg/kg bolus, then 0.01μg/kg/min and increase by 0.005 μg/kg/min (after 1 μg/kg bolus) no sooner than every 3 h Range: 0.01–0.03 μg/kg/min	0	0	++ Recombinant human B-type natriuretic peptide	Use limited to acutely decompensated HF with dyspnea with minimal activity Should not be used for intermittent outpatient infusion, scheduled repetitive use, to improve renal function, to enhance diuresis, or as primary therapy for cardiogenic shock
Nitroglycerin 0.25–4 μg/kg/min (20–300 μg/min)	0	0	++	Predominantly reduces preload; increases venous capacitance Useful in patients with ischemia due to direct coronary vasodilation Contraindicated with sildenafil and other PDE 5 inhibitors
Nitroprusside Initial: 0.2 μg/kg/min (10–15 μg/min) Usual: 1–4 μg/kg/min Max: 10 μg/kg/min	0	0	++++	Preload and afterload reduction (venous and arterial vasodilation) Useful for acute management of low cardiac output states Methemoglobin levels should be monitored and elevated or rising levels are indications for discontinuing

BP, blood pressure; HF, heart failure; HR, heart rate; NTG, nitroglycerin; PDE, phosphodiesterase

TABLE 3.9. Antiarrhythmic Agents

Agents (Listed by Vaughan Williams Classification)	Indications	Dosage	Comments
Class IA (Infrequently Used)			
Procainamide	Malignant ventricular ectopy; conversion of A fib and A flutter to NSR; WPW	12–17 mg/kg at 20–30 mg/min IV, then 2–5 mg/min (or 500–1,000 mg PO q4–6h)	N-acetyl procainamide is active metabolite and tends to accumulate in renal failure; lupuslike syndrome; fever; rash; agranulocytosis; QT interval prolongation; mild negative inotropy
Quinidine sulfate	Malignant ventricular ectopy; conversion of A fib and A flutter to NSR; WPW	6–10 mg/kg at 20 mg/min IV, then 1–3 mg/min (or 200–400 mg PO q6h)	Diarrhea; thrombocytopenia; hemolysis; fever; hepatitis; rash; cinchonism; QT interval prolongation; increased digoxin level; IV causes hypotension; PO route preferred
Disopyramide	Malignant ventricular ectopy; conversion of A fib and A flutter to NSR; WPW	100–200 mg PO q6h	Anticholinergic effects; negative inotropy; QT interval prolongation
Class IB (Infrequent Use Except Lidocaine)			
Lidocaine	Malignant ventricular ectopy; WPW	1–1.5 mg/kg IV over 2 min IV May repeat 0.5–0.75 mg/kg IV to a max 3 mg/kg, then infusion 1–4 mg/min	Seizures; paresthesias; delirium; levels increased by cimetidine; minimal hemodynamic effects
Mexiletine	Malignant ventricular ectopy; less effective than IA and IC agents	150–300 mg PO q6–8h with food	Nausea; tremor, dizziness; delirium; hepatitis; dose-related bradycardia, but minimal hemodynamic effects; levels increased by cimetidine

(continued)

TABLE 3.9. *(continued)* **Antiarrhythmic Agents**

Agents (Listed by Vaughan Williams Classification)	Indications	Dosage	Comments
Class IC			
Flecainide	Life-threatening ventricular arrhythmias refractory to other agents	100–200 mg PO q12h IV formulation not available in the U.S.	Proarrhythmic effects; moderate negative inotropy; dizziness; conduction abnormalities Contraindicated if conduction abnormalities, coronary disease, HF Avoid if electrolyte abnormalities or liver disease
Propafenone	Life-threatening ventricular arrhythmias refractory to other agents Used for supraventricular arrhythmias	IV formulation not available in the U.S. 150–300 mg PO q8h 600 mg po single dose used for cardioversion of recent onset A fib	Proarrhythmic effects; negative inotropy; dizziness; nausea; bronchospasm; conduction abnormalities Avoid if structural heart disease, conduction abnormalities, or abnormal electrolytes
Class IA/IB (Hybrid Electrophysiologic Effects, Rarely Used)			
Moricizine	Life-threatening ventricular arrhythmias refractory to other agents	100–300 mg PO q8h	Proarrhythmic effects; dizziness; nausea; rash; headache
Class II (β-Blocking Agents)			
Metoprolol	Slowing ventricular rate in A fib, A flutter, SVT, and MAT	5 mg q5min IV up to 15 mg, then 25–100 mg PO q8–12h	Cardioselective at low doses; hypotension; negative inotropy
Esmolol	Slowing ventricular rate in A fib, A flutter, SVT, and MAT	250–500 μg/kg over 1 min IV, then 50 μg/kg/min; rebolus and increase q5min by 50 μg/kg/min to maximum of 300 μg/kg/min	Cardioselective at low doses; hypotension; negative inotropy; very short half-life Use 100 mg vial for loading dose
Propranolol	Slowing ventricular rate in A fib, A flutter, and SVT; suppression of PVCs	Up to 0.15 mg/kg over 20 min IV, then 3 mg/h (or 10–80 mg PO q6h)	Not cardioselective; hypotension; bronchospasm; negative inotropy

(continued)

TABLE 3.9. *(continued)* **Antiarrhythmic Agents**

Agents (Listed by Vaughan Williams Classification)	Indications	Dosage	Comments
Class III			
Amiodarone	Life-threatening ventricular arrhythmias refractory to other agents Used for atrial arrhythmias Drug of choice for reduced LV function	PO: 800–1600 mg qd for 1–3 wk, then 600–800 mg qd for 4 wk, then 100–400 mg qd IV: 150 mg over 10 min, then 1 mg/min for 6 h, then 0.5 mg/min maintenance infusion; switch to PO when possible; for recurrent ventricular arrhythmias, supplement with infusions of 150 mg over 10 min IV: 300 mg for VF refractory to 1–2 shock-CPR cycles and one vasopressor agent	Half-life >50 days; pulmonary fibrosis; corneal microdeposits; hypo/hyperthyroidism; bluish skin; hepatitis; photosensitivity; conduction abnormalities; mild negative inotropy; increased effect of warfarin sodium; increased digoxin level ARDS has been reported With IV administration, hypotension, bradycardia, and AV block can occur
Ibutilide	Conversion of A fib and A flutter to NSR	≥60 kg: 1 mg IV over 10 min; wait 10 min; then if needed, another 1 mg IV over 10 min <60 kg: same protocol, using 0.01 mg/kg doses	Can cause QT interval prolongation, torsade, and transient heart block Avoid if abnormal electrolytes, prolonged QT interval Use with caution in patients with EF <35%
Sotalol	Life-threatening ventricular arrhythmias; conversion of A fib and A flutter to NSR	PO: 80 mg q12h; may increase up to 160 mg PO q8h IV formulation not available in the U.S.	β-blocker with Class III properties; proarrhythmic effects; QT interval prolongation, torsade de pointes
Class IV (Calcium Channel Antagonists)			
Verapamil	Conversion of SVT to NSR; slowing ventricular rate in A fib, A flutter, and MAT	5–10 mg IV over 2–3 min (repeat in 30 min prn), then 0.1–5 μg/kg/min IV (or 40–160 mg PO q6h)	Hypotension; negative inotropy; conduction disturbances; increased digoxin level; contraindicated in WPW; avoid combination with β-blockade, digoxin, amiodarone

(continued)

TABLE 3.9. *(continued)* Antiarrhythmic Agents

Agents (Listed by Vaughan Williams Classification)	Indications	Dosage	Comments
Diltiazem	Conversion of SVT to NSR; slowing ventricular rate in A fib, A flutter, and MAT	0.25 mg/kg IV over 2 min (may repeat once in 15 min with 0.35 mg/kg IV), then 5–15 mg/h (or 30–90 mg PO q6h)	Hypotension; less negative inotropy than verapamil; conduction disturbances; rare hepatic injury; contraindicated in WPW; avoid combination with β-blockade, digoxin, amiodarone
Miscellaneous Agents			
Adenosine	Conversion of SVT, to NSR	6 mg rapid IV bolus; if ineffective, 12 mg rapid IV bolus 2 min later; follow bolus with saline flush; use smaller doses (3 mg) if giving through central venous line	Flushing; dyspnea; nodal blocking effect increased by dipyridamole and decreased by theophylline and caffeine; very short half-life ($\approx$10 s)
Atropine	Initial therapy for symptomatic bradycardia	0.5 mg IV bolus; repeat q5min prn to total of 3 mg IV	May induce tachycardia and ischemia
Digoxin	Slowing AV conduction in A fib and A flutter	0.5 mg IV bolus, then 0.25 mg IV q2–6h up to 1 mg; maintenance 0.125–0.375 PO/IV qd	Heart block; arrhythmias; nausea; yellow vision; numerous drug interactions; generally contraindicated in WPW Monitor level
Isoproterenol	Rarely used for torsade de pointes	Start at 2 μg/min, increase as needed (usually $\leq$10 μg/min)	Tachycardia; ischemia; hypotension
Magnesium sulfate	Torsade de pointes; adjunct for VT and VF	2 g IV over 10 min, then 1 g IV q6h	Can cause conduction disturbances; mild hypotension; flaccidity; optimal dose uncertain

A fib, atrial fibrillation; A flutter, atrial flutter; ARDS, acute respiratory distress syndrome; AV, atrioventricular; CPR, cardiopulmonary resuscitation; HF, heart failure; IV, intravenous; MAT, multifocal atrial tachycardia; NSR, normal sinus rhythm; PO, by mouth; PVC, premature ventricular contraction; SVT, supraventricular tachycardia; VF, ventricular fibrillation; VT, ventricular tachycardia; WPW, Wolff-Parkinson-White

TABLE 3.10. Antiarrhythmics of Choice

Rhythm	Treatment	Prevention of Recurrence
Paroxysmal supraventricular tachycardia	*If unstable, electrical cardioversion* initially 100 J monophasic synchronized, or biphasic equivalent *If stable* 1st choice: vagal maneuvers such as carotid sinus massage 2nd choice: IV adenosine Alternatives: IV verapamil; IV diltiazem; IV β-blocker If reduced LVEF, amiodarone preferred to calcium channel antagonists Consider electrical cardioversion; rapid atrial pacing, or IV ibutilide if normal LVEF	Assess need for drug therapy 1st choice: PO β-blocker, PO verapamil, or PO diltiazem 2nd choice: PO digoxin 3rd choice: Class IA/C or Class III drugs If reduced EF, amiodarone preferred
Atrial flutter or fibrillation	*If unstable, electrical cardioversion* A flutter, initially 50 J monophasic synchronized or biphasic equivalent; A fib, initially 100 J monophasic synchronized or biphasic equivalent *If stable* *For rate control:* IV diltiazem, β-blocker, amiodarone, or digoxin depending on clinical setting *For restoring sinus rhythm:* 1st choice: IV/PO Class IC or Class III drugs Class IA drugs rarely used If CAD, sotalol preferred over Class IC If HF, amiodarone preferred over Class IC	Determine whether rate control only or rhythm control is necessary; correct electrolyte abnormalities Rate control with oral drugs: β-blockade, verapamil, diltiazem, digoxin, or amiodarone Rhythm control with oral drugs: Class III or Class IC or Class IA (rarely used) drugs depending on clinical setting Prophylactic warfarin and/or aspirin should be prescribed for paroxysmal or chronic A fib/flutter unless contraindicated *Notes: (1) If A fib persists >24–48 h, anticoagulate prior to conversion; (2) use type IA antiarrhythmic agents only after blocking the AV node with digoxin or a calcium channel or β-blocker; (3) prior to cardioversion, consider whether TEE or several weeks anticoagulation is necessary*
Multifocal atrial tachycardia	1st choice: Treat the underlying condition, e.g., metabolic or electrolyte abnormalities or rarely digoxin toxicity 2nd choice: IV diltiazem or IV verapamil 3rd choice: IV esmolol or IV metoprolol (use caution despite β-1 selectivity)	Avoid hypoxemia; correct metabolic derangements; avoid aminophylline and theophylline if possible β-blockade may be contraindicated because of pulmonary disease *Note: Digitalis and electrical cardioversion are both ineffective for this rhythm*
Wolff-Parkinson-White syndrome with atrial fibrillation or flutter	1st choice: electrical cardioversion (initially 100 J monophasic synchronized or biphasic equivalent)	1st choice: catheter ablation of accessory pathway 2nd choice: PO, Class IC, or Class III agents

(continued)

TABLE 3.10. *(continued)* **Antiarrhythmics of Choice**

Rhythm	Treatment	Prevention of Recurrence
	2nd choice: IV procainamide, amiodarone, ibutilide, or flecainide	*Note: If wide complex (antidromic), avoid drugs that block AV node such as adenosine, β-blockers, calcium channel antagonists, and digoxin*
Paroxysmal junctional tachycardia	May respond to Class II, III, or IC Catheter ablation may be necessary	Rare arrhythmia
Nonparoxysmal junctional tachycardia	Correct underlying abnormality, e.g., digoxin toxicity, electrolyte abnormalities, myocardial ischemia, hypoxia	Rarely consider β-blockade or calcium channel antagonists
Ventricular tachycardia	***If unstable, defibrillation*** Initially 200 J unsynchronized monophasic or biphasic equivalent ***If stable with pulse*** Drug choices: 1st: IV amiodarone 2nd: IV lidocaine 3rd: IV procainamide 4th: β-blockade, Mg Electrical: Synchronized cardioversion	Consider electrophysiologic assessment and need for defibrillator Drug therapy should be tailored to circumstance. It may include β-blockade, amiodarone, sotalol, or LV remodeling regimen in heart failure Other antiarrhythmic agents may be proarrhythmic *Note: Symptomatic ventricular tachycardia requires evaluation and treatment. Asymptomatic ventricular arrhythmias may require evaluation especially if reduced LV function. Therapy is not usually needed for premature ventricular contractions.*
Torsade de pointes	***If unstable, defibrillation*** Initially 200 J unsynchronized monophasic or biphasic equivalent ***If stable*** 1st choice: IV magnesium sulfate 2nd choice: increase heart rate with atrial pacing, isoproterenol, or atropine	Discontinue precipitating drugs (e.g., type IA agents, tricyclic antidepressants, nonsedating antihistamines, phenothiazines)
Ventricular fibrillation	Per ACLS algorithm, shock-CPR (2min) sequences (200/300/360 J monophasic or biphasic equivalent), followed by vasopressor such as epinephrine or vasopressin	Give drugs while continuing CPR After 1–2 shocks, consider epinephrine 1 mg IV at 3–5 min intervals. May give vasopressin 40 U IV once, instead of 1st or 2nd dose epinephrine Consider amiodarone 300 mg IV over 10 min Other possible drugs include IV lidocaine, procainamide, or Mg

A fib, atrial fibrillation; A flutter, atrial flutter; ACLS, advanced cardiac life support; CAD, coronary artery disease; IV, intravenous; HF, heart failure: LVEF, left ventricular ejection fraction; PO, by mouth

TABLE 3.11. Parenteral Antihypertensive Agents—Pharmacologic Characteristics
(See Table 3.12 for Therapy of Specific Conditions)

Agent	Dosage/Onset/Duration	Comments
Parenteral Vasodilators		
Nitroprusside	Dosage: IV Infusion 0.2–10 μg/kg/min Onset: <1 min Duration: 1–10 min	Thiocyanate toxicity (serum level >10 mg/dL) usually occurs after >48 h especially in presence of renal dysfunction; treat with sodium thiosulfate Methemoglobinemia Cyanide toxicity
Nitroglycerin	Dosage: IV infusion 0.25–4 μg/kg/min (20–300 μg/min) Onset: 1–2 min Duration: 3–10 min	Tachyphylaxis, headache, methemoglobinemia
α and β Adrenergic Blocker		
Labetalol	Dosage: 20 mg IV over 2 min, then 40–80 mg IV q10min to a total of 300 mg or IV infusion starting at 0.5–2 mg/min; titrate to effect, max 4 mg/min Onset: 5 min Duration: 2–12 h	Bronchospasm, conduction disturbances, bradycardia
α Adrenergic Blocker		
Phentolamine	Dosage: IV infusion 1–5 mg/min or IV bolus 5–10 mg q5–15min Onset: 1–2 min Duration: 3–10 min	Indicated for pheochromocytoma Tachycardia, GI stimulation, hypoglycemia
β Adrenergic Blockers • Side-effects include bronchospasm, negative inotropy, HF, conductive disturbances		
Metoprolol	Initial: 5 mg IV Range: 5–15 mg IV Onset: 5–10 min Duration: 3–6 h	
Esmolol	Dosage: IV 250–500 μg/kg over 1 min then 50 μg/kg/min; rebolus and increase q5min by 50 μg/kg/min to max of 300 μg/kg/min Onset: 1–3 min Duration: 1–2 min for β-blockade	Careful BP monitoring because hypotension is common The bolus dose should be withdrawn from the 100-mg vial Infusion doses >300 μg/kg/min have not been studied
Propranolol	Dosage: IV 1–10 mg load then 3 mg/h Onset: IV 2–3 min Duration: 1–6 h	
Angiotensin Converting Enzyme Inhibitor		
Enalaprilat	Dosage: IV 0.625–5 mg slowly over 5 min q6h Onset: 15 min Duration: 4–6 h	Effective in renin-dependent hypertension Initial dose in pt on diuretics: 0.625 mg

(continued)

TABLE 3.11. *(continued)* **Parenteral Antihypertensive Agents—Pharmacologic Characteristics**

Agent	Dosage/Onset/Duration	Comments
Calcium Channel Antagonists		
Nicardipine	Initial: 5 mg/h IV Titrate: 2.5 mg/h every 5–15 min Range: 5–15 mg/h Onset: 1–5 min Duration: 30 min	IV substitute for PO nicardipine therapy: 20 mg PO q8h = 0.5 mg/h 30 mg PO q8h = 1.2 mg/h 40 mg PO q8h = 2.2 mg/h
Diltiazem	IV: 0.25 mg/kg over 2 min (typically 15–20 mg IV) (may repeat once in 15 min with 0.35 mg/kg, typically 25 mg IV) then 5–15 mg/h	Compared to verapamil, relatively more vasodilator potency and less antiarrhythmic potency
Dopamine-1 Receptor Agonist		
Fenoldopam	Initial: 0.1–0.3 μg/kg/min; increase by 0.05–0.1 μg/ kg/min; maximum 1.6 μg/kg/min	Increases renal blood flow Tachycardia; monitor for hypokalemia q6 Can worsen glaucoma; contains sulfites; effect of dialysis unknown; avoid in intracranial hypertension
Central Sympatholytic		
Methyldopa	Dosage: IV 250–1000 mg q6h Onset: 4–6 h Duration: 10–16 h	Sedation, CNS depression

BP, blood pressure; CNS, central nervous system; GI, gastrointestinal; HF, heart failure; IV, intravenous; PO, by mouth

TABLE 3.12. Antihypertensive Therapy

- For hypertension associated with neurologic disorders, see chapter 9
- Rate of BP reduction and final BP goal depends on diagnosis. In general BP should not be reduced more than 10% to 15% over 4–6 hours and then a more gradual reduction over the ensuing days. Rapid control of BP is indicated in aortic dissection. Diuretic only for patient with clinically evident fluid overload.

Type	Recommended Therapy	Comments
Central/Peripheral Nervous System		
Hypertensive encephalopathy	1°: Nitroprusside Alt: Labetalol Alt: Calcium channel blocker	Drugs to avoid: methyldopa, clonidine, other central nervous system depressants
Aortic dissection	1°: β-blocker and then add nitroprusside Alt: Labetalol	Increases in heart rate, cardiac output, and dP/dT could be deleterious; so always give β-blocker first Drugs to avoid: hydralazine, minoxidil, nifedipine
Postcardiopulmonary bypass	1°: Nitroprusside + narcotics	First exclude postoperative pain/distress as reason for hypertension/tachycardia
Post-major vascular surgical procedure	1°: Nitroprusside Alt: Labetalol	First exclude postoperative pain/distress as reason for hypertension/tachycardia
Malignant Hypertension		
Grade III or IV fundoscopic changes	1°: Nitroprusside and β-blocker or labetalol Alt: Calcium channel blockers	Drugs to avoid: clonidine, methyldopa
Eclampsia (BP >140/90 mm Hg, edema, proteinuria, seizures in pregnancy)	1°: Hydralazine + delivery Alt: Labetalol Alt: Calcium channel blockers	Drugs to avoid: trimethaphan, diuretics, "pure β-blockers"; nitroprusside has potential risk to fetus and is reserved for refractory hypertension
Renal		
Renal parenchymal disease; Renovascular hypertension; Vasculitis	1°: Nitroprusside and β-blocker or labetalol Alt: Calcium channel blockers Alt: ACE inhibitors	Avoid ACE inhibitors if renal artery stenosis suspected, or significant renal insufficiency
Endocrine		
Pheochromocytoma	1°: Phentolamine or phenoxybenzamine β-blockers *after* α-blockade Alt: Labetalol Alt: Nitroprusside	*Must* provide α-blockade first and then β-blockade
Drug-induced		
Monoamine oxidase inhibitors	1°: Phentolamine Alt: Nitroprusside Alt: Labetalol	
Sympathomimetics (cocaine, amphetamines, phencyclidine, tricyclics, diet pills)	1°: Labetalol or nitrates Alt: Phentolamine Alt: Nitroprusside	
Withdrawal of centrally acting antihypertensive (clonidine, β-blockers)	1°: Labetalol Alt: Nitroprusside Alt: Phentolamine Alt: Resume clonidine or β-blocker	Restart agent that was discontinued if possible

ACE, angiotensin converting enzyme; BP, blood pressure; ICP, intracranial pressure

TABLE 3.13. Treatment of Pulmonary Arterial Hypertension

- This form includes familial and idiopathic ("primary") PAH and PAH associated with congenital systemic-to-pulmonary shunts, portal hypertension, collagen vascular diseases (e.g., scleroderma), certain drugs and toxins (e.g., anorexic agents), HIV disease, and hemoglobinopathies (e.g., sickle cell disease). IPAH has a mPAP >25 mm Hg at rest and a PCWP or LA pressure ≤15 mm Hg.
- Treatments below are not being recommended for PH due to postcapillary etiologies (e.g., left-sided heart disease), hypoxic etiologies (e.g., sleep disordered breathing, chronic high altitude), airway or parenchymal lung diseases (e.g., COPD, ILD), and chronic thrombotic and embolic etiologies.
- Progressive evaluation may include EKG, chest x-ray, echocardiogram, 6-minute walk, pulmonary function studies, chest CT, polysomnogram, serologies (e.g., ANA, RF, Scl 70, HIV), liver sonogram, VQ scan, pulmonary angiography, and RHC.
- Anticoagulant therapy based on risk benefit analysis should be considered to reduce risk of pulmonary thrombo-embolism or systemic embolism.
- Consider lung transplant evaluation or balloon atrial septostomy in appropriate refractory candidates.

Agent	Dosage	Comments
Oxygen	Inhaled (l/min) to maintain SaO_2 >90%	Controversial in patients with PAH associated with large right-to-left shunts due to congenital heart disease (Eisenmenger physiology)
Spironolactone	Range 25–200 mg/d PO in single or divided doses (max 400 mg/d)	For symptoms of right heart volume overload Monitor serum K and renal function
Nitric oxide (NO)	Range 5–80 ppm inhaled Vasoreactivity testing: 10 or 20 ppm inhaled (2–3 sets of baseline hemodynamics over 1 h then NO dose given over 6–10 min with hemodynamics determined) Doses >20 ppm increase risk of methemoglobinemia; monitor methemoglobin levels prior to and at 1 and 6 h after initiating prolonged therapy and after each dose increase, otherwise daily. NO dose should be reduced for methemoglobin concentration ≥5%	An endogenous chemical messenger acting via guanylate cyclase to cause vasodilatation Used to test pulmonary vasoreactivity in IPAH: Positive response = decrease of ≥10 mm Hg in mPAP to mPAP ≤40 mm Hg without a decrease in CO May be useful as continuous inhalation therapy in ventilated patients with PH and right HF Interruptions in delivery during chronic administration or large dose reductions may cause symptoms of rebound PAH May increase bleeding risk due to inhibitory effects on platelet aggregation
Calcium Channel Blocker • Reserved for IPAH with a positive vasodilator test (see NO above). • Maintenance of response defined as NYHA Class I–II and near normal resting hemodynamics should be re-evaluated in 6 months. If response not maintained then patient should be considered for therapy with prostanoids or an endothelin-1 receptor antagonist. • There are limited data on dose ranges and optimal dosing.		
Nifedipine (immediate release)	Initial: 10 mg PO q8 Usual IPAH range 30–180 mg ÷ q8h	Preferred over diltiazem if HR ≤100 Should be up titrated cautiously

(continued)

TABLE 3.13. *(continued)* **Treatment of Pulmonary Arterial Hypertension**

Agent	Dosage	Comments
Diltiazem (regular release)	Initial: 30–60 mg PO q6–8 Usual IPAH range: 120–720 mg ÷ q6–8h	Preferred over nifedipine or amlodipine if HR >100 Should be up titrated cautiously
Amlodipine	Initial: 2.5–5 mg PO qd Usual IPAH range: 2.5–30 mg PO qd	Diltiazem preferred if HR >100 Limited data and should be up titrated cautiously

Prostanoids

- Epoprostenol is produced in the vascular endothelium. Treprostinil and iloprost are stable analogues of epoprostenol. These agents are vasodilators with platelet antiaggregating properties.
- Adverse reactions associated with initiation and up titration of prostanoid therapy include jaw pain, flushing, headache, nausea, diarrhea, rash, anxiety, hypotension, and musculoskeletal pain. In addition epoprostenol therapy carries the risk of catheter-related infections and thromboembolic events, treprostinil can cause pain and induration at the infusion site, and iloprost has been associated with trismus and cough.

Agent	Dosage	Comments
Epoprostenol	Initially 2 ng/kg/min IV with increases of 1–2 ng/kg/min no faster than hourly or until unacceptable (dose-limiting) pharmacologic effects occur Average discharge dose after a 3-d initial titration was 6.5 ng/kg/min Adjustments: Increases or decreases of 1–2 ng/kg/min are usually based on symptoms or excessive side effects "Plateau" dose usually 20–40 ng/kg/min	Recommended for NYHA Class III–IV PAH with advanced disease; considered first line therapy for NYHA Class IV PAH Chronic overdosing can result in high-output HF Requires a central venous catheter for administration; interruptions in delivery or large dose reductions may cause symptoms of rebound PAH
Treprostinil	Initially: 1.25 ng/kg/min SC infusion; (decrease to 0.625 ng/kg/min if not tolerated) Adjustments: increase by ≤1.25 ng/kg/min per wk for the first 4 wk then ≤2.5 ng/kg/min per wk based on symptoms; similar decreases are made based on excessive side effects	Reserved for NYHA Class III–IV PAH, particularly those without significant benefit on oral therapy Limited data with >40 ng/kg/min Avoid interruptions in delivery Liver disease: initial dose should be decreased to 0.625 ng/kg/min and increased cautiously
Iloprost	Initially: 2.5 μg inhaled; if tolerated, increase to 5 μg 6–9 times per day (≥q2h) while awake, according to need and tolerability; max dose studied, 45 μg daily (5 μg 9 times per d)	Reserved for NYHA Class III–IV PAH, and may be useful as adjunct to oral therapy Liver disease: give 2.5 μg at intervals ≥3 h to max of 6 times daily; dose may be cautiously increased or given more frequently per patient response

(continued)

TABLE 3.13. *(continued)* **Treatment of Pulmonary Arterial Hypertension**

Agent	Dosage	Comments
Endothelin Receptor Antagonist		
• Endothelin-1 is a vasoconstrictor and smooth muscle mitogen. • Bosentan may cause hepatotoxicity. If elevated AST or ALT with symptoms or Bili of ≥2 × UNL, then stop. If AST or ALT >3 and ≤5 × UNL, then reduce or hold and monitor AST/ALT; if levels return to pretherapy values, then continue or reintroduce (starting dose); and monitor levels. If ALT or AST >5 and ≤8 × UNL, then stop and monitor levels; if levels return to pretherapy values, then consider reintroduction (starting dose) and monitor levels. If ALT or AST >8 × UNL, then stop and should avoid reintroducing.		
Bosentan	Initial, 62.5 mg PO q12h for 4 wk Maintenance, up to 125 mg PO q12h Adults <40 kg: initial and maintenance, 62.5 mg PO q12h (monitor liver function [monthly] and hemoglobin [1 mo, 3 mo, every 3 mo]) Should avoid if elevated AST or ALT >3 × the UNL at baseline	Reserved for NYHA Class III–IV PAH Adverse reactions include hepatotoxicity, anemia, edema, headache, hypotension, nausea, emesis, dyspepsia, palpitations, and flushing
Phosphodiesterase (Type-5) Inhibitor		
• Limited data on long-term efficacy and safety alone or in combination with prostanoids or bosentan.		
Sildenafil	Range 25–100 mg q8–12h Dose increases of 25 mg q8–12h every 2–4 wk, based on symptoms (limited data on dosing, particularly maximal efficacious dose) Increased plasma levels can occur in the elderly (age >65) and with renal impairment (Cr clearance <30 mL/min), hepatic impairment and concurrent use of cytochrome P450 inhibitors	Reserved for NYHA Class III PAH Inhibitor of cGMP specific phosphodiesterase; lengthens and enhances effects of inhaled NO Hypotension can result with the coadministration of nitrates Adverse reactions include headache, flushing, periorbital edema, and priapism

ALT, alanine aminotransferase; AST, aspartate aminotransferase; Bili, bilirubin; CO, cardiac output; COPD, chronic obstructive pulmonary disease; CT, computed tomography; EKG, electrocardiogram; HF, heart failure; ILD, interstitial lung disease; IPAH, idiopathic pulmonary arterial hypertension; K, potassium; LA, left atrium; mPAP, mean pulmonary artery pressure; NO, nitric oxide; NYHA, New York Heart Association; PAH, pulmonary arterial hypertension; PCWP, pulmonary capillary wedge pressure; PH, pulmonary hypertension; PO, by mouth; RHC, right heart catheterization; SaO_2, arterial oxygen saturation; UNL, upper normal limit; VQ, ventilation-perfusion

TABLE 3.14. Drugs Associated with QT Interval Prolongation[a]

Antiarrhythmic Agents
Sotalol
Ibutilide, dofetilide, sematilide
Disopyramide
Procainamide
Quinidine
Amiodarone[b]
Nonantiarrhythmic Agents
Erythromycin, clarithromycin, telithromycin, azithromycin
Ketoconazole, itraconazole
Quinolones (sparfloxacin, moxifloxacin, gatifloxacin, gemifloxacin, levofloxacin)
Phenothiazines (chlorpromazine, droperidol, haloperidol, thioridazine)
Fosphenytoin
Methadone
Pentamidine
Probucol
Quetiapine
Risperidone
Arsenic trioxide
Astemazole[c]
Bepridil, mibefradil
SSRI (venlafaxine)
Terfinadine[c]
Tricyclic antidepressants
Trimethoprim-sulfamethoxazole

[a]Additional information available at www.qtdrugs.org.
[b]Risk of torsade is low.
[c]Not available in the U.S.

Pulmonary Therapies

TABLE 4.1. Asthma—Therapeutic Options

Agents	Dosage
Inhaled β Agonists	
Albuterol	2.5 mg (0.5 ml) diluted in 2–3 ml 0.9% NaCl q2–6h 10–15 mg/h (2–3 ml) diluted to a minimum of 4 ml at gas flow of 6–8 L/min (see Table 4.4)
Levalbuterol	0.63–1.25 mg q2–6h
Subcutaneous β Agonists	
Epinephrine	0.3 mg (0.3 ml)
Terbutaline	0.25 mg (0.25 ml)
Anticholinergic Agents	See Tables 4.2 and 4.3
Theophylline	See Table 4.5
Corticosteroids	
Methylprednisolone *or*	60–125 mg q6–8h
Hydrocortisone *or*	2 mg/kg q4h
Hydrocortisone	2 mg/kg *then* 0.5 mg/kg/h
Inhaled Corticosteroids	
Beclomethasone	40–160 μg twice daily
Budesonide	200–800 μg twice daily
Flunisolide	500–1,000 μg twice daily
Fluticasone	MDI: 88–220 μg twice daily PWD: 100–1,000 μg twice daily
Triamcinolone	200 μg 3 to 4 times daily or 400 μg twice daily

IV, intravenous; MDI, metered dose inhaler; PO, by mouth; PWD, powder

Route	Formulation	Comment
Nebulized	0.5% solution	The frequency of intermittent β agonist administration will vary with the severity of illness of the patient; in severely ill patients, the initial interval may be hourly
Continuous nebulization	0.5% solution	
Nebulized	0.63 mg/3 ml 1.25 mg/3 ml	No greater benefit over albuterol in acutely ill, critically ill, or mechanically ventilated patients; clinical effects similar to albuterol
Subcutaneous	1:1000 solution	May be considered in patients who do not respond to inhaled β agonists; may repeat dose every 15 min as needed up to 3 doses
Subcutaneous	1 mg/ml	A second dose may be given after 20 min if necessary
IV/PO		
IV	40, 62.5 mg/ml	
IV	50 mg/ml	
IV		
Continuous infusion		
MDI	MDI: 40, 80 μg/puff	May be considered as an adjunct to systemic steroid therapy initially; initial dose may be higher
MDI	MDI: 200 μg/puff	
MDI	MDI: 250 μg/puff	
MDI, Rotadisk	MDI: 44, 110, 220 μg/puff	
Diskus	PWD: 50, 100, 250 μg/puff	
MDI	MDI: 100 μg/puff	

TABLE 4.2. Antibronchospastic Agents—Metered Dose Inhalers

Agent	β_2/β_1 Potency	Dose Per Actuation	Recommended Dosage/Interval
Inhaled β-Adrenergic Agents			
Albuterol	++++/±	90 μg*	1–2 puffs q2–6h
Salmeterol[a]	See note		
Anticholinergic Agents			
Ipratropium bromide	—	18 μg	2–4 puffs q2–6h
Albuterol and	++++/±	90 μg*	2 puffs, 4× daily
ipratropium	—	18 μg	
Tiotropium	—	18 μg	One capsule, inhaled once daily Individual capsules used for each dose

The dosing interval may vary depending on the severity of illness of the patient. The dose may need to be higher for patients on mechanical ventilation (i.e., 4–8 puffs q2–6h).
[a] *Salmeterol is indicated for prophylactic use in chronic stable asthma and is not recommended for the treatment of acute bronchospasm.* For maintenance of bronchodilatation and prevention of the symptoms of asthma, the usual dose is 2 puffs (42 μg) twice (in the morning and evening) daily.
*Dose delivered in terms of 90 μg of albuterol base.

TABLE 4.3. Antibronchospastic Agents—Nebulized Drugs

Agent	β_2/β_1 Potency	Formulations	Dosage
β-Adrenergic Agents[a]			
Albuterol	++++/±	0.5% solution	2.5–5 mg diluted in 2–3 ml 0.9% NaCl q2–6h Continuous nebulization; see Table 4.4
Levalbuterol	++++/±	0.63 mg/3 ml 1.25 mg/3 ml	0.63–1.25 mg q2–6h
Anticholinergic Agents			
Ipratropium bromide	—	0.02% solution	500 μg diluted in 2–5 ml 0.9% NaCl q6–8h
Albuterol and Ipratropium	++++/± —	Ipratropium 0.5 mg and albuterol 3 mg/3 ml	3 ml q6h
Atropine Sulfate	—	1 mg/ml injectable preparation	2.5–5 mg diluted in 2–3 ml 0.9% NaCl q3–5h
Glycopyrrolate	—	0.2 mg/ml injectable preparation	2 mg diluted in 2–3 ml 0.9% NaCl q6h

[a]Dosing interval depends on the status of the patient, but in severe asthma it may be as frequent as q1–2h under medical supervision.

TABLE 4.4. Antibronchospastic Agents—Continuous Nebulization

Use the guidelines below (±20%) for 1 hour of nebulization. For prescribed dose of 10 mg/h at 15 L/min flow, add 2 mL albuterol (5 mg/mL) to 48 mL saline for 50 mL/h output. For multiple hours of operation, multiply by the number of hours desired.

Continuous Nebulizer—HEART®

	High Flow					
Desired dose (mg/h)	5	10	15	5	10	15
Albuterol 5 mg/mL (mL)	1	2	3	1	2	3
Saline (mL)	29	28	27	49	48	47
Flow rate = Output	10 L/min = 30 mL/h			15 L/min = 50 mL/h		

Continuous Nebulizer—UniHEART—IV™

	Low Flow					
Desired dose (mg/h)	5	10	15	5	10	15
Albuterol 5 mg/mL (mL)	1	2	3	1	2	3
Saline (mL)	3	2	1	8	7	6
Flow rate = Output	2 L/min = 4 mL/h			4 L/min = 9 mL/h		

Continuous Nebulizer—MiniHEART®

	Very Low Flow					
Desired dose (mg/h)	2.5	5	7.5	10	12.5	15
Albuterol 5 mg/mL (mL)	0.5	1	1.5	2	2.5	3
Saline (mL)	7.5	7	6.5	6	5.5	5
Flow rate = Output	2 L/min = 8 mL/h					

TABLE 4.5. Theophylline/Aminophylline—Dosing

	Theophylline	Aminophylline	Comments
Loading Doses			
No prior theophylline or aminophylline	5 mg/kg IV over 30 min	6 mg/kg IV over 30 min	Theophylline = 80% × aminophylline Loading dose administered over 30 min
Prior theophylline or aminophylline	Estimate	Estimate	Theophylline 1 mg/kg IV/PO increases the serum concentration 2 mg/L; aminophylline 1.2 mg/kg IV/PO increases the serum concentration 2 mg/L; therapeutic range 10–20 mg/L
Maintenance Infusion			
Adults (smokers)	0.72 mg/kg/h	0.9 mg/kg/h	Maximum doses: theophylline 900 mg/d, aminophylline 1,080 mg/d
Adults (nonsmokers)	0.48 mg/kg/h	0.6 mg/kg/h	
Adults (heart failure, liver disease, cor pulmonale)	0.24 mg/kg/h	0.3 mg/kg/h	Maximum doses: theophylline 400 mg/d, aminophylline 480 mg/d

IV, intravenous; PO, by mouth

TABLE 4.6. Theophylline/Aminophylline–Drug Interactions

Drugs that Decrease Theophylline/Aminophylline Clearance/Metabolism (Serum Levels Rise)	Drugs that Increase Theophylline/Aminophylline Clearance/Metabolism (Serum Levels Fall)	Drugs whose Activity is Decreased by Theophylline/ Aminophylline
Amiodarone	Carbamazepine	Adenosine
Cimetidine	Pentobarbital	Benzodiazepines
Ciprofloxacin	Phenobarbital	Hydantoins
Clarithromycin	Phenytoin	Nondepolarizing neuromuscular blocking agents
Disulfiram	Rifampin	
Enoxacin	Rifabutin	
Erythromycin	Ritonavir	
Fluvoxamine	Ticlopidine	
Interferon		
Ketoconazole		
Mexiletine		
Norfloxacin		
Oral contraceptives		
Propranolol		
Troleandomycin		
Verapamil		

TABLE 4.7. Upper Airway Obstruction—Nonspecific Therapies

Therapy	Indication	Dosage/Route	Comments
Helium 80%–oxygen 20% mixture	Partially obstructed airway	Inhalation	Limits FiO_2 to maximum O_2 concentration in mixture Decreases turbulence of airflow Helium/oxygen also available in helium 70%—oxygen 30% mixture
Dexamethasone	Decreases airway edema	4–10 mg IV q6h	Antitumor effect on certain anterior mediastinal tumors Prophylactic for postextubation trauma, surgical trauma; efficacy controversial
Radiation	Shrinks tumor		Anterior mediastinal tumors; tissue diagnosis may be required
Racemic epinephrine	Decreases swelling of airway mucosa	0.5 ml of 2.25% solution in 2–5 ml 0.9% NaCl inhaled q1–4h prn	Vasoconstrictor; may precipitate angina
Endotracheal intubation	Fully obstructed airway Partially obstructed airway and respiratory failure Prohibitively increased work of breathing	Oral or nasal endotracheal intubation Surgical access: cricothyroidotomy (for rapid access) or tracheostomy	Technique of choice depends on experience of operator, although surgical access may be required Caution: sedatives, anesthetics, or neuromuscular blockade may convert a partially obstructed airway to a totally obstructed airway

TABLE 4.8. Mucolytic Agents

Agent	Formulations	Dosage/Interval/Comments
N-acetylcysteine	10%, 20% solutions	Nebulization: 3–5 ml of 20% solution or 6–10 ml of 10% solution tid or qid Instillation: 1–2 ml of 10% or 20% solution tid or qid Administer after aerosolized β agonist to prevent bronchospasm 20% solution of N-acetylcysteine should be diluted 1:1 with normal saline
Dornase α recombinant	2.5 ml ampule containing 1 mg/ml	Nebulization: 2.5 ml qd using a recommended nebulizer. (Hudson T Up-draft II and disposable jet nebulizer, Marquest Acorn II in conjunction with Pulmo-Aide compressor, Pari LC Jet$^+$ nebulizer in conjunction with the Pari PRONEB compressor) The effects of dornase α on respiratory tract infections in cystic fibrosis patients >21 years old may be smaller than younger patients, and twice daily dosing may be required in these patients Dornase α may be continued or initiated during acute respiratory exacerbations, although the benefit of dornase α during acute respiratory exacerbations is unknown
Saturated solution of potassium iodide (SSKI)	1 g/ml	0.3–0.6 ml (300–600 mg) PO tid or qid
Guaifenesin	100 mg/5 ml, 200 mg/5 ml solutions	100–400 mg PO qid

PO, by mouth

TABLE 4.9. Sclerosing Agents for Pleurodesis

Agent	Dosage	Dilution	Comments/Side Effects
Doxycycline	500–1,000 mg	0.9% NaCl 25–100 ml	Fever, chest pain
Talc insufflation	2–10 g		Pain, fever, hypotension; talc insufflation may be done in conjunction with thoracoscopy
Antineoplastic Agents			
Bleomycin	60 U	0.9% NaCl 50–100 ml	Do not exceed 40 U/m^2 in elderly patients, significant systemic absorption, GI side effects, pain, fever
Cisplatin and cytarabine	Cisplatin 100 mg/m^2 and cytarabine 1,200 mg (mixed together)	0.9% NaCl 250 ml	Use depends on antineoplastic activity rather than on irritative properties; myelosuppression; GI side effects
Doxorubicin	10–100 mg	0.9% NaCl 10–100 ml	Increased toxicity compared with tetracyclines, pain, fever, nausea, vomiting
Fluorouracil	2–3 g	0.9% NaCl 50–100 ml	Leukopenia 7–10 d after instillation
Mechlorethamine	10–30 mg	0.9% NaCl 10–100 ml	Increased toxicity compared with tetracyclines, nausea, vomiting, pain, fever, leukopenia
Thiotepa	0.6–0.8 mg/kg	0.9% NaCl 50–100 ml	Less irritating than other agents

GI, gastrointestinal
Local anesthetics such as 1% lidocaine may be added to the sclerosing solution to reduce pain (up to a total dose of 400 mg).

TABLE 4.10. Loculated Pleural Effusion—Thrombolytic Therapy

Agent	Dosage	Comments
Alteplase, recombinant	2–50 mg in 50–120 ml 0.9% NaCl	Pleuritic chest pain may be treated with analgesics Risk of bleeding complications, avoid concurrent anticoagulation Most common adult dose is 50 mg

Directions for use:

1. The optimal dosage of thrombolytic agent, duration of therapy, and effectiveness remain to be determined.
2. The volume of agent administered should be adjusted based on the size of the effusion.
3. After the agent is instilled into the pleural space, the chest tube should be clamped and the patient rotated in several positions to permit adequate drug distribution throughout the pleural space.
4. The chest tube should remain clamped for 0.5 to 4 hours.
5. After the chest tube is unclamped, the chest tube should be put on suction and the contents of the pleural space evacuated.
6. The volume of the fluid returned should be determined. (Note: the volume of the dose instilled must be subtracted from the volume returned.)

TABLE 4.11. Pulmonary Embolism—Therapy

Agent	Loading Dosage	Maintenance Dosage	Comments
Anticoagulants			
Heparin sulfate	80 U/kg IV bolus	18 U/kg/h for at least 7 d	Check aPTT 6 h after therapy initiated; maintain aPTT 1.5–2.5 × baseline Heparin clearance is increased in pulmonary embolism compared with deep venous thrombosis Contraindicated in patients with active bleeding or heparin-induced thrombocytopenia and thrombosis See Table 8.7 for weight-based dosing.
Warfarin	5–10 mg/d	2–7.5 mg/d	Therapy may start on the 2nd day of heparinization Dosage should be adjusted to maintain PT 1.5–2 × baseline PT (INR 2–3) Use for 3–6 m to prevent recurrent pulmonary emboli unless there are persisting risk factors for hemorrhage Contraindicated in patients with active bleeding and in pregnancy Decrease loading and maintenance in presence of liver disease. See Table 8.6
Enoxaparin	—	1 mg/kg q12h	Warfarin therapy started on day 1 of therapy No need to monitor aPTT Equally effective with less risk of bleeding compared with unfractionated heparin
Tinzaparin	—	175 anti-Xa U/kg daily	Treatment for at least 5 d until anticoagulated with warfarin
Thrombolytics[a]			Indications include severe hypoxemia or hemodynamic instability See Table 8.7
Recombinant tissue plasminogen activator (rtPA)	100 mg IV over 2 h		Contraindicated in patients with active bleeding, severe hypertension, trauma, recent stroke or surgery, or any hemorrhagic disease

aPTT, activated partial thromboplastin time; INR, international normalization ratio; IV, intravenous; PT, prothrombin time

[a]The conventional indication for thrombolytic therapy is "massive" pulmonary embolism, characterized by one or more of the following abnormalities: (a) angiographic evidence of pulmonary artery occlusion of at least 40%; (b) hypotension with systolic arterial pressure <90–100 mm Hg; (c) syncope; (d) echocardiographic evidence of right ventricular dysfunction.

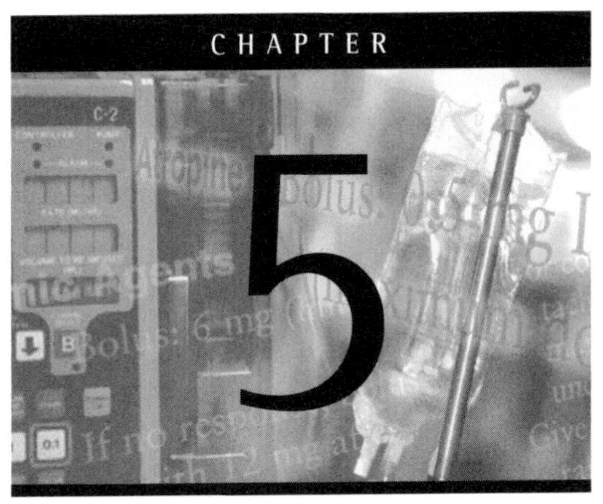

Renal, Electrolyte, and Acid Base Disturbances

TABLE 5.1. Hypernatremia

Therapy	Dosage	Comments
5% dextrose in water (D5W) or 0.45% NaCl	By calculation: see comment	Free water replacement is based on formula for calculating water deficit: Water deficit (L) = normal total body water − estimated total body water Water deficit = (0.5 × body weight [kg]) − [(0.5 × body weight [kg]) × (140/actual serum Na^+)] Replace half of water deficit in the first 24 h and the remainder over the following 2–3 d Monitor serum Na^+ q1–2h to ensure gradual correction Correcting too rapidly may produce cerebral edema, seizures, and death
Desmopressin (DDAVP)	Intranasal: 0.1–0.4 ml (10–40 μg) qd	Can be administered as a single daily dose or divided into 2 doses
	SC/IV: 0.5–1 ml (2.0–4.0 μg) qd	When switching from the intranasal to IV route, the comparable antidiuretic dose is approximately 1/10 of the intranasal dose
Vasopressin	SC/IM: 5–10 U bid-tid	Low cost; however, complications include hypertension and sterile abscesses IV administration not usually recommended

IM, intramuscular; IV, intravenous; SC, subcutaneous

- Homeostasis of extracellular fluid is more dominant mechanism than maintenance of osmolality. Hypernatremia may be associated with low, normal, or excessive body water.
- If thirst mechanism is intact, vasopressin replacement is a matter of convenience.
- Excessive or rapid correction is particularly dangerous if hypernatremia has persisted for more than 24 hours because there is increased central nervous system intracellular osmolality. In this setting, secondary cerebral edema may produce seizures or death.

TABLE 5.2. Hyponatremia

Therapy	Dosage	Comments
Furosemide	20–200 mg IV q4–6h	Treatment usually required if serum sodium <110 mEq/L or patient is symptomatic Aim to bring serum sodium up to 120–125 mEq/L, but raise no more than 12 mEq/L in the first 24 h
0.9% NaCl (154 mEq Na^+/L)	By calculation (see comment)	Calculation: Na^+ deficit (mEq) = 0.60 × lean body wt (kg) × (120 – measured Na^+)
3% NaCl (513 mEq Na^+/L)	By calculation (see comment above)	Only for severe neurologic derangements or seizures Administer very cautiously as overly rapid correction can cause CNS toxicity (central pontine myelinolysis) or volume overload
Demeclocycline	300 mg PO q12h	For patients with SIADH Antagonizes ADH action in the distal nephron

ADH, antidiuretic hormone; CNS, central nervous system; PO, by mouth; SIADH, syndrome of inappropriate antidiuretic hormone release

- Important to exclude "spurious" hyponatremia caused by hyperglycemia. This occurs because the osmotically active solute, glucose, causes a shift of water from the intracellular compartment to the extracellular compartment and dilutes extracellular sodium. For every 62 mg/dl rise in glucose, there is a 1 mEq/L fall in sodium.
- The rate of correction of hyponatremia should be proportional to its rate of occurrence. Acute correction of hyponatremia should not exceed a 20 mEq/L rise in concentration of serum sodium in the first 48 hours of therapy.
- Osmolality (mOsm/kg) = $2(Na^+ + K^+) + (BUN/2.8) + (glucose/18)$.

TABLE 5.3. Hyperkalemia

Therapy	Dosage	Onset/Duration	Comments
Acute Management			
Sodium bicarbonate ($NaHCO_3$)	1 mEq/kg IV over 3–5 min	Onset: 15–30 min Duration: 1–2 h	Can cause sodium overload and hyperosmolality
Calcium gluconate 10% (100 mg/ml = 9 mg/ml elemental Ca^{+2}, 0.46 mEq/ml)	5–10 ml IV over 2–5 min	Onset: 1–5 min Duration: 1–2 h	Rapid onset, but short-lived Not compatible with $NaHCO_3$; must flush line between infusions Can augment digoxin toxicity
Calcium chloride 10% (100 mg/ml = 27.2 mg/ml elemental Ca^{+2}, 1.36 mEq/ml)	5–10 ml IV over 2–5 min	Onset: 1–5 min Duration: 1–2 h	Rapid onset, but short-lived Not compatible with $NaHCO_3$; must flush line between infusions Can augment digoxin toxicity Preferred preparation when volume is an issue because it contains more elemental calcium per g than calcium gluconate
Dextrose and insulin	Dextrose 0.5 g/kg with 0.3 U regular insulin per g dextrose	Onset: 10–15 min Duration: 3 h	Usual dosing is 25 g dextrose with 6–10 U regular insulin Insulin should be given IV to avoid delayed hypoglycemia that can follow SC insulin; important to administer glucose concurrently
Albuterol	10–20 mg via nebulized aerosol	Onset: 30 min Duration: 2 h	Mechanism is intracellular shunting of potassium by β 2-adrenergic agonists Beware of possible angina
Subacute and Chronic Management			
Sodium polystyrene sulfonate (SPS)	PO: 15–60 g in 100–200 ml 20% sorbitol q4h PR: 50 g in 50 ml 70% sorbitol added to 100–200 ml water	Onset: PO: 2 h PR: 1 h Duration: 4 h	Resin exchanges sodium for potassium in the gut PO SPS removes 1 mEq KCl/g, PR SPS removes 0.5 mEq KCl/g Be aware of sodium load in patients with heart failure

IV, intravenous; PO, by mouth; PR, per rectum; SC, subcutaneous
If conservative methods of therapy fail, up to 50 mEq/h of potassium can be removed by hemodialysis. Peritoneal dialysis removes approximately 10 mEq/h.

TABLE 5.4. Hypokalemia

Therapy	Dosage	Comments
Potassium chloride (KCl)	See sliding scale for IV infusion (Table 5.5) Maximum infusion rate of 40 mEq/h IV through a central line with continuous cardiac monitoring Solutions should be prepared in non-dextrose containing fluids (i.e., NS or 0.45% NaCl)	Life-threatening hypokalemia usually is caused by gastrointestinal losses (diarrhea) or genitourinary losses (diuretics) Magnitude of deficit can only be approximated Loss of 200–400 mEq of potassium lowers plasma potassium by 1 mEq/L Clinical manifestations are rare when potassium level is ≥2.5 mEq/L, the exception being patients with cardiac disease The most serious complications are conduction disturbances and arrhythmias; muscle weakness can occur Cautious replacement in oliguric or anuric patients Peripheral IV administration can be painful; pain is less if solutions contain less than 60 mEq KCl/L Rapid IV replacement (greater than 20 mEq/h) warrants continuous cardiac monitoring Check magnesium and supplement if below lower limit of normal
Potassium citrate and citric acid	40–60 mEq PO bid to qid	Solution of 1,100 mg potassium citrate and 334 mg citric acid monohydrate per 5 ml; equivalent to 2 mEq potassium and 2 mEq bicarbonate per ml Dose may be adjusted based on urine pH Useful in renal tubular acidosis, when replacement of both potassium and bicarbonate is required Aggressive treatment of acidosis with bicarbonate alone may aggravate coexisting hypokalemia

NS, normal saline (0.9%); NaCl, sodium chloride.
Potassium sparing diuretics may be considered in patients with severe renal losses of potassium; however, they should not be used in patients with renal insufficiency or in conjunction with aggressive potassium supplementation.

TABLE 5.5. Sliding Scale Algorithm for Potassium Chloride (KCl) Infusion

K^+ (mEq/L)	KCl Infusion Rate (mEq/h)
<2.5	20–40
2.5–3.0	15–20
3.1–3.5	10
3.6–4.0	5
>4.1	—

Potassium level should be checked frequently—i.e., every 4 to 6 hours, during IV infusion. Patients receiving ≥15 mEq/h should have cardiac monitoring. Doses ≥15 mEq/h should ideally be delivered via central vein because of pain with peripheral administration. (Maximum recommended concentration is 0.4 mEq/ml of solution.)

TABLE 5.6. Hypercalcemia

Therapy	Dosage	Comments
0.9% NaCl	250–500 ml/h	With or without furosemide 20 mg IV q4–6h Volume expansion in patients with normal renal function leads to urinary calcium losses Calcium loss up to 2 g/24 h Need to monitor magnesium, phosphorus, and potassium
Calcitonin-salmon	Initial: 4 IU/kg SC/IM q12h Repeat: 8 IU/kg SC/IM q12h	Perform skin test for allergy before first dose in patients with suspected sensitivity to calcitonin-salmon Decreases bone reabsorption, but effect is limited and diminishes after several days Maximum dose 8 IU/kg q6h if no response to lower doses May be added to bisphosphonate to achieve normal calcium levels within a few days
Zoledronic acid	4 mg IV as a single dose over at least 15 min	Minimum time period for retreatment is 7 d
Pamidronate disodium	60 mg (for moderate hypercalcemia) or 90 mg (for severe hypercalcemia) as a single IV infusion (diluted in 1 L 0.9% NaCl or D5W) over 24 h	Moderate hypercalcemia: corrected serum calcium 12–13.5 mg/dl; severe hypercalcemia: corrected serum calcium >13.5 mg/dl A minimum of 7 d should elapse to assess response before re-treatment If retreating, dosage is same as initial dose Osteonecrosis of the jaw may occur in patients with cancer
Gallium nitrate	100 mg/M^2 IV (for mild hypercalcemia), 150 mg/M^2 IV (moderate hypercalcemia), or 200 mg/M^2 IV (severe hypercalcemia) in 1 L 0.9% NaCl or D5W infused over 24 h × 5 d	If serum calcium is lowered to normal range in less than 5 d, treatment may be discontinued Potential for nephrotoxicity
Hydrocortisone	1 mg/kg IV q8h	Especially effective in patients with sarcoidosis, breast carcinoma, and hematologic malignancies Equivalent doses of other glucocorticoids (dexamethasone or methylprednisolone) may be used (see Table 6.1)

IM, intramuscular; IV, intravenous; SC, subcutaneous

TABLE 5.7. Hypocalcemia

Therapy	Dosage	Comments
Acute Therapy		
Calcium gluconate 10% (100 mg/ml = 9 mg/ml elemental Ca^{+2}, 0.46 mEq/ml)	Initial: 1 g (10 ml) IV over 10 min Infusion: 100 mg/h	Treat as medical emergency if symptomatic (seizures, confusion, tetany, laryngospasm, arrhythmias, hypotension) Therapy of acidosis with bicarbonate lowers ionized serum calcium further Calcium infusion should be continued until elemental calcium level reaches 8–9 mg/dL, then monitor levels and administer as needed Concomitant magnesium supplementation is often required to maintain calcium level
Calcium chloride 10% (100 mg/ml = 27.2 mg/ml elemental Ca^{+2}, 1.36 mEq/ml)	Initial: 1 g (10 ml) IV over 10 min Infusion: 100 mg/h	Preferred preparation when volume is an issue because it contains more elemental calcium per g than calcium gluconate Increased bioavailability in hepatic failure
Chronic Therapy		
Calcium carbonate	1.25–5 g PO daily in 3–4 divided doses	1.25 g calcium carbonate contains 500 mg elemental calcium
Ergocalciferol (vitamin D_2)	25,000 to 150,000 U/d PO	Used for the treatment of chronic hypocalcemia, rickets, familial hypophosphatemia, and hypoparathyroidism Start therapy with oral calcium Slow acting preparation Long duration of action; if hypercalcemia develops, it may not resolve for weeks Inexpensive
Dihydrotachysterol	0.125–1 mg PO qd	Used for the treatment of chronic hypocalcemia, acute, chronic and latent forms of postoperative tetany and idiopathic tetany, and hypoparathyroidism Fast onset; expensive
Calcitriol	0.5–2 μg PO qd	Acute hypocalcemia Rapid onset If hypercalcemia occurs, it is not long lasting
Calcifediol	50–100 μg PO gd	Used for the treatment and management of metabolic bone disease or hypocalcemia in patients on chronic renal dialysis Intermediate duration of action
Doxercalciferol	10 μg PO 3 times weekly	Used for the management of secondary hyperparathyroidism in patients undergoing chronic renal dialysis Maximum dose 20 μg 3 times weekly Intermediate duration of action

(continued)

TABLE 5.7. *(continued)* **Hypocalcemia**

Therapy	Dosage	Comments
Paricalcitol	0.04–1 μg/kg IV every other day during hemodialysis	Used for the management of secondary hyperparathyroidism in patients undergoing chronic renal dialysis Intermediate duration of action

IV, intravenous; PO, by mouth

- Clinically significant hypocalcemia is an uncommon problem, but it may occur after multiple rapid transfusions, parathyroidectomy, thyroidectomy, or severe pancreatitis.
- Correction for calcium in the setting of hypoalbuminemia: total serum calcium will fall 0.8 g/dl for every 1 g decrease in serum albumin.
- Consider obtaining measurement of ionized calcium to most accurately determine degree of calcium deficit.
- Calcium preparations should be diluted to prevent phlebitis and to limit tissue necrosis if extravasated.
- Do not administer calcium in solutions with either bicarbonate or phosphate; insoluble salts can form.

TABLE 5.8. Hyperphosphatemia

Therapy	Dosage	Comments
Aluminum hydroxide	30–120 ml PO q4–6h	Can cause constipation
Hemodialysis or peritoneal dialysis		
Acetazolamide	15 mg/kg q3–4h	
NS infusion		

NS, normal saline (0.9%); PO, by mouth

Acute, severe hyperphosphatemia in association with symptomatic hypocalcemia can be life threatening. Hyperphosphatemia is associated with tumor lysis, rhabdomyosis, exogenous phosphate administration, lactic, or ketoacidosis.

TABLE 5.9. Hypophosphatemia

Therapy	Dosage	Comments
Potassium phosphate (K_2PO_4) or sodium phosphate (Na_2PO_4)	For mild to moderate hypophosphatemia (PO_4 = 1.6–3.0 mg/dL): 0.16–0.32 mmol/kg IV over 6–8 h For severe hypophosphatemia (PO_4 = <1.5 mg/dL): 0.64 mmol/kg IV over 6–8 h	Muscle weakness caused by hypophosphatemia can precipitate or exacerbate heart failure, respiratory failure, and neurologic symptoms Intravenous replacement warranted for serum phosphate levels less than 1 mg/dl Be cautious of IV therapy in patients with hypercalcemia because metastatic calcification may occur Maximum phosphate infusion rate is 10 mmol/h (Ann Pharmacother 1997;31:683) Important metabolic replacement in hyperalimentation solutions 1 mmol phosphate = 31 mg phosphate Each ml of potassium phosphate contains phosphate 3 mmol and potassium 4.4 mEq; beware of hyperkalemia and follow potassium levels Each ml of sodium phosphate contains phosphate 3 mmol and sodium 4 mEq
Potassium and sodium phosphate for oral solution	250–500 mg (8–16 mmol) PO qid	Oral therapy is preferred when serum phosphate levels approach 2 mg/dL May require days to replenish intracellular stores of phosphorus, even after serum levels normalize Each capsule/packet contains K^+ 7 mEq and Na^+ 7 mEq

IV, intravenous; PO, by mouth

TABLE 5.10. Acidosis

Drug	Dosage	Indications	Comments
Sodium bicarbonate ($NaHCO_3$)	By calculation (see comment below)	Severe nonanion gap metabolic acidosis or hyperkalemia	Generally not given unless pH <7.20 or HCO_3^- <10 mEq/L Usual rate of administration is 2–5 mEq/h Can cause chemical phlebitis or cellulitis Many drug incompatibilities; flush line after use After cardiac arrest, reversal of acidosis results from adequate ventilation and blood flow. May consider use upon return of spontaneous circulation after long arrest interval (1 mEq/kg IV). Not recommended for routine use after cardiac arrest. May be associated with paradoxical mixed venous acidosis Can cause sodium overload and hyperosmolality Treatment of underlying etiology (i.e., sepsis, hypoperfusion, poisoning) is essential to reverse acidosis

- Decision to treat is controversial and depends on clinical situation; indications vary with etiology such as bicarbonate responsive acidosis (e.g., diabetic ketoacidosis).
- Bicarbonate deficit, an approximation of the amount of bicarbonate replacement needed to return bicarbonate concentration to normal:

  HCO_3^- deficit = body weight (kg) × 0.4 × (desired $[HCO_3^-]$ – measured $[HCO_3^-]$)
- In patients with chronic metabolic acidosis caused by chronic renal failure, replace with bicarbonate when bicarbonate concentration is less than 15 mEq/L to prevent osteomalacia.
- Treatment of lactic acidosis should be directed to the underlying etiology.

TABLE 5.11. Alkalosis

Therapy	Dosage	Indications	Comments
Potassium chloride (KCl)	Mild alkalosis: 100–150 mEq/d Severe alkalosis: Up to 300 mEq/d	Chloride-responsive alkalosis	Will replete not only chloride, but also potassium deficit, which may be substantial, especially with diuretic-induced alkalosis Spironolactone or potassium-sparing diuretics may be useful in hypokalemic patients
Sodium chloride (NaCl)	Mild alkalosis: 100–150 mEq/d Severe alkalosis: Up to 300 mEq/d	Chloride-responsive alkalosis	Alternative to KCl Use with caution in patients with HF
Acetazolamide	5 mg/kg qd up to qid (PO/IV)	Works well in edematous patients with cirrhosis or HF	Carbonic anhydrase inhibitor; impairs renal sodium and renal bicarbonate resorption, thus reducing net acid excretion Will have diuretic effect and may cause potassium losses
Hydrochloric acid (HCl)	0.1 N HCl by calculation (see comment)	For rapid correction of severe metabolic alkalosis	Concentration is 100 mEq HCl per 1 L sterile water Must administer via a central venous line Amount of H^+ needed to correct deficit can be determined by formula: H^+ (mEq) = 0.5 × weight (kg) × (103 – serum chloride)
Ammonium chloride	By calculation (see comment)	Metabolic alkalosis due to significant chloride losses	Ammonium ions are converted to urea in the liver with the generation of hydrogen and chloride ions Should not be given to patients with hepatic failure H^+ (mEq) = 0.5 × weight (kg) × (103 – serum chloride)

HF, heart failure; IV, intravenous; PO, by mouth
Correct volume, potassium, and chloride depletions.

TABLE 5.12. Tumor Lysis Syndrome

Complication	Intervention	Comments
Associated with rapidly growing malignancies (eg. leukemias, lymphomas) that are highly chemo or radio sensitive. Therapy initiated before administration of chemotherapy. Syndrome characterized by increases in uric acid, potassium, phosphate, and decreases in calcium that may result in renal failure, arrhythmias, seizures, or sudden death.		
Pretreatment Evaluation and Preparation		
Volume loading and diuresis	Hypotonic fluids (D5W/0.45% NaCl) 3,000 ml/M2/day	Loop diuretics if necessary to maintain urinary output
Evaluate renal function	Monitor weight, intake and output, and electrolytes	Ultrasound Attempt to relieve obstructive uropathy if present
Control uric acid	Increase clearance (diuresis), prevent uric acid synthesis, increase degradation	Allopurinol 200–400 mg/m^2/d IV (max. 600 mg/d) until serum uric acid is normal Rasburicase 0.15–0.2 mg/kd qd × 5 d Correct acidosis Alkalinize urine (pH >7.0) with $NaHCO_3$ (100–150 mEq in 1 L D5W or sterile water) is controversial and may promote Ca_2PO_4 deposition in the kidney, heart, and other organs if hyperphosphatemia is present Alkalinization is not required with a uricase Dialyze if urate nephropathy presents with oliguria
Control phosphate	Initiate oral phosphate binders (aluminum hydroxide) if adequate GI function	
Delay chemotherapy if necessary	Until good urine output established and uric acid controlled	Initiate hemodialysis if indicated; oliguria due to acute uric acid nephropathy is very responsive to dialytic therapy
Postchemotherapy Management		
Volume replacement and diuresis	Maintain forced diuresis	Omit $NaHCO_3$ from IV solutions because of phosphate crystallization in urine
Monitor electrolytes	Monitor every 4–6 h depending on tumor burden and/or rate of biochemical changes	Monitor ECG for hyperkalemia and/or hypocalcemia
Control uric acid	Allopurinol 200–400 mg/M^2/day PO for the first 3 d of chemotherapy, then 200 mg/M^2/d PO maintenance Rasburicase 0.15–0.2 mg/kd qd × 5 d	

(continued)

TABLE 5.12. *(continued)* **Tumor Lysis Syndrome**

Complication	Intervention	Comments
Renal failure	Hemodialysis	Indications: Oliguria/azotemia Uncontrolled hyperkalemia Symptomatic hypocalcemia Uric acid nephropathy or rapidly rising uric acid Phosphate nephropathy or rapidly rising phosphate Iatrogenic volume overload in the face of oliguria Continuous arterial or venovenous hemofiltration or hemodiafiltration will control volume status but may not maintain rapid efficient clearance of potassium if tumor lysis is overwhelming

ECG, electrocardiogram; GI, gastrointestinal; IV, intravenous; PO, by mouth

TABLE 5.13. Diuretics

Site of Action	Type of Diuresis, Onset, and Duration	Usual Dosage	Comments
Loop of Henle	K^+ and Na^+ wasting, hypo-osmotic or isosmotic urine		Ototoxicity with bumetanide, furosemide, and torsemide in high doses; clinically effective when GFR <25 ml/min
Bumetanide	Onset: PO: 30 min IV: <10 min Duration: PO: 5–6 h IV: 4 h	Bolus: 0.5–1.0 mg q2–3 h prn Infusion: 0.08–0.3 mg/h PO: 0.5–2 mg tid-qd	Bumetanide 1 mg ≈ furosemide 40 mg Doses >10 mg PO or 20 mg IV may be required in patients with renal failure or in the management of edema or hypertension IV loading dose may be used before starting infusion
Furosemide	Onset: PO: 60 min IV: 5 min Duration: PO: 6 h IV: 2 h	Bolus: 20–80 mg q1–2h prn Infusion: 3–12 mg/h PO: 20–80 mg q6–8h prn	IV doses of 400 mg per bolus or 3–7 g total per day have been used in some patients IV bolus doses are usually doubled until a maximum dose of 400 mg is reached An IV loading dose may be used before starting infusion Furosemide IV dose = 60% to 70% PO dose
Torsemide	Onset: PO: 60 min IV: 15 min Duration: PO: 6–8 h IV: 6–8 h	Bolus: 25 mg Infusion: 3–10 mg/h PO: 5–40 mg qd	Inject IV dose over 2 min Dose can be titrated upward by doubling the dose until therapeutic effect achieved or maximum dose of 200 mg is attained, although 400–800 mg may be required in patients with acute renal failure Torsemide IV dose = PO dose Torsemide 10–20 mg = furosemide 40 mg = bumetanide 1 mg Patients with CrCl 15–20 ml/min and HF may require an initial infusion rate of 10 mg/h IV loading dose may be used before starting an infusion
Distal Tubule ± Proximal Tubule	Moderate natriuresis and potassium wasting		May be ineffective when GFR <25 ml/min Commonly used in combination with loop diuretics to enhance efficacy
Chlorothiazide	Onset: PO: 60 min IV: 15 min Duration: PO: 6–8 h IV: 6–8 h	IV bolus or PO: 500–1,000 mg bid-qid	

(continued)

TABLE 5.13. *(continued)* **Diuretics**

Site of Action	Type of Diuresis, Onset, and Duration	Usual Dosage	Comments
Hydrochlorothiazide	Onset: PO: 2 h Duration: PO: 12–18 h	PO: 25–100 mg qd	
Metolazone	Onset: PO: 1 h Duration: PO: 12–24 h	PO: 5–20 mg qd	Thiazide type diuretic Administer 30 min before IV diuretic
Collecting Duct (Potassium Sparing)			Weak diuretics; risk of hyperkalemia is relative contraindication
Triamterene	Onset: PO: 2–4 h Duration: PO: 12–16 h	PO: 100–200 mg qd	Maximum dose 300 mg/d
Amiloride	Onset: PO: 2 h Duration: PO: 24 h	PO: 5–20 mg qd	
Spironolactone	Onset: PO: >24 h Duration: PO: 48–72 h	PO: 25–200 mg/d given qd or bid	Gradual onset of diuresis with maximal effect on 3rd day
Proximal Tubule			
Acetazolamide	Onset: PO: 30 min IV: 5 min Duration: PO: 6–8 h IV: 4–5 h	For alkalosis: 5 mg/kg/d mg IV/PO qid-qd × 2–4 d For edema: 5 mg/kg/d IV/PO divided bid-qid	Carbonic anhydrase inhibitor, causes bicarbonaturia and potassium wasting

CrCl, creatinine clearance; GFR, glomerular filtration rate; HF, heart failure; IV, intravenous; PO, by mouth

TABLE 5.14. Electrolyte Composition of Common IV Solutions

	mEq/L							
	Na^+	Cl^-	K^+	HCO_3^-	Mg^{+2}	Ca^{+2}	Osm	Calories
Crystalloid								
0.9% NaCl (NS)	154	154	—	—	—	—	292	—
0.9% NaCl & 5% dextrose in water (D5W/NS)	154	154	—	—	—	—	565	170
0.45% NaCl (1/2 NS)	77	77	—	—	—	—	146	—
0.45% NaCl & 5% dextrose in water (D5W-1/2NS)	77	77	—	—	—	—	420	170
0.2% NaCl & 5% dextrose (D5W-1/4 NS)	34	34	—	—	—	—	330	170
5% dextrose in water (D5W)	—	—	—	—	—	—	274	170
10% dextrose in water (D10W)	—	—	—	—	—	—	548	340
Ringer's lactate (RL)	130	109	4	28[a]	—	3	277	—
3% NaCl (hypertonic saline)	513	513	—	—	—	—	960	—
Colloid								
Hetastarch 6%	154	154	—	—	—	—	310	—
Hetastarch 6% in lactated electrolyte injection	143	124	3	28[a]	9	3	307	340
5% albumin (5 g/100 ml)	145	145		—		—	—	—
25% albumin (25 g/100 ml)	145	145		—		—	—	—

[a]Present in solution as lactate, which is metabolized to bicarbonate (HCO_3^-).

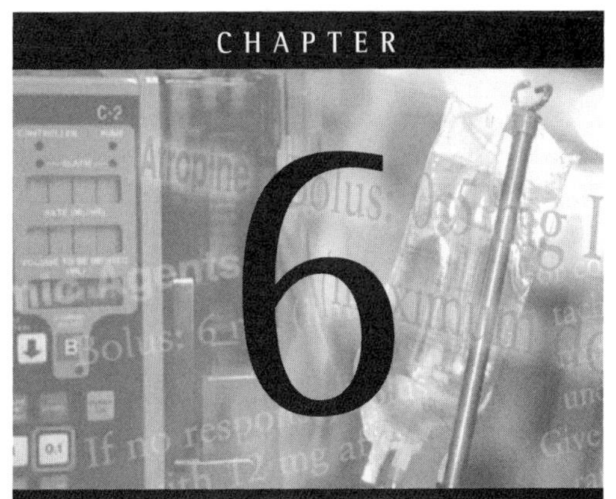

CHAPTER

6

Endocrine Therapies

TABLE 6.1. Corticosteroid Potencies

Agent	Equivalent Dose	Relative Mineralocorticoid Effect[a]	Biologic Half-Life
Short-Acting			
Cortisone	25 mg	++	8 h
Hydrocortisone	20 mg	++	8 h
Intermediate-Acting			
Prednisone	5 mg	+	18 h
Prednisolone	5 mg	+	18 h
Methylprednisolone	4 mg	0	18 h
Long-Acting			
Dexamethasone	0.75 mg	0	36 h

[a]Range of mineralocorticoid effect is from ++ (highest) to 0 (none).

TABLE 6.2. Thyroid, Pituitary, and Adrenal Hormonal Replacement

Agent	Indications	Dosage	Comments
Thyroid			
Levothyroxine (T4, L-thyroxine)	Hypothyroidism, myxedema coma	Initial replacement: 25–50 μg PO qd Maximum replacement: 200 μg PO qd In critically ill with myxedema coma: 200–500 μg IV/day slowly	Converted to T_3 in periphery Follow TSH for normalization and patient's clinical status For stupor or coma, treat with 200–500 μg IV bolus followed by 75 μg/day; consider hydrocortisone 50–100 mg IV q8h × 5 d as adjunctive therapy for hypocortisolism Half-life: euthyroid, 6 d; hypothyroid, 8 d; hyperthyroid, 3 d IV dose = 75% of PO dose (for replacement therapy) Preferred over T_3 for critically ill patients Many experts prefer the lower doses initially for safety, especially in the elderly, comatose, and those with heart disease May precipitate angina or arrhythmias
Liothyronine (T_3, triiodothyronine)	Hypothyroidism, myxedema coma	Replacement: 25–75 μg PO qd Myxedema coma: 12.5–25 μg IV q6h	Assessment of therapy is more difficult; wait at least four hours after IV dose Half-life: euthyroid, 24 h; hypothyroid, 38 h; hyperthyroid, 17 h
Pituitary/Adrenal			
Synthetic ACTH (cosyntropin)	Screening test for adrenal insufficiency	250 μg (25 units) IV/IM	Some authors recommend using smaller doses such as 1 μg for assessment of HPA axis Normal function is indicated by control cortisol level >5 μg/dl and 30 min post level >18 μg/dl with an increase of ≥7 μg/dl above control Small doses of prednisone will not affect cortisol response Dexamethasone does not affect cortisol response
Fludrocortisone	Mineralocorticoid replacement in primary adrenal insufficiency	50–200 μg PO qd	Titrated to achieve normal serum potassium and blood pressure Not required in secondary adrenal insufficiency

(continued)

TABLE 6.2. *(continued)* **Thyroid, Pituitary, and Adrenal Hormonal Replacement**

Agent	Indications	Dosage	Comments
Hydrocortisone	Replacement	25 mg IV/PO q AM and 12.5 mg IV/PO q PM	For equivalent corticosteroid dosages, see Table 6.1
	Stress	50–100 mg IV/PO q8h	For treatment of adrenal insufficiency complicating critical illness, maximum dose of glucocorticoid should be equivalent to hydrocortisone 300 mg/d
	Preoperative	1 d preoperatively: 25 mg IV/PO at 6 PM and midnight Day of operation: 50 mg IV during surgery Postoperative: 50 mg IV q8h × 24 h, then 25 mg IV/PO q8h × 24–48 h	For patients who may have adrenal insufficiency
Desmopressin	Diabetes insipidus	Intranasal: 10–40 μg in 1–3 divided doses daily SC/IV: 2–4 μg in 2 divided doses daily	May cause hypertension, water retention, headache, abdominal cramps; swelling and burning may occur at the injection site after SC administration

HPA, hypothalamic-pituitary-adrenal; IM, intramuscular; IV, intravenous; PO, by mouth; SC, subcutaneous; TSH, thyroid stimulating hormone

TABLE 6.3. Therapy for Thyrotoxicosis

Drug	Indication	Dosage/Route	Comment
Thiourea Agents	Used when radioisotopes are NOT indicated: e.g., children, young adults, pregnancy, mild thyrotoxicosis, small goiters Preparing hyperthyroid patients for surgery and elderly patients for radioactive iodide treatment		Inhibit thyroid hormone synthesis Low incidence of posttreatment hypothyroidism Complications: agranulocytosis (0.1% to 0.4% of patients) Definitive therapy required; relapses after these agents discontinued
Propylthiouracil		100–300 mg PO q6–8h (<200 mg/d during pregnancy)	Drug of choice during pregnancy Complication (rare): hepatic necrosis
Methimazole		80–120 mg PO qd	Less frequent dosing than propylthiouracil Lower incidence of hepatitis
Iodide	Thyroid storm		Inhibits thyroid hormone release
Lugol's solution (7 mg I/drop)		3–10 gtts PO tid	Cannot be used as sole therapy
SSKI (35 mg I/drop)		5 gtts PO qid	
Other Agents			
Radioactive iodine (I^{131})	Generally used in older patients (>25 years) because of theoretical risk of carcinogenesis		Destroys cells that concentrate iodine Never used in pregnant patients
Propranolol	Antagonism of peripheral effects of hormone Symptomatic relief of tremor, tachycardia, etc. Initial treatment of choice for thyroid storm	10–40 mg PO q6–8h 1 mg IV aliquots up to 0.15 mg/kg 3–5 mg/h infusion	Dose adjusted to response in heart rate (goal is ≤100 beats/min) Other β-blockers may be equally effective
Dexamethasone	Thyroid storm	2 mg IV q6h	Inhibits thyroid hormone release

IV, intravenous; PO, by mouth

TABLE 6.4. Ketoacidosis and Hyperosmolar Coma

Syndrome	Situation	Therapy	Comments
Diabetic ketoacidosis	Fluid deficit	Initially isotonic fluids, 1 L rapidly, then 1 L/h after clinical response of patient	Rate and type of fluid is adjusted according to laboratory results and patient response 0.45% NaCl can be alternated with 0.9% NaCl Dextrose may be added to the IV fluids when the blood glucose falls below 300 mg/dl
	Hyperglycemia	Regular insulin 6–10 U/h IV infusion	Blood glucose must be monitored every 2 h Insulin infusion rate should be titrated to reduce blood glucose by 60–100 mg/dl/h to glucose of 300 mg/dl
	Hypokalemia	Potassium 10–40 mEq/h	Serum potassium may be elevated acutely in the presence of acidosis, but total body potassium is reduced Correction of acidosis and insulin administration will reduce serum potassium levels Administration should begin when the measured potassium level is in the normal range Administer with caution to patients with renal insufficiency Administer as the chloride or phosphate salt
	Acidosis	Bicarbonate	Usually unnecessary unless pH <6.9 or arrhythmias are present
	Hypophosphatemia	Potassium phosphate or sodium phosphate	Guide by serum phosphate level
Hyperosmolar nonketotic coma	Dehydration	1 L 0.45% NaCl rapidly, then 1 L/h for several h	A major free water deficit is usually present Rehydration is the major therapy Neurologic status should be monitored frequently because of the possibility of cerebral edema from too rapid a fall in serum osmolality
	Hyperglycemia	Regular insulin 3–5 U/h IV infusion	Goal of insulin therapy is to achieve a blood glucose of 250–300 mg/dl Patients are quite sensitive to the effects of insulin; blood glucose should be lowered at a rate of 60–100 mg/dl/h Because blood glucose can fall precipitously, insulin infusion rates should be more conservative than in patients with diabetic ketoacidosis
Alcoholic Ketoacidosis			Usually when PO intake stopped Management is correction of fluid, electrolyte, and acid-base abnormalities that affect the chronic alcoholic Blood glucose usually is <200 mg/dl

IV, intravenous; PO, by mouth

TABLE 6.5. Insulin Preparations

Preparation	Onset	Peak	Duration	Comments
Short-Acting				
Regular	IV: 10–30 min SC: 30–60 min	IV: 30 min SC: 2–3 h	IV: 1 h SC: 5–7 h	Preferred for ketoacidosis and other conditions with rapidly changing requirements Only form of insulin that can be given IV
Semilente	SC: 30–90 min	SC: 4–10 h	SC: 12–16 h	Not for IV administration
Lispro	SC: 0.25 h	SC: 0.5–1.5 h	SC: 2.5–5 h	Not for IV administration
Insulin aspart	SC: 0.25 h	SC: 1–3 h	SC: 3–5 h	Not for IV administration
Insulin glulisine	—	SC: 0.5–1.5 h	SC: 1–2.5 h	Not for IV administration
Intermediate-Acting				
NPH	SC: 1–2 h	SC: 4–12 h	SC: 18–24 h	Not for IV administration
Lente	SC: 1–2.5 h	SC: 7–15 h	SC: 18–24 h	Not for IV administration
Long-Acting				
Protamine zinc	SC: 6–8 h	SC: 18–24 h	SC: 36 h	Not for IV administration
Ultralente	SC: 4–8 h	SC: 10–30 h	SC: ≥36 h	Not for IV administration

IV, intravenous; SC, subcutaneous

TABLE 6.6. Hyperglycemia: Regular Insulin Sliding Scales

Subcutaneous (SC) Dosing

Blood glucose concentration (mg/dL)	SC regular insulin (units)
<180	—
180–240	2
240–300	4
300–360	6
360–400	8
>400	10–12

IV Continuous Dosing

Blood glucose concentration (mg/dL)	IV infusion rate (U/h)
<120	—
120–179	0.5–1
180–240	1–2
241–300	2
301–360	3
361–400	4
>400	6–8

Administer insulin not more than every 4 hours.
Not for patients with shock or other hypoperfusion states.
Monitor serum glucose every 2 to 4 hours; may alternate with finger stick glucose measurements.

TABLE 6.7. Amylin Analog

Conversion of Pramlintide to Insulin Unit Equivalents

Prescribed Pramlintide Dose (μg)	Insulin Unit Equivalents Using U-100 Syringe (Units)	Corresponding Volume (ml)
15	2.5	0.025
30	5	0.05
45	7.5	0.075
60	10	0.1
120	20	0.2

Pramlintide is an adjunct treatment in patients who use mealtime insulin therapy and who have failed to achieve desired glucose control despite optimal insulin therapy. Pramlintide is not indicated for acute glucose management in critically ill patients and should be discontinued in this setting. Pramlintide therapy should only be restarted after the patient's critical illness has resolved, and the patient is consuming a stable caloric intake. Titration of the patients's insulin dose, oral hypoglycemic dose, and pramlintide may be required in this setting. Patients should be monitored at regular intervals to assess the effect on blood glucose.

Pramlintide Dosage and Administration

Pramlintide should be administered using a 0.3 ml, U-100 insulin syringe.

The pramlintide dose may be prescribed in micrograms, but it will be administered in Units indicated on the U-100 insulin syringe.

Table 6.7 outlines the conversion of the pramlintide dose prescribed in micrograms to the administration dose in Units.

TABLE 6.8. Oral Hypoglycemic Agents

Agent	Starting Dosage	Onset/Duration	Comments
Sulfonylurea			
Glimepiride	1–2 mg PO qd	Onset: 2–3 h Duration: 24 h	Lower dosage in elderly and those with hepatic or renal disease because of risk of hypoglycemia
Glipizide	5 mg PO qd	Onset: 1 h Duration: 10–24 h	As potent as glyburide Contraindicated in patients with renal or hepatic impairment
Glyburide	2.5 mg PO qd	Onset: 1.5 h Duration: 18–24 h	Prolonged biologic effect despite short half-life (1–2 h)
α-Glucosidase Inhibitor			
Acarbose	25 mg PO tid	Onset: unknown Duration: unknown	Delays glucose absorption from GI tract Not recommended in patients with renal impairment GI side effects
Miglitol	25–100 mg PO tid	Onset: unknown Duration: unknown	Delays glucose absorption from GI tract Not recommended in patients with renal impairment GI side effects
Bioguanide			
Metformin	500 mg PO bid	Onset: 1–3 h Duration: 24 h	May increase serum levels of cimetidine May decrease absorption of vitamin B_{12} and folic acid causing deficiencies May cause lactic acidosis, especially in patients with renal impairment; stop drug in setting of excessive ethanol ingestion, hypoxemia, shock, hepatic failure or surgery GI side effects
Meglitinides			
Repaglinide	0.5–4 mg PO tid before meals	Onset: unknown Duration: unknown	Take 15–30 min before meals Starting dose in patients with severe renal function is 0.5 mg
Nateglinide	60–120 mg PO tid before meals	Onset: unknown Duration: unknown	Take 15–30 min before meals Use with caution in patients with chronic liver disease
Thiazolidinedione			
Pioglitazone	15–45 mg PO qd	Onset: unknown Duration: unknown	Usually used in combination with sulfonylureas, metformin, or insulin Check LFT before beginning therapy Contraindicated in liver disease when ALT >2.5 × ULN Can cause fluid retention and may exacerbate HF Drug interactions with CYP450 3A4 substrates

(continued)

TABLE 6.8. *(continued)* **Oral Hypoglycemic Agents**

Agent	Starting Dosage	Onset/Duration	Comments
Rosiglitazone	2–8 mg PO qd	Onset: unknown Duration: unknown	Usually used in combination with sulfonylureas, metformin, or insulin Check LFT before beginning therapy Contraindicated in liver disease when ALT >2.5 × ULN Contraindicated in renal impairment Can cause fluid retention and may exacerbate HF

ALT, aminotransferase; GI, gastrointestinal; HF, heart failure; LFT, liver function tests; PO, by mouth; ULN, upper limit of normal

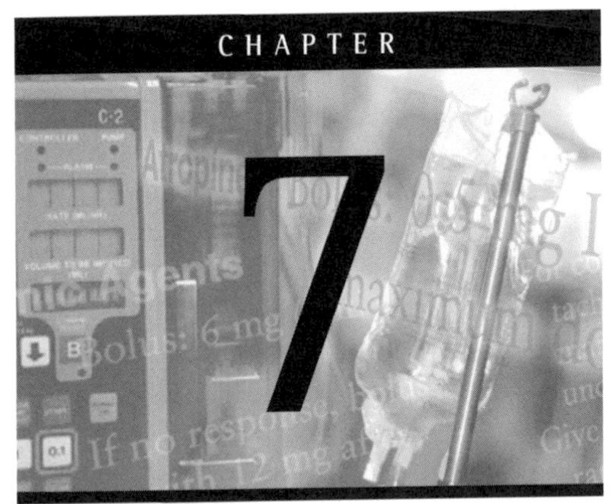

Gastroenterology, Liver, and Nutrition Therapies

TABLE 7.1. Gastrointestinal Hemorrhage—Available Therapies

Clinical Setting	Suggested Therapy	Dosage	Comments
Acute Treatment			
Acute upper GI hemorrhage	Omeprazole	40 mg PO/NG q8–12h × 5 d	Omeprazole is a sustained-release capsule that may be opened, but the contents must not be crushed before administration; the powder for oral suspension should be used in this setting
	Pantoprazole	40–80 mg IV bolus followed by 8 mg/h for 2–3 d	
	H_2 antagonists or Vasopressin	H_2 antagonists: (see Table 7.4) Vasopressin: 0.2–0.3 U/min IV, maximum 0.9 U/min	Monitor ECG; use nitroglycerin prophylactically in patients at risk for cardiac ischemia
Acute variceal hemorrhage	Octreotide	50–100 μg bolus, followed by continuous infusion at 50–100 μg/h for 24–48 h	More effective in controlling bleeding than vasopressin with less side effects (e.g., headache, chest pain, abdominal pain)
	Vasopressin	0.2–0.3 U/min IV, maximum 0.9 U/min	See acute upper GI hemorrhage
Acute lower GI hemorrhage	Vasopressin	0.2–0.3 U/min IV, maximum 0.9 U/min	See acute upper GI hemorrhage
Prophylaxis			
Prophylaxis against stress gastritis	H_2 antagonists, Sucralfate, proton pump inhibitors, or antacids	H_2 antagonists: see Table 7.4 Sucralfate: 1–2 g PO/NG q4–6h Lansoprazole 30 mg IV qd Pantoprazole 40 mg IV qd Esomeprazole 20 mg IV qd Omeprazole 20 mg PO/NG qd	H_2 antagonists and antacids: titrate pH >4; may predispose to nosocomial pneumonia Sucralfate: no effect on pH Limited data supporting the use of proton pump inhibitors for stress ulcer prophylaxis Omeprazole is a sustained-release capsule that may be opened but the contents must not be crushed before administration; the powder for oral suspension should be used in this setting

(continued)

TABLE 7.1. *(continued)* **Gastrointestinal Hemorrhage—Available Therapies**

Clinical Setting	Suggested Therapy	Dosage	Comments
Prevention of recurrent upper GI hemorrhage	H_2 antagonists or antacids	H_2 antagonists: see Table 7.4 Antacids: 30 ml PO/NG q2h (or continuously at 0.5 ml/min)	See stress gastritis
Prevention of recurrent variceal hemorrhage	β-blockers	Propranolol 10 mg PO qid	Titrate to 25% reduction in resting heart rate Consider sclerotherapy or surgery

ECG, electrocardiogram; GI, gastrointestinal; IV, intravenous; NG, nasogastric; PO, by mouth

TABLE 7.2. Hepatic Encephalopathy—Therapies

Clinical Setting	Dosage	Comments
Acute hepatic encephalopathy[a]	Lactulose: 30–45 ml PO/NG q1h until laxative effect occurs, then 30–45 ml tid Neomycin: 1.5–6 g/d PO/NG divided q6–8h	Lactulose retention enema: 300 ml lactulose in 700 ml water or saline PR for 30–60 min q4–6h
Chronic hepatic encephalopathy	Titrate dose to 2–3 soft stools/day	

PO, by mouth; PR, per rectum; NG, nasogastric
[a]Electrolyte correction, avoidance of sedatives and narcotics, and attention to volume status, nutrition, intracranial pressure, and infection are also indicated.

TABLE 7.3. Antacids

Composition/ Preparation	Content per 15 ml Al+2	Mg+2	SMC	Acid Neutralizing Content (mEq per ml)	Sodium Content (mg per 15 ml)	Dosage
Aluminum Hydroxide Plus Magnesium Hydroxide[a,b]						
Maalox TC	1,800	900	0	5.44	2.40	5–10 ml qid
Maalox	675	600	0	2.66	4.20	10–20 ml qid
Aluminum Hydroxide Plus Magnesium Hydroxide[a,b] Plus Simethicone						
Mylanta	600		60	2.54	2.04	10–20 ml 4–6 × d
Mylanta Double Strength	1,200	1,200	120	5.08	3.42	10–20 ml tid
Extra Strength Maalox Plus	1,500	1,350	120	5.8		10–20 ml qid
Aluminum Hydroxide[c,d]						
AlternaGel	1,800	0	0	3.2	7.50	15–30 ml 3–6 × d
Amphojel	960	0	0	2	6.90	10 ml 4–6 × d
Magaldrate (Aluminum and Magnesium Oxides)						
Riopan Plus[e]	0	0	0	3	0.30	15–30 ml qid

SMC, simethicone

[a]Magnesium containing antacids may cause diarrhea.

[b]Hypermagnesemia may occur in patients with renal failure who receive magnesium containing antacids.

[c]Aluminum containing antacids may cause constipation.

[d]Aluminum containing antacids may cause hypophosphatemia.

[e]Contains the equivalent of 29% to 40% magnesium oxide and 18% to 26% aluminum oxide.

TABLE 7.4. Nonantacid Therapies for Gastritis

Therapy	Usual Dosage	Comments
H_2 Antagonists		
Cimetidine	Intermittent: 300 mg IV q6–8h Infusion: 37.5 mg/h PO/NG: 300 mg q6h	Adverse effects: altered mental status, thrombocytopenia, elevated liver enzymes, many drug interactions
Famotidine	Intermittent: 20 mg IV q12h Infusion: not applicable PO/NG: 20 mg q12h	Adverse effects: altered mental status, thrombocytopenia, elevated liver enzymes
Ranitidine	Intermittent: 50 mg IV q6–8h Infusion: 6.25 mg/h PO/NG: 150 mg q12h	Adverse effects: altered mental status, thrombocytopenia, elevated liver enzymes
Proton Pump Inhibitors		
Esomeprazole	PO/NG: 20–40 mg qd	Enteric-coated granules in capsule form may be opened, but contents must not be crushed before administration NG administration: Empty capsule contents into 60 ml syringe and mix with 50 ml water; vigorously shake syringe for 15 s; flush NG tube with additional water after administering granules; do not administer if pellets have dissolved or disintegrated Do not administer with meals Adverse effects: headache, nausea, vomiting, diarrhea, abdominal pain, potential drug interactions
Lansoprazole	PO/NG: 15–30 mg qd	Enteric coated granules in capsule form may be opened, but contents must not be crushed before administration The contents of the capsule can be emptied into 60 ml of tomato, apple, or orange juice and swallowed immediately The contents of the oral suspension packet should be mixed with 30 ml of water The oral disintegrating tablet should be placed on the tongue and allowed to disintegrate with or without water; the tablet should dissolve within a minute and should not be swallowed intact or chewed. Alternatively a 15-mg tablet may be placed into an oral syringe with 4 ml of water or a 30 mg tablet with 10 ml of water; gently shake to allow quick dispersal; after tablet dispersal administer contents; refill syringe with 2 ml water, shake gently, and administer remaining contents Do not administer with meals
Omeprazole	PO/NG: 20 mg qd	Sustained-release capsule may be opened, but contents must not be crushed before administration; the powder for oral suspension should be used in this setting Do not administer with meals
Pantoprazole	PO: 40 mg qd	Swallow tablets whole, with or without food Do not split, chew, or crush tablets
Rabeprazole	PO: 20 mg qd	Swallow tablets whole, with or without food Do not split, chew, or crush tablets

(continued)

TABLE 7.4. *(continued)* **Nonantacid Therapies for Gastritis**

Therapy	Usual Dosage	Comments
Other Agents		
Sucralfate (a sulfated disaccharide)	PO/NG: 1 g qid	Sucralfate has no effect on gastric pH Available as suspension 1 g/10 ml Tablets may be crushed and dissolved in 30 ml of water for administration through an NG tube Adverse effects: constipation, hypophosphatemia, bezoar formation especially in patients receiving tube feedings
Other Conditions		
Helicobacter pylori	Bismuth subcitrate 2 × 262 mg qid + metronidazole 250 mg tid + amoxicillin 500 mg qid or 1 g bid or Tetracycline 500 mg qid × 14 d	Alternative regimen: Clarithromycin 500 mg tid + omeprazole 40 mg qd × 14 d
Misoprostol (prostaglandin) PGE_1	Prevention of NSAID-induced ulcers: 200 μg PO bid-qid Gastric or duodenal ulcer: 100–200 μg PO bid-qid	Contraindicated in pregnant women Adverse effects: diarrhea, nausea, abdominal pain

IV, intravenous; NG, nasogastric tube; NSAID, nonsteroidal anti-inflammatory drug; PO, by mouth

TABLE 7.5. Antiemetics

Agent	Usual Indication	Dosage	Comments
Phenothiazines			
Prochlorperazine	Postoperative; chemotherapy	PO/IM/IV: 5–10 mg q6–8h PR: 25 mg q12h	Extrapyramidal effects, drowsiness, blurred vision Not effective for motion-induced nausea and vomiting
Promethazine	Postoperative; motion-induced	PO/IM/IV/PR: 12.5–50 mg q4–6h	Drowsiness, dry mouth, confusion, blurred vision
Antihistamines			
Hydroxyzine	Postoperative; motion-induced	IM/IV: 25–100 mg q4–6h	Drowsiness, dry mouth, confusion, blurred vision
Trimethobenzamide	Postoperative	PO: 250 mg tid or qid IM/PR: 200 mg tid or qid	Parkinson-like symptoms, drowsiness, blurred vision, hypotension Less effective than phenothiazines
5-HT$_3$-antagonists			Should not be used for routine nausea and vomiting; traditional antiemetics are the preferred agents
Dolasetron	Chemotherapy-induced nausea and vomiting resistant to standard antiemetic regimens	IV/PO: 100 mg 30–60 min before chemotherapy	Serotonin antagonist Side effects include diarrhea, headache, constipation Use for prophylaxis of chemotherapy-induced nausea and vomiting; not effective once vomiting starts
	Postoperative	IV: 12.5 mg 15 min before cessation of surgery or as soon as nausea and vomiting presents	Conventional antiemetic agents should be tried if single dose ineffective
Ondansetron	Chemotherapy-induced nausea and vomiting resistant to standard antiemetic regimens	IV: 16–32 mg as a single dose administered 30 min before chemotherapy PO: 8 mg 30 min before chemotherapy regimens; repeat doses 4 h and 8 h after chemotherapy; then 8 mg tid for 1–2 d	Serotonin antagonist Side effects include diarrhea, headache, constipation Use for prophylaxis of chemotherapy-induced nausea and vomiting; not effective once vomiting starts Fewer treatment failures with single dose compared to multiple dose
	Postoperative	IV: 4–8 mg as a single dose	Conventional antiemetic agents should be tried if single dose ineffective
Granisetron	Chemotherapy-induced nausea and vomiting resistant to standard antiemetic regimens	IV: 10 μg/kg IVP starting 30 min before the emetogenic drug PO: 1 mg bid	Side effects include headache, asthenia, somnolence, diarrhea, and constipation May not be effective for delayed onset nausea and vomiting

(continued)

TABLE 7.5. *(continued)* **Antiemetics**

Agent	Usual Indication	Dosage	Comments
	Postoperative	IV: 20–40 μg/kg as a single dose	Conventional antiemetic agents should be tried if single dose ineffective
Others			
Metoclopramide	Chemotherapy	PO/IV: 1–2 mg/kg before chemotherapy, followed by 2 mg/kg q2h × 2, then q3h × 3	Dopamine receptor antagonist Extrapyramidal effects, drowsiness, fatigue
Scopolamine	Prophylaxis against motion-induced nausea and vomiting	Topical: 1 patch q72h	Belladonna alkaloid Dry mouth, drowsiness, mental status changes
Dexamethasone	Chemotherapy-induced nausea and vomiting resistant to standard antiemetic regimens	IV: 10–20 mg before chemotherapy, then 4–8 mg IV/PO q8h × 1–5 d postchemotherapy	Side effects include mood changes, anxiety, euphoria, hyperglycemia
Lorazepam	Chemotherapy-induced nausea and vomiting resistant to standard antiemetic regimens	IV: 0.5–1.5 mg/M^2 total dose before chemotherapy	Useful for anticipatory nausea and vomiting Side effects include drowsiness, sedation, disorientation, hallucinations, amnesia

IM, intramuscular; IV, intravenous; IVP, IV push; PO, by mouth; PR, per rectum

TABLE 7.6. Antidiarrheals

Agent	Composition	Dosage/Adverse Effects	Actions/Interactions/ Comments
Imodium	Loperamide 2 mg capsule, 1 mg/5 ml liquid, 1 mg/ml liquid	4 mg initially, then 2 mg after each loose stool up to 8 mg/d	Drug action: decreases GI motility, may possess antisecretory activity
		Bloating, abdominal pain, drowsiness, dizziness, dry mouth, nausea, vomiting	Drug interactions:[a,b] Comments:[c]
Donnagel, Parepectolin	Attapulgite 600 mg per 15 ml	30 ml after each loose bowel movement up to 7 × d Constipation	Drug action: absorbs bacteria and toxins, reduces water loss Drug interactions:[d] Comments:[c]
Kaopectate advanced formula	Attapulgite 750 mg per 15 ml	30 ml after each loose bowel movement up to 7 × d Constipation	Drug action: absorbs bacteria and toxins, reduces water loss Drug interactions: [d] Comments:[c]
Lomotil	Diphenoxylate 2.5 mg and atropine 25 μg per tablet or per 5 ml syrup	1–2 tabs or 5–10 ml qid Bloating, abdominal pain, drowsiness, dry mouth, blurred vision, nausea vomiting, urinary retention	Drug action: reduces GI motility Drug interactions:[a,b] Comments:[c]
Deodorized tincture of opium (DTO)	Opium 10%	0.6 ml qid Constipation, drowsiness	Drug action: reduces GI motility Comments:[c] Contains 10 mg of anhydrous morphine per 1 ml
Paregoric	Camphorated tincture of opium	5–10 ml qid-qd Constipation, drowsiness	Drug action: reduces GI motility Comments:[c] Contains 10 mg of anhydrous morphine per 5 ml
Octreotide	Synthetic analogue of endogenous somatostatin	100–600 μg/d SC bid-qid Nausea, cramping, and pain at injection site	Drug action: blocks release of serotonin and other active peptides; especially useful in watery diarrhea syndromes such as carcinoid tumors and vasoactive intestinal peptide-secreting tumors (VIP-omas)

(continued)

TABLE 7.6. *(continued)* **Antidiarrheals**

Agent	Composition	Dosage/Adverse Effects	Actions/Interactions/ Comments
Pepto-Bismol	Bismuth subsalicylate 262 mg per 15 ml	30 ml q30min–1h, up to 8 doses/d Salicylate toxicity, dark Hemoccult-negative stools	Drug action: unknown Drug interactions:[d,e]

CNS, central nervous system; GI, gastrointestinal; ICU, intensive care unit; SC, subcutaneous
Note: Should be used with caution in any ICU setting until pathogenesis clearly established.
[a]Added CNS depressant effects.
[b]Added anticholinergic effects.
[c]Should not be administered in the presence of pseudomembranous colitis.
[d]Decreased digitalis absorption.
[e]May have additive platelet inhibitory effects.

TABLE 7.7. Infectious Diarrhea—Agents of Choice for Common Treatable Pathogens

Organism	Primary Therapy	Alternative Therapy	Comments
Aeromonas hydrophila	TMP-SMX 1 DS tablet PO bid × 5 d	Ciprofloxacin 500 mg PO bid × 5 d	
Campylobacter jejuni	Erythromycin 250–500 mg PO qid × 7 d	Ciprofloxacin 500 mg PO bid × 7 d, or Doxycycline 100 mg PO bid × 7 d Azithromycin 500 mg PO qd × 3 d	Therapy should begin early in the course of the disease
Clostridium difficile	Metronidazole 250–500 mg PO tid × 7–14 d	Vancomycin 125 mg PO qid × 7–14 d, or Bacitracin 25,000 U PO qid × 7 d Vancomycin 1 g IV q12h	Relapses should be treated with longer courses of vancomycin
Escherichia Coli			
Enterotoxigenic (ETEC)	Bismuth subsalicylate 60 ml PO qid × 5 d	Trimethoprim 200 mg PO bid × 5 d	
Entero-adherent (EAEC)	TMP-SMX 1 DS tablet PO bid × 5 d	Ciprofloxacin 500 mg PO bid × 5 d, or Doxycycline 100 mg PO bid × 5 d	
Enterohemorrhagic (EHEC)	Ciprofloxacin 500 mg PO bid × 5 d		
Entero-invasive (EIEC)	Ampicillin 500 mg PO or 1 g IV qid × 5 d		
Enteropathogenic (EPEC)	TMP-SMX 1 DS tablet PO bid × 5 d	Neomycin 100 mg/kg/d PO × 3–5 d	
0157-H7	None		TMP-SMX may be contraindicated
Food Poisoning *(C. perfringes, S. aureus, B. cereus, Listeria)*	None		Self-limited disease; does not require antibiotic therapy
***Salmonella* species**			
Uncomplicated enterocolitis	None		
Enteric fever (nontyphoid salmonella)	TMP-SMX 1–2 DS tablets PO bid × 14 d	Ampicillin 2–6 g/d IV/ PO × 14 d, or Ciprofloxacin 500 mg PO bid × 14 d, or Ceftriaxone 1 g IV q12h × 14 d, or Cefotaxime 4–8 g/d IV × 14 d, or Chloramphenicol 3–4 g/d IV × 14 d	

(continued)

TABLE 7.7. *(continued)* **Infectious Diarrhea—Agents of Choice for Common Treatable Pathogens**

Organism	Primary Therapy	Alternative Therapy	Comments
Shigella	Ciprofloxacin 500 mg PO bid × 3–5 doses	Norfloxacin 400 mg PO bid 3–5 d, or TMP-SMX 1 DS tablet PO bid × 3–5 d, or Ampicillin 0.5–1 g IV/PO qid × 3–5 d	Preferred agents are ciprofloxacin, norfloxacin, or TMP-SMX
Vibrio cholera	Doxycycline 300 mg PO × 1 d	Ciprofloxacin 1 g PO × 1 d	
Vibrio parahemolyticus	None		
Yersinia enterocolitica	Ciprofloxacin 500 mg PO q12h × 3 doses	Ceftriaxone 2 g IV qd	

DS, double strength; IV, intravenous; PO, by mouth; TMP-SMX, trimethoprim-sulfamethoxazole

TABLE 7.8. Energy Expenditure Calculations

Method	Equation	Comments
Indirect calorimetry	Patient-specific energy expenditure	Requires metabolic cart for determinations
General recommendations	Low stress (UUN 5–10 g/d): 20 kcal/kg/d Moderate stress (UUN 10–15 g/d): 25–30 kcal/kg/d High stress (UUN >15 g/d): 35 kcal/kg/d	Simple starting point for most patients Fat 10 kcal/kg/day = 1 g/kg/day Protein 1.5 g/kg/day or adjusted for level of renal function Maintain glucose infusion rate <5 mg/kg/min
American College of Chest Physicians Guidelines	25 total calories/kg/day Glucose: 30% to 70% of total calories Fat: 15% to 30% of total calories Protein: 10% to 15% of total calories	Calories based on usual body weight Glucose: keep blood glucose <225 mg/dl Fat: keep triglyceride <500 mg/dl Protein: 1.2–1.5 g/kg/day, keep BUN <100 mg/dl
Hemodynamic equations	Energy expenditure (kcal/d) = 95.18 (hemoglobin × cardiac output × ($SaO_2 - SvO_2$)	Equation has not been validated prospectively in critically ill patients. Values of SaO_2 and SvO_2 are expressed as a decimal
Harris-Benedict equation	BEE (kcal/d) Male = 66 + (13.7 × wt in kg) + (5 × ht in cm) – (6.8 × age in yr) Female = 655 + (9.6 × wt in kg) + (1.7 × ht in cm) – (4.7 × age in yr)	Equations tend to underpredict energy expenditure while addition of activity and stress factors tend to overpredict energy expenditure in critically ill patients
	Activity Factors	
	Confined to bed	1.2
	Ambulatory	1.3
	Fever factor	1.13/°C >37°
	Injury Factor	
	Surgery	1.1–1.2
	Infection	1.2–1.6
	Trauma	1.1–1.8
	Sepsis	1.4–1.8

BEE, basal energy expenditure; BUN, blood urea nitrogen; UUN, urine urea nitrogen
Nitrogen balance calculation:
Nitrogen balance = Nitrogen in – (nitrogen out + insensible losses)
1 g nitrogen = 6.25 g protein
Nitrogen out = UUN
Insensible losses = 3–4 g/d (increased with diarrhea)
Nitrogen in = protein/6.25

TABLE 7.9. Fuel Sources (Enteral and Parenteral Formulations)

Fuel	Caloric Density	Respiratory Quotient (RQ)	Comments
Carbohydrate	3.4 kcal/g	1.0	30% to 60% of total nonprotein calories Maximum infusion rate: 5 mg/kg/min
Fat	9.0 kcal/g	0.7	20% to 40% of nonprotein calories Usual daily dose: 1 g/kg/d
Protein	4.0 kcal/g	0.8	Usually not counted as a calorie source

TABLE 7.10. Parenteral Nutrition Guidelines

I. Determining Nonprotein Calorie Requirement

A. General guidelines (30 nonprotein kcal/kg/day)

Fat calories 10 kcal/kg/day × ___ kg = ___ fat kcal/day (= 1 g/kg/day)
Dextrose calories 20 kcal/kg/day × ___ kg = ___ dextrose kcal/day (= 4.1 mg/kg/min),[a]

OR

B. Indirect calorimetry ___ kcal/day RQ*___

0.33 × ___ kcal/day = ___ fat kcal/day
0.67 × ___ kcal/day = ___ dextrose kcal/day
*Adjust percentage of fat and dextrose calories to achieve an RQ value between 0.8–0.9

II. Determining Protein (Amino Acid) Requirement

A. General guidelines

1.5 g/kg/day × ___ kg = ___ g protein/day **OR**

B. Disease specific guidelines based on renal function (keep BUN < 100 mg/dl)

___ g/kg/day × ___ kg = ___ g protein/day

Normal renal function	1.5 g/kg/day
Acute renal failure	0.5g/kg/day
Intermittent hemodialysis	1.0 g/kg/day
Continuous renal replacement therapy	1.5 g/kg/day

III. Solution Formulations

A. Fat volume (20% solution = 2 kcal/ml)

___ kcal/___ kcal/ml = ___ ml 20% fat solution*
*All volumes should be rounded off to the nearest 50 ml

B. Dextrose dose (dextrose 3.4 kcal/g) from Section I above

___ kcal/3.4 kcal/g = ___ g dextrose solution

C. Protein dose

___ g/d from Section II above

IV. Daily Electrolyte Requirements in Patients with Normal Renal Function

Na 35–150 mEq; K 40–120 mEq; Chloride 100–150 mEq; PO_4 15–30 mmol[b]; Mg 8–24 mEq; Ca Glu 5–20 mEq

V. Additional Additives

Multivitamins, trace elements, regular insulin as needed, H_2 blockers, vitamin K as needed

[a]To avoid hyperglycemia, order one-half of the total dextrose calories on the first day and advance to full dextrose calories on the second day as tolerated.
[b]Each ml of sodium phosphate contains 3 mmol PO_4^{-2} and 4 mEq Na^+. Each ml of potassium phosphate contains 3 mmol PO_4^{-2} and 4.4 mEq K^+.

TABLE 7.11. Enteral Nutrition Solutions

Enteral Solution	Prot (g/L)	Carb (g/L)	Fat (g/L)	Na mEq/L	K mEq/L	mOsmOs/ kg H_2O	Cal/ ml	Comments
Criticare HN	38	220	5.3	27	34	650	1.06	Lactose free
Impact	56	130	28	48	33	375	1	Lactose free
Isocal	34	135	44	23	34	270	1.06	Lactose free
Isocal HN	44	123	45	40	41	270	1.06	Lactose free
Osmolite	37	143	37	27	26	300	1.06	Lactose free
Osmolite HN	44	140	35	40	40	300	1.06	Lactose free
Vivonex TEN	38.2	205	2.77	20	20	630	1	Lactose free
Peptamen	40	127.2	39.2	22	32	270	1	For GI impairment
Pulmocare	62	104	92	56	44	475	1.5	For pulmonary patients
Respalor	75	146	70	54	37	580	1.5	For pulmonary patients
Stresstein	70	170	28	56.5	56.4	901	1.2	For moderately and severely stressed patients
TraumaCal	83	195	69	52	36	490	1.5	For moderately and severely stressed patients
Amin-Aid	6.6	124.3	15.7	5	N/A	700	2	For acute or chronic renal failure
Hepatic-Aid II	15	57.3	12.3	5	UK	560	1.2	For chronic liver disease
Travasorb Hepatic	29.4	215.2	14.7	10.2	22.6	600	1.1	For hepatic failure

N/A, Not applicable; UK, unknown

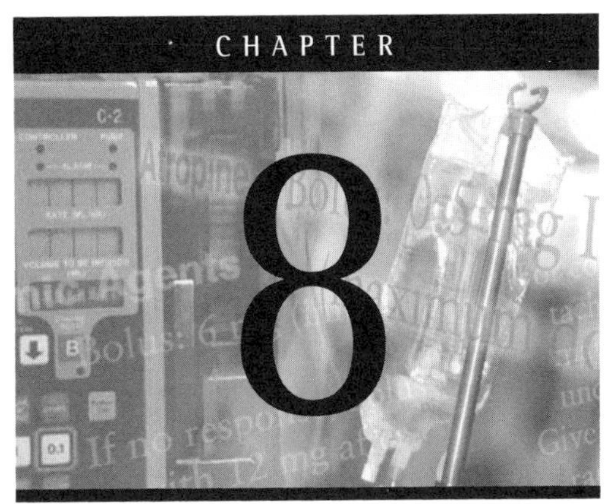

Hematologic Therapies

TABLE 8.1. Blood Component Therapies

Preparation	Indications	Dosage	Comments
Whole blood[a–d]	Acute massive blood loss Increases O_2 carrying capacity Increases intravascular volume	Volume of 1 unit is approximately 500 ml (450 ml blood plus anticoagulant) with hematocrit of 38%	RBCs and plasma After storage, few if any platelets and no factors V or VIII No major advantage over component therapy
Packed red blood[a–e]	Acute massive blood loss Increases O_2 carrying capacity Increases intravascular volume	Volume of 1 unit is approximately 250 ml with hematocrit of 65% to 70%	1 unit increases hematocrit by approximately 3% Leukocyte-poor blood prevents fever by lowering exposure to HLA and other antigens In emergency (risk of exsanguination) group O negative blood can be given. After 2–4 units of O negative blood, subsequent transfusions during the acute episode should continue with O negative to prevent hemolysis
Platelets[a–c]	Bleeding due to thrombocytopenia or abnormal platelet function Post-op bleeding, platelets $<100{,}000/mm^3$ Bleeding patient, platelets $<50{,}000/mm^3$ Prophylaxis, platelets $<20{,}000/mm^3$ [f]	Volume of 1 unit is approximately 50 ml Usual transfusion 6–8 units Final volume approximately 300 ml	ABO compatibility desirable but not necessary 1 unit raises platelet count approximately 5,000–7,000/cu mm Potential complications: fever, sepsis, DIC, uremia, allo- or autoantibodies If alloimmunization present (poor 1 h posttransfusion count), HLA match can improve platelet survival; IVIG may also be useful May need anti-D IgG if Rh negative and given Rh positive platelets

(continued)

TABLE 8.1. *(continued)* **Blood Component Therapies**

Preparation	Indications	Dosage	Comments
Granulocytes[a–d]	<500 granulocytes/mm^3 Fever, progressive infection despite antibiotics, hypoplastic marrow Qualitative function abnormalities (e.g., chronic granulomatous disease)	Volume of usual unit 300–500 ml with 0.5–2 × 10^{10} cells	Hematocrit approximately 10% to 20% Fever, chills, dyspnea, leukoagglutination reactions common Questionable efficacy in neutropenia/sepsis and most other clinical situations

DIC, disseminated intravascular coagulation; HLA, human leukocyte antigen; IVIG, IV immunoglobulin; RBC, red blood cells

[a]Potential for infectious disease transmission.

[b]Potential for alloimmunization.

[c]Potential for transfusion reaction.

[d]

Recipient's Blood Group	*Transfused Blood Compatibility*
O	O
A	A or O
B	B or O
AB	AB, A, B, or O

[e]*Typing* (ABO and Rh compatible) alone results in 99.8% chance of compatible transfusion, requires 5–10 minutes *screen* (testing recipients serum against common antigens associated with transfusion reactions) results in 99.94% chance of a compatible transfusion; requires 45 minutes to 1 hour *major cross match* (tests recipients serum against donor's RBCs) results in 99.95% chance of compatibility; >1 hour to perform.

[f]Prophylaxis in an afebrile patient, not on antibiotics, with no invasive procedures planned, who is not bleeding or has stable platelet counts >10,000/cu mm; may elect to transfuse at a higher platelet count in patients who are febrile, on antibiotics, or have rapidly falling counts.

TABLE 8.2. Clotting Component Preparations

Preparation	Indications	Dosage	Comments
Fresh frozen plasma[a]	Replace multiple factor deficiency in bleeding patient (e.g., severe liver disease, DIC, reversal of warfarin, dilutional coagulopathy after massive transfusions) After transfusion of 10 units PRBCs in patient with excessive bleeding Bleeding in any patient with elevated PT or aPTT, prolonged thrombin time, or fibrinogen <100 mg/dl Antithrombin III deficiency requiring heparin therapy C_1-esterase deficiency with life-threatening laryngeal edema	Volume of 1 unit is approximately 250 ml	Usual replacement 1–2 units 1 unit has near normal amounts of all coagulation factors and approximately 400 mg fibrinogen Adequate hemostasis achieved with factor levels of approximately 30% normal 2 units increase levels of factors by approximately 20% ABO compatibility desirable but not necessary[b] 1 ml FFP contains 1 unit of each coagulation factor
Cryoprecipitate[a]	Hypofibrinogenemia (<100 mg/dl) Hemophilia A Von Willebrand disease Factor XIII deficiency Uremic bleeding DIC	6–10 units in 250 ml q8–10h	Each 10–40 ml bag contains 250 mg fibrinogen, approximately 100 units factor VIII procoagulant and von Willebrand factor, and 75 units factor XIII Does not contain factors II, VII, IX, or X
Recombinant activated coagulation factor VII (rFVIIa)	Bypass inhibitors to FVIII and factor IX in hemophilia A and B, congenital factor VII deficiency Off-label use: Surgical or traumatic bleeding with acquired FVII deficiency Warfarin-associated bleeding Coagulopathy of severe liver dysfunction Management of acute intracerebral hemorrhage	90 μg/kg IV bolus, may be repeated 90–120 μg/kg IV bolus, may be repeated q2h alternatively 15–30 μg/kg IV q12h (warfarin) 2–120 μg/kg IV (hepatic coagulopathy)	Binds tissue factor and activated platelets at site of injury, promotes conversion of prothrombin to thrombin Generally does not cause systemic thrombosis Reports of venous thrombosis, myocardial infarction, cerebral sinus thrombosis in patients treated with rFVIIa but cause and effect unclear
Recombinant human factor VIII	Hemophilia A	Major surgery or life threatening hemorrhage; antihemophilic factor 100% (50 IU/kg) repeat q6–12h until healing complete or threat resolved[c]	Several preparations available, some with human albumin (theoretical infectious risk)

(continued)

TABLE 8.2. *(continued)* Clotting Component Preparations

Preparation	Indications	Dosage	Comments
Factor VIII (plasma derived)	Hemophilia A	Major trauma, surgery or life-threatening hemorrhage, required peak pre- and postsurgery level 80% to 100% (40–50 IU/kg), administer q6–24h until healing complete[c] Refractory bleeding due to inhibitor (<50 Bethesda units/mL) 100–150 porcine units/kg IV	If bleeding not controlled with adequate dose, test for inhibitor, if titers elevated consider antihemophilic factor (porcine)
Factor IX complex[a] (prothrombin complex concentrate)	Hemophilia B Factor IX deficiency Warfarin overdose Factor X deficiency Hemophilia A (factor VIII inhibitors) Factor VIII deficiency (Proplex T only) Factor II deficiency	Major trauma or surgery, levels of factor IX needed 25% to 50%, initial load <75 U/kg, repeat q18–30h prn measured factor IX levels[d] For warfarin overdose, give 15 U/kg	Contains factors II, VII, IX, and X Thromboembolic problems are common with administration; 5–10 units heparin added to each ml of reconstituted complex Patients with liver disease or antithrombin III deficiency should not receive complex Fresh frozen plasma is usually preferred because of clotting problems with factor IX complex; primarily used to control bleeding from warfarin overdose or factor II, VII, IX, or X deficiencies
Purified factor IX concentrate	Hemophilia B Factor IX deficiency	Units required = body weight × 1 unit/kg × desired factor IX increase (in % of normal)	20-fold purer than prothrombin complex Essentially no factors II or VII; <10 units factor X per 100 units factor IX For serious hemorrhage, factor IX should be increased to 30% to 50%; for surgery, factor IX should be maintained at 30% to 50% for 1 wk postoperatively
Recombinant factor IX	Hemophilia B	Major surgery, trauma or life-threatening hemorrhage, circulating factor IX activity required 50% to 100% (see empiric dosing in comments) duration of therapy 7–10 d	Empirical dosing's body weight (kg) × desired % increase in plasma factor IX × 1.2 IU/kg

(continued)

TABLE 8.2. *(continued)* **Clotting Component Preparations**

Preparation	Indications	Dosage	Comments
Antithrombin III concentrate[a]	Congenital antithrombin III deficiency (level <75% of normal)	Dosage units = [desired – baseline level AT-III(%)] × wt (kg)	Dosage must be individualized 1 IU/kg raises level of AT-III by 1% to 2% Levels should be measured before and 30 min after dose After 1st dose, level should be >120% of normal and then maintained at >80% of normal with q24h dosing If administering heparin, lower dose after administering concentrate to prevent excessive bleeding
Fibrin glue (fibrinogen concentrate)	Use with topical thrombin as sealant for vascular grafts, plastic surgery, neurosurgery, bronchopleural fistula	1 unit	Recipient may make antibody to bovine thrombin, leading to false prolongation of coagulation values; glue should not be injected blindly because arterial clots may occur

aPTT, activated partial thromboplastin time; DIC, disseminated intravascular coagulation; FFP, fresh frozen plasma; PRBC, packed red blood cells; PT, prothrombin time

[a]Potential for infectious disease transmission.

[b]

Recipient Blood Group	*Transfused Plasma Compatibility*
O	O, A, B, AB
A	A, AB
B	B, AB
AB	AB

[c]Dose (IU factor VIII) for rFVIII or plasma-derived FVIII = body weight (kg) × 0.5 IU/kg × desired factor VIII increase (%).

[d]To raise blood level % (factor IX complex): (a) determine plasma volume = wt (kg) × 70 ml/kg (adult) × [1-Hct (in decimals)]; (b) determine number of units needed = desired – actual level × plasma volume (mL).

TABLE 8.3. Hematologic Growth Factors

Agent/Indications	Dosage	Comments
Epoetin Alfa (Erythropoietin Human Glycoform α)		
To correct anemia of chronic renal failure	Initial: 50–100 U/kg IV or SC 3 × /wk Maintenance: 25 units/kg IV or SC 3 × /wk	Switch to maintenance when hematocrit >30% Ensure adequate iron stores Maintenance dose can range from 12.5–525 units/kg 3 × /wk, adjusted by increments of 10–25 units/kg Most frequent adverse effects in chronic renal failure (e.g., hypertension, seizures) are related to the rate and extent of increase in erythrocyte count and hematocrit
Cancer chemotherapy (nonmyeloid malignancies)	150 units/kg IV/SC 3 × wk × 8 wk Maintenance 300 units/kg 3 × wk	Use if baseline serum erythropoietin level is less than 200 mU/mL
HIV disease	Initial: 100 units/kg IV or SC 3 × /wk × 8 wk then increase dose by 50–100 units/kg every 4–8 wk until adequate response	Indication: serum erythropoietin <500 mU/ml Increase dose after 8 wk
Darbepoetin		
Anemia associated with chronic renal failure, cancer	0.45 μg/kg IV or SC q w, can be adjusted at 4-w intervals by 25% Decrease dose by 25% if hemoglobin approaches 12 g/dL or increases by greater than 1 g/dL in 2-wk period	Half-life 2–3 times longer than epoetin alfa Clinical equivalent to epoetin alfa Preferred for outpatient therapy rather than inpatient therapy; long half-life offers no advantage for inpatient therapy May increase blood pressure in chronic renal failure Rapid increase in hemoglobin (>1 g/dL in a week) increases risk of vascular access thrombosis, stroke, myocardial infarction
Filgastrim (Granulocyte-Colony Stimulating Factor, G-CSF)		
To decrease risk of infectious complications of febrile neutropenia in patients with nonmyeloid malignancies receiving myelosuppressive therapy	5–10 μg/kg SC qd × 2 wk	Dosage regimens may vary with investigational protocols May be given until absolute neutrophil count reaches 10,000/cu mm Side effects: fever, bone pain, headache, rash
To accelerate myeloid recovery after chemotherapy and autologous bone marrow transplantation	5–10 μg/kg IV over 30 min or 1–20 μg/kg SC qd × 2–4 wk	Administration continued until absolute neutrophil counts greater than 1000/cu mm × 3 d, then dose reduced
HIV-associated or drug-induced neutropenia	60 μg/kg IV over 30 min or 1–20 μg/kg SC qd × 2–4 wk	

(continued)

TABLE 8.3. *(continued)* **Hematologic Growth Factors**

Agent/Indications	Dosage	Comments
Pegfilgastrim		
Prevention of febrile neutropenia in patients with nonmyeloid malignancies	6 mg SC injection	Pegylated granulocyte colony stimulating factor which delays renal clearance Preferred for outpatient therapy rather than inpatient therapy; long half-life offers no advantage for inpatient therapy Side effects similar to filgastrim Increase risk of chemotherapy-related myelosuppression if given 14 d before and 1 d after each chemotherapy cycle Do not use if weight <45 kg
Sargramostim (Granulocyte/Macrophage-Colony Stimulating Factor, GM-CSF)		
Myeloid reconstitution after autologous bone marrow transplantation	250 mg/M^2 IV over 2 h qd × 21 d	Side effects include capillary leak syndrome, flulike syndrome
Failure or engraftment delay in autologous bone marrow transplantation	250 mg/M^2 IV over 2 h qd × 14 d	Repeat in 7 d if engraftment has still not occurred; a third course of 500 mg/M^2/d for 14 d may be tried after another 7 d off therapy

IV, intravenous; SC, subcutaneous

TABLE 8.4. Transfusion Reactions—Therapy

Complication	Etiology	Management
Urticaria, pruritus	Antibodies to donor plasma protein (mild)	Interrupt transfusion; give diphenhydramine 25–100 mg PO or IV; if problem resolves, resume transfusion
Febrile nonhemolytic reactions (fever, chills, urticaria, agitation, headache, dyspnea, and/or palpitations)	Antibodies to donor plasma proteins, leukocytes or platelets, rarely bacterial contamination	Stop transfusion Check for clerical errors Return blood to blood bank with fresh blood and urine samples to check for hemoglobin, bilirubin, and haptoglobin Antipyretics Leukocyte-poor blood as alternative
Acute hemolytic reaction (agitation, confusion, chest pain, chills, fever, tachycardia, flank pain, shock, hematuria, and/or hemorrhage)	Antibodies to red cell antigens	Stop transfusion and return blood to blood bank with fresh blood and urine samples to check for hemoglobin, bilirubin, and haptoglobin Antipyretics Leukocyte-poor blood as alternative Supportive care Maintain urine output with furosemide, mannitol; alkalinize urine
Anaphylaxis (anxiety, chest pain, wheezing, shock)	Antibodies to donor plasma protein (severe), especially congenital IgA deficiency (total IgA or IgA subclass deficiency)	Stop the transfusion Epinephrine 0.3 ml (1:1,000) SC or, if reaction is severe (e.g., shock), 0.5–1.0 ml (1:10,000) IV push Support circulation Oxygen Bronchodilators See Table 11.2

Ig, Immunoglobin; IV, intravenous; PO, by mouth; SC, subcutaneous

TABLE 8.5. Immune Globulin Preparations

Preparation	Indications	Dosage	Comments
Cytomegalovirus[a] (CMV) immune globulin	For attenuation of primary CMV disease associated with kidney transplantation (i.e., CMV seronegative transplant recipient who receives kidney from CMV seropositive donor)	150 mg/kg IV within 72 hrs of transplant, then 100 mg/kg at 2, 4, 6, 8 wk after transplant, then 50 mg/kg at 12 and 16 wk after transplant	IgG preparation (5% to 6% solution) with standardized amount of antibody to CMV from pooled adult human plasma Infusion rate: 15 mg/kg/h for 15 min; if no adverse reactions, then 30 mg/kg/h for 15 min; then increase to maximum infusion rate of 60 mg/kg/h (volume not to exceed 75 ml/h)
	Prophylaxis of CMV disease (seropositive donor to seronegative recipient) in liver, heart, lung, or pancreas transplantation	150 mg/kg IV within 72 hrs of transplant, then 150 mg/kg at 2, 4, 6, 8 wk after transplant, then 100 mg/kg at 12 and 16 wk after transplant	CMV prophylaxis in organ transplants (other than kidney) use with ganciclovir If patient develops nausea, back pain, or flushing during infusion slow rate or temporarily stop infusion
	Severe CMV pneumonia	400 mg/kg IV with ganciclovir on days 1, 2, 7 or 8 followed by 200 mg/kg CMV-IVIG on days 14 and 21	Discontinue if blood pressure falls or anaphylaxis Can precipitate and worsen renal insufficiency Aseptic meningitis may occur within 2–48 h of therapy
Hepatitis B immune globulin[a]	Passive immunity for individuals exposed to hepatitis B virus or HBsAg-positive material Postexposure prophylaxis following percutaneous bites, direct mucous membrane contact, ingestion, or intimate contact	0.06 ml/kg or 3–5 ml IM	Administer within 24 h but not later than 7 d after exposure Derived from plasma from individuals with high HBsAb titers (10% to 18% protein) Should be combined with active immunization with hepatitis B vaccine at separate site if not previously vaccinated May be repeated 1 mo later in known vaccine nonresponders

(continued)

TABLE 8.5. *(continued)* **Immune Globulin Preparations**

Preparation	Indications	Dosage	Comments
Immune serum globulins[a] (ISG)	IM immune globulins are used to provide passive immunity for susceptible individuals exposed to infectious diseases when no vaccine is available or there is insufficient time for active immunization.		16% solution of immune globulins May cause local pain and tenderness at the injection site for several days
	Hepatitis A	0.02 ml/kg IM	As soon as possible and within 2 wk of exposure
	Non-A, non-B hepatitis	0.06 ml/kg IM	As soon as possible
	Measles (rubeola)	0.25 ml/kg IM (maximum 15 ml) for normal host; 0.5 ml/kg IM for immunosuppressed host	Measles virus vaccine live within 72 h of exposure is preferred Use IgIM when vaccine contraindicated (<1 y of age, pregnancy, immunocompromised) Not given concurrently with live measles virus vaccine
	Rubella (1st trimester exposure)	0.55 ml/kg IM	Efficacy in preventing disease is poor
	Varicella zoster	0.06–0.12 ml/kg IM	Alternative to Varicella-zoster Ig
IV immuno-globulin[a] (IVIG)	Congenital agammaglobulinemia or hypogammaglobulinemia	100–200 mg/kg monthly	5% to 6% solution Contraindicated in patients with selective IgA deficiencies; however, some preparations are low in IgA and can be used
	Idiopathic thrombocytopenic purpura	Refer to manufacturers' instructions	
	Kawasaki syndrome	400 mg/kg/d × 4 d or 2 g/kg × 1 dose	Most adverse reactions are related to the infusion rate (i.e., anaphylaxis and hypotension) Specific infusion rates according to manufacturers' instructions
	Patients refractory to platelet transfusions who are bleeding or need surgery	400 mg/kg/d × 4 d or 2 g/kg × 1 dose	
Rh immune globulin[a]	Block immune response in obstetrics to small amounts of Rh incompatible blood exposure during delivery, ectopic pregnancy, or abortion When Rh positive blood components are given to Rh negative recipients of childbearing age	50–300 mg IM	50 mg dose is protective for abortion, miscarriage, ectopic pregnancy, vaginal hemorrhage, or abdominal trauma during first 12 wk of pregnancy 300 mg dose is given to Rh negative mothers after exposure to 15 ml fetal blood caused by delivery, abortion, or ectopic pregnancy, or after amniocentesis

(continued)

TABLE 8.5. *(continued)* **Immune Globulin Preparations**

Preparation	Indications	Dosage	Comments
Rh_0-D immune globulin IV[a]	To prevent Rh isoimmunization in Rh-negative women exposed to Rh-positive fetal red blood cells at 28 weeks gestation, at term, and after invasive intrauterine procedures such as amniocentesis	300 μg IV at 28 weeks and 102 μg IV at delivery	Preparation is IgA-depleted and unlikely to cause anaphylactic reaction in women with IgA deficiency and anti-IgA antibodies Vial should not be shaken because it can damage protein and cause aggregate formation that increases risk of adverse reaction
	Treatment of ITP in Rh positive patient who has not had a splenectomy	25–50 μg/kg IV initial dose, then maintenance therapy with 25–60 μg/kg IV	For ITP, hemolysis is the dose-limiting toxicity Hgb decrease >2 g/dl in 5% to 10% In ITP, fever can be treated with acetaminophen, diphenhydramine, or prednisone If Hgb <10, reduced dose (25–40 μg/kg) should be given Frequency and dose of maintenance therapy determined by clinical response, including platelet counts, red cell counts, Hgb, and reticulocyte levels
Tetanus immune globulin (TIG)[a]	Prophylaxis	250 units IM (standard) 500 units IM (severe exposure or delayed administration)	Used in conjunction with active immunization with tetanus toxoid (separate site) in individuals with less than 3 doses of tetanus toxoid or if immunization status unknown TIG does not interfere with immune response to tetanus toxoid
	Treatment of tetanus	3,000–6,000 units IM	Used in treatment of tetanus in conjunction with antibiotics, sedation, and supportive care

(continued)

TABLE 8.5. *(continued)* **Immune Globulin Preparations**

Preparation	Indications	Dosage	Comments
Varicella-zoster immune globulin (VZIG)[a]	Prophylaxis after exposure of immunodeficient patient to varicella zoster (See comments)	125 units/10 kg body weight IM, max dose 625 U (5 vials), min dose 125 U	Purified human immune globulin (5%) High risk patients: immunocompromised state, pregnant women, neonates, premature infants Antiviral treatment (acyclovir) can be considered for adolescents and adults if illness occurs Investigational new drug available under expanded access protocol (FFF Enterprises, Temecula, CA, 24h telephone 800-843-7477). Requires informed consent and possibly local IRB approval
Rabies immune globulin (RIG)[a]	Pre-exposure immunization	RIG not recommended for pre-exposure immunization	Pre-exposure immunization with human diploid cell rabies vaccine (HDCRV, 1 ml/dose IM on d 0, 7, 21, and 28 or 0.1 ml/dose intradermally on d 0, 7, 21, and 28) does not eliminate the need for postexposure prophylaxis
	Postexposure immunization	20 IU/kg IM previous immunization 1 ml/dose IM on d 0 and 3	Should always include both immunization with RIG and vaccination (HDCRV, 1 ml/dose IM on d 0, 3, 7, 14, and 28) Patients with adequate rabies antibody titer should receive only the vaccine RIG may be given up to the 8th day after the 1st dose of vaccine is given

HDCRV, human diploid cell rabies vaccine; Hgb, hemoglobin; Ig, immunoglobulin; ITP, idiopathic thrombocytopenia purpura; IV, intravenous; ISG, immune serum globulin

[a]Potential for infectious disease transmission.

TABLE 8.6. Venous Thrombosis—Prophylaxis

Drug	Indication	Dosage	Comments
Dextran sulfate	High-risk surgery patients at risk for thromboembolism	Dextran 40 (10% solution) 500 ml IV q3d during prolonged bedrest	More costly than other antithrombotic agents Inhibits platelet function and fibrin polymerization Contraindicated in established venous thromboembolism and in patients with heart failure or dextran hypersensitivity No more effective than warfarin or heparin in general surgery patients
Heparin sodium	Venous thrombosis (general) Venous thrombosis (perioperatively for most abdominal, thoracic, or urologic procedures)	Fixed low dose 5,000 U SC q8–12h Fixed low dose 5,000 U SC 2 h prior to surgery, then 5,000 U SC q8–12h × 5–7 d, or Continuous infusion 1 U/kg/h at surgery, then for 3–5 d after surgery	
	Maintaining patency of indwelling venous catheters	1 ml (10–100 U/ml) after each use of catheter or q4–8h	Withdraw at least 1 ml from catheter prior to flush
Dalteparin sodium	For prevention of postoperative deep vein thrombosis in patients undergoing abdominal surgery who are at moderate to high risk[a–c] of thromboembolic complications	Moderate–high risk[a,b]: 2,500 units daily deep SC (not IM) 1–2 h prior to surgery, then qd for 5–10 d High-very high risk[b,c]: initial dose—5,000 units SC prior to surgery or 2,500 units 1–2 h prior to surgery, followed 12 h later by 2,500 units SC After initial dose, 5,000 units SC qd × 5–10 d	Low molecular weight heparin, porcine derived, each mg = 156.25 anti-Factor Xa International Units Dosage adjustment and routine monitoring of coagulation parameters are not necessary At recommended doses does not affect platelet aggregation fibrinolysis, prothrombin time, thrombin time, activated partial thromboplastin time Pharmacology differs from heparin or other low molecular weight heparins and is not interchangeable on a unit-for-unit basis Dosage adjustments in renal and hepatic disease have not been established; use with caution Use with care in patients receiving oral anticoagulants and/or platelet-aggregation inhibitors

Enoxaparin sodium	For prevention of postoperative deep-vein thrombosis in patients undergoing hip replacement surgery	30 mg deep SC bid, initial dose given as soon as possible after surgery but not more than 24 h postoperatively Given for 7–10 d	Low molecular weight heparin; porcine-derived Daily monitoring of the therapeutic effect is not necessary during therapy if laboratory indices of coagulation are normal prior to hip surgery At recommended doses, does not affect platelet aggregation or global-clotting tests (PT, aPTT) Pharmacology differs from heparin or other low molecular weight heparins and is not interchangeable on a unit-by-unit basis Adjust dose in renal disease Dosage adjustment in hepatic disease has not been established Use with care in patients receiving oral anticoagulants and/or platelet-aggregation inhibitors
Fondaparinux	Prevention of deep venous thrombosis after hip fracture surgery or hip replacement	2.5 mg daily SC, usually started 4–8 h postoperatively and treated for 5–9 d	Synthetic heparin analog that increases factor Xa inhibition without neutralizing thrombin Does not bind platelet factor IV, does not cause immune-mediated thrombocytopenia No effect on PT, aPTT time, bleeding time, or platelet function Renal clearance Not recommended if creatinine clearance <30 mL/min, platelets below 100,000/μL, or weight <50 mg Bleeding most common adverse effect especially if given less than 6 h after surgery
Warfarin			
Therapy and prophylaxis	Venous thrombosis and pulmonary embolism	10–15 mg PO qd $\times$ 2–5 d, then 2–10 mg PO qd Coagulation end point for therapy: 1.3–1.5 $\times$ control PT (INR 2–3)[d]	Indirect anticoagulant; alters synthesis of vitamin K dependent coagulation factors II, VII, IX, and X; use for follow-up anticoagulation after heparin Requires 2–7 d of therapy to deplete coagulation factors and to initiate anticoagulant effect; should overlap with heparin therapy by 4–5 d Multiple drug interactions (see Table 13.2)

(continued)

TABLE 8.6. *(continued)* **Venous Thrombosis—Prophylaxis**

Drug	Indication	Dosage	Comments
Warfarin (*continued*)			*Cautions:* (a) hemorrhage: if minor, hold and reduce dose; if moderate or severe, reverse with phytonadione, fresh frozen plasma, factor IX complex and/or rF*VIIa* (Table 8.2); (b) necrosis of skin or other tissues (especially in females and in protein C deficiency): treat with phytonadione and heparin
	Rheumatic mitral valve disease		
	• if history of systemic embolism, or paroxysmal or chronic atrial fibrillation, or sinus rhythm with left atrium diameter >5.5 cm	INR target 2.5 (range 2.0–3.0)	
	• if recurrent systemic embolism despite adequate warfarin	INR target 2.5 (range 2.0–3.0) and aspirin PO 80–100 mg/d or INR 2.5–3.5 and dipyridamole PO 400 mg/d or clopidogrel	
	Mitral valvuloplasty	Warfarin for 3 wks prior to procedure and 4 wks after the procedure. INR target 2.5 (range 2.0–3.0)	
	Mitral valve prolapse		
	• with documented but unexplained TIA	Aspirin 50–162 mg/d	
	• with systemic embolism, chronic or paroxysmal atrial fibrillation, or recurrent TIAs despite aspirin therapy	INR target 2.5 (range 2.0–3.0)	
	Mitral annular calcification with non-calcific embolism and associated atrial fibrillation	INR target 2.5 (range 2.0–3.0)	

Aortic valve disease		Low incidence of systemic embolism unless concomitant mitral valve disease, atrial fibrillation, or history of systemic emboli
Aortic valve disease with mobile aortic atheromas and aortic plaques >4mm by TEE	Consider warfarin therapy	
Prosthetic heart valves/mechanical heart valves	All patients with mechanical heart valves should receive warfarin Unfractionated heparin or LMWH should be used until the INR is stable and therapeutic for 2 consecutive days	
St. Jude Medical bileaflet valve (aortic position)	INR target 2.5 (range 2.0–3.0)	
Tilting disk valves and bileaflet mechanical valves (mitral position)	INR target 3.0 (range 2.5–3.5)	
CarboMedics bileaflet valve or Medtronic Hall tilting disk mechanical valves (aortic position, normal left atrium size, sinus rhythm)	INR target 2.5 (range 2.0–3.0)	
Mechanical valve and additional risk factors (atrial fibrillation, myocardial infarction, left atrial enlargement, endocardial damage, low ejection fraction)	INR target 3.0 (range 2.5–3.5) with low dose aspirin, 75–100 mg/d	
Caged ball or caged disk valves	INR target 3.0 (range 2.5–3.5) with low dose aspirin, 75–100 mg/d	
Mechanical valves with systemic thromboembolism despite therapeutic INR	INR target 3.0 (range 2.5–3.5) with low dose aspirin, 75–100 mg/d	
Mechanical valves in whom warfarin must be discontinued	LMWH or aspirin 80–100 mg/d	
Bioprosthetic valve replacement	Heparin or LMWH until INR stable for 2 consecutive days	

(continued)

TABLE 8.6. *(continued)* **Venous Thrombosis—Prophylaxis**

Drug	Indication	Dosage	Comments
Warfarin *(continued)*	First 3 months after valve insertion		
	mitral position	Warfarin INR target 2.5 (2.0–3.0 range)	
	aortic position	Warfarin INR 2.5 target (2.0–3.0 range) or aspirin 80–100 mg/d	
	bioprosthetic valves with a history of systemic embolism	Warfarin for 3 to 12 months	
	bioprosthetic valve with evidence of left atrial thrombus at surgery	INR target 2.5 (range 2.0–3.0)	
	Bioprosthetic valve with atrial fibrillation; long-term treatment	INR target 2.5 (range 2.0–3.0)	
	Bioprosthetic valves with sinus rhythm; long-term treatment	Aspirin 75–100 mg/d	
	PFO and atrial septal aneurysm with unexplained systemic embolism or TIAs and venous thrombosis, or pulmonary embolism	INR target 2.5 (2.0–3.0 range) until venous interruption or closure of PFO	
	Antithrombotic therapy in atrial fibrillation		Risk factors for thrombosis are: previous TIA or stroke, hypertension, heart failure, diabetes, clinical coronary artery disease, mitral stenosis, prosthetic heart valves, or thyrotoxicosis
	• if age < 60 y with no risk factors[d]	Aspirin 325 mg/d	
	• if age < 60 y with heart disease and no risk factors	Aspirin 325 mg/d	
	• if age > 60 y with no risk factors	Aspirin 325 mg/d	
	• if age > 60 y with diabetes or coronary disease	INR 2.0–3.0 with optional addition of aspirin 81–162 mg/d	

• if heart failure ejection fraction <.35, thyrotoxicosis, hypertension	INR 2.0–3.0	
• if age > 75 y, especially women, with or without risk factors	INR 2.0–3.0	
• with cardioversion if atrial fibrillation more than 2 d in duration	INR 2.0–3.0 for 3 w before elective cardioversion and then continued for 4 weeks	
Infective endocarditis • in patients with mechanical prosthetic valves		Continue anticoagulant therapy because of high frequency of systemic thromboembolism but increase risk of intracranial hemorrhage
Nonbacterial thrombotic endocarditis • with systemic or pulmonary emboli	Heparin therapy (see above)	
Disseminated cancer with aseptic vegetations	Full dose unfractionated heparin	

aPTT, activated partial thromboplastin time; INR, International Normalized Ratio; ISI, International Sensitivity Index; IV, intravenous; IM, intramuscular; PFO, patent foramen ovale; PO, by mouth; PT, prothrombin time; SC, subcutaneous; TIA, transient ischemic attacks; TEE, transesophageal echo

Recommendations based in part on 7th ACCP Conference on Antithrombotic and Thrombolytic Therapy. Chest 2004;126:3(Suppl):457S – 482S.

[a] Patients at risk for thromboembolic complications who are undergoing abdominal surgery are ≥40 years of age, obese, or in whom surgical procedure requires general anesthesia greater than 30 minutes in duration.

[b] Additional risk factors include malignancy, history of deep-venous thrombosis, or pulmonary embolism.

[c] Other risk factors: prolonged immobility or paralysis, varicose veins, heart failure, myocardial infarction, fractures of the pelvis, hip, or leg, possibly high-dose estrogen therapy, and hypercoagulable states.

[d] The International Normalized Ratio (INR) is used to monitor warfarin therapy. The INR is intended to standardize prothrombin time (PT) reporting by minimizing the variability that can result from differences in the sensitivity of the thromboplastin reagent used to perform the PT test. The sensitivity of the thromboplastin reagent is measured by the ISI, which is referenced to a World Health Organization (WHO) reference standard. The INR is calculated as follows: $(\text{patient PT/mean normal control})^{ISI}$. The INR adjusts for differences in sensitivity of the thromboplastin reagent and reflects the result that would be obtained with the WHO reference thromboplastin.

TABLE 8.7. Anticoagulant Therapy

Drug	Indication	Dosage	Comments
Heparin sodium	Acute pulmonary embolism Proximal deep venous thrombosis Acute myocardial infarction Acute arterial occlusion Cerebral embolism or transient ischemic attack Embolism associated with mitral valve disease and/or atrial fibrillation	80 U/kg IV load and then 18 U/kg/h maintenance infusion	Measure aPTT at 6 h, then adjust per weight-based dosing (see table below) (aPTT 1.5–2.5 × control) Follow hematocrit, platelet count, and fecal occult blood See also Table 4.11, re: anticoagulation and thrombolytic therapy Start warfarin therapy on day 1 if long-term anticoagulation anticipated, then stop heparin after 4–7 d of joint therapy and INR 2–3 without heparin (see below) With acute MI, begin with or after rtPA therapy and administer with aspirin (325 mg PO qd) Nondose-related thrombocytopenia occurs with bovine lung heparin (15%) and porcine intestinal heparin (5%); when thrombocytopenia develops with one preparation, it may be useful to switch to the other; discontinue heparin if platelet count <100,000/cu mm; heparin is rarely associated with thrombosis (usually arterial) and irreversible in vivo platelet aggregation (white clot syndrome)
	Continuous arteriovenous or venovenous hemofiltration	Bolus 15–25 U/kg IV, then 5–15 U/kg/h, follow aPTT (35–45 sec) or maintain ACT 150–200 s	Dose individualized for patients who are critically ill or who have preexisting coagulopathy
Enoxaparin	Deep venous thrombosis Treatment -inpatient with and without pulmonary embolism -outpatient treatment in patients without pulmonary embolism	1 mg/kg/dose SC q12h or 1.5 mg sid	Start warfarin within 72 h and continue enoxaparin until INR is between 2.0–3.0 (usually 7 d) Renal impairment Clcr <30 ml/min 1mg/kg SC qd Not approved for dialysis patients
	Unstable angina Percutaneous coronary interventions Acute coronary syndrome	1 mg/kg SC q12h in conjunction with aspirin 100–325 mg PO sid	

(continued)

TABLE 8.7. *(continued)* **Anticoagulant Therapy**

Drug	Indication	Dosage	Comments
Dalteparin	Acute treatment of unstable angina or non-Qwave MI	120 IU/kg SC q12h for 5–8 d with concurrent aspirin therapy	Dosage adjustment and routine monitoring of anticoagulation not necessary
Argatroban	Heparin-induced thrombocytopenia	Initial dose (normal hepatic function) 2 μg/kg/min IV adjusted to keep aPTT 1.5–3 times normal If hepatic dysfunction present, start 0.5 μg/kg bolus and increase infusion to 30 μg/kg/min	Direct-thrombin inhibitor Steady state anticoagulated effect after 1–3 h, monitored by aPTT Decrease dose with hepatic dysfunction aPTT returns to normal within 2 h of discontinuation 10% to 15% incidence of hematuria, allergic reactions–dyspnea/cough, or rash No adjustment for renal failure Conversion to warfarin, no load, start at expected daily dose
	Percutaneous intervention	Start 25 μg/kg/min and administer bolus of 350 μg/kg over 3–5 min with goal of ACT >300 s If ACT <300 s, give 150 μg/kg bolus and increase infusion to 30 μg/kg/min If ACT >450 sec, decrease infusion to 15 μg/kg/min	
Lepirudin	Heparin-induced thrombocytopenia	Initial dose (if normal renal function) 0.4 mg/kg IV bolus (15–20 s) followed by continuous infusion at 0.15 mg/kg/h	Direct thrombin inhibitor Monitor aPTT 4 h after infusion starts (range 1.5–2.5 ratio) If aPTT is below target, increase infusion by 20%, if aPTT is too high, decrease infusion by 50% Repeat aPTT after any dosing change

(continued)

TABLE 8.7. *(continued)* **Anticoagulant Therapy**

Drug	Indication	Dosage	Comments
Lepirudin (*continued*)	Concomitant use with thrombolytic therapy	Initial dose 0.2 mg/kg IV bolus (15–20 s) followed by continuous infusion at 0.1 mg/kg/h	All patients with Clcr <60 or serum Cr >1.5 mg/dL require dosage reduction Dosing with renal failure: -Clcr 45–60 mL/min, Scr 1.6–2.0 mg/dL; 50% std infusion rate or 0.075 mg/kg/h -Clcr 30–44, Scr 2.1–3.0; 30% std infusion rate or 0.045 mg/kg/h -Clcr 15–29, Scr 3.1–6.3; 15% std infusion rate or 0.0225 mg/kg/h -Clcr <15, Scr >6.0 avoid or stop infusion Over dosage with life threatening bleeding, blood transfusion and hemofiltration or dialysis with high flux dialysis membrane, e.g., AN 69, may be useful
Tinzaparin	Treatment of acute symptomatic deep venous thrombosis with or without pulmonary embolism in conjunction with warfarin	175 anti-Xa IU/kg SC qd, duration of therapy at least 6 d while warfarin therapy initiated	Low molecular weight heparin derived from porcine heparin Decreased clearance with severe renal failure, use with caution
Bivalirudin	IV anticoagulation, alternative to heparin in patients with unstable angina or undergoing percutaneous coronary intervention	1 mg/kg bolus IV then 2.5 mg/kg/h IV for 4 h, then 0.2 mg/kg/h for 14–20 h Alternative 0.75 mg bolus IV, then 1.75 mg/kg/h for duration of procedure, then D/C	Hirudin derivative, direct thrombin inhibitor Use in conjunction with aspirin Not associated with immune thrombocytopenia

Body Weight-Based Dosing of IV Heparin

Initial Dose: 80 U/kg load then 18 U/kg/h maintenance with aPTT at 6 h

aPTT	Dose Change U/kg/h	Additional Action	Next aPTT
<35 s (1.2 × control)	+4	Rebolus with 80 U/kg	After 6 h
35–45 s (1.2–1.5 × control)	+2	Rebolus with 40 U/kg	After 6 h
46–70 s (1.5–2.5 × control)	0	0	Within first 24 h, check every 6 h, then daily
71–90 s (2.3–3.0 × control)	–2	0	After 6 h
>90 s (>3 × control)	–3	Stop infusion × 1 h	After 6 h

ACT, activated clotting time; aPTT, activated partial thromboplastin time; INR, International Normalized Ratio; IV, intravenous; MI, myocardial infarction; PO, by mouth; SC, subcutaneous

TABLE 8.8. Preoperative and Postoperative Anticoagulation

Indication for Patients Who Are Taking Oral Anticoagulants	Before Surgery	After Surgery
Acute venous thromboembolism		
Month 1	IV heparin[a]	IV heparin[a]
Months 2 and 3	No change[b]	IV heparin
Recurrent venous thromboembolism[c]	No change[b]	SC heparin
Acute arterial embolism		
Month 1	IV heparin	IV heparin[d]
Mechanical heart valve	No change[b]	SC heparin
Nonvalvular atrial fibrillation	No change[b]	SC heparin

[a] A vena caval filter should be considered if acute venous thromboembolism has occurred within 2 weeks or if the risk of bleeding during intravenous heparin therapy is high.
[b] If patients are hospitalized, subcutaneous heparin may be administered, but hospitalization is not recommended solely for this purpose.
[c] The term refers to patients whose last episode of venous thromboembolism occurred more than 3 months before evaluation but who require long-term anticoagulation because of a high risk of recurrence.
[d] Intravenous heparin should be used after surgery only if the risk of bleeding is low.

TABLE 8.9. Reversal of Anticoagulants

Agent	Indications	Dosage	Comments
Heparin Reversal			
Protamine	Heparin overdose or heparin-associated hemorrhage	Dose required decreases with elapsed time after heparin discontinued	If heparin was given SC, some clinicians load with protamine 25–50 mg IV and then infuse calculated dose over 8–16 h
		0–29 min: 1–1.5 mg protamine/100 U heparin	Monitor effect with ACT or aPTT Can cause hypotension, bradycardia, dyspnea, allergic reactions
		30–60 min: 0.5–0.75 mg/100 U heparin >120 min: 0.25–0.375 mg/100 U heparin Infuse protamine slowly IV, rate not to exceed 50 mg in 10 min (50 mg protamine in 5 ml sterile water = 10 mg/ml)	Relatively contraindicated in diabetics who have received NPH insulin because of risk of hypersensitivity
	Reversal of extracorporeal heparinization	1.5 mg protamine/100 U of heparin	
Fresh frozen plasma			See Table 8.2
Hemostasis			
Aminocaproic acid	Treatment of life-threatening hemorrhage from systemic hyperfibrinolysis and urinary fibrinolysis (e.g., cardiac surgery, portacaval shunt, abruptio placenta, liver transplantation, prostatectomy)	4–5 g IV infusion over 1 h, then 1 g/h for 8 h or until hemorrhage controlled PO dose same as IV dose	Can be used with heparin to treat selected cases of DIC Do not exceed 30 g/d Adverse effects: muscle necrosis with prolonged administration, cardiac myocyte injury, intrarenal or ureteral thrombosis Reduce dose in renal, cardiac, or hepatic disease
Conjugated estrogens	Hemorrhage associated with uremia	0.6 mg/kg/d × 5 d	Infuse over 30 min Effects last 7–14 d
Desmopressin (DDAVP)	Hemorrhage associated with uremia Hemophilia A von Willebrand disease Cardiac surgery	0.3 μg/kg qd	Infuse over 30 min Effects last 8–12 h Side effects: facial flushing, conjunctival erythema, headache, blood pressure reduction, tachycardia

(continued)

TABLE 8.9. *(continued)* **Reversal of Anticoagulants**

Agent	Indications	Dosage	Comments
Recombinant activated coagulation factor VII (rFVIIa)	Warfarin-associated bleeding	15–30 μg/kg IV q12h (warfarin)	Binds tissue factor and activated platelets at site of injury, promotes conversion of prothrombin to thrombin Generally does not cause systemic thrombosis Reports of venous thrombosis, myocardial infarction, cerebral sinus thrombosis in patients treated with rFVIIa but cause and effect unclear
Topical thrombin	Hemostasis (when oozing from capillaries and small venules is visible and accessible)	General: 100 U/ml applied topically Profuse bleeding: 1,000–2,000 U/ml applied topically	Final concentration is a function of indication for use
Tranexamic acid	To reduce or prevent hemorrhage in patients with hemophilia; reduce need for replacement therapy after dental extraction	Immediately before surgery, 10 mg/kg IV then 25 mg/kg PO 3–4 ×/d for 2–8 d	Competitive inhibitor of plasminogen activation and at higher concentration noncompetitive inhibitor Contraindicated in patients with acquired defective color vision and subarachnoid hemorrhage; if patients are going to be treated for more than several days, a full ophthalmologic examination is required Dose adjusted for moderate to severe renal failure

ACT, activated clotting time; aPTT, activated partial thromboplastin time; DIC, disseminated intravascular coagulation; IV, intravenous; NPH, neutral protamine Hagedorn; PO, by mouth; SC, subcutaneous

TABLE 8.10. Antiplatelet Drugs

Drug	Indication	Dosage	Comments
Aspirin	Prevention of strokes and transient ischemic attacks; prevention and treatment of MI Adjunct with thienopyridine in PCI	81–325 mg PO qd	Inhibits platelet conversion of arachidonic acid to thromboxane for 5–7 d after exposure Enteric-coated preparations may be better tolerated by some patients 5% to 45% of patients with coronary artery disease may be relatively resistant to antiplatelet effects
Dipyridamole	Used in combination with warfarin for post-operative thromboembolic complications of cardiac valve replacement	75–100 mg PO qid	
Clopidogrel	Acute coronary syndrome PCI including the prevention of myocardial infarct poststent placement	300–600 mg PO then 75 mg PO qd Initiated 2–6 h prior to PCI	A thienopyridine that inhibits adenosine diphosphate receptor-mediated platelet activity Often used in combination with aspirin Thrombotic thrombocytopenia purpura rare
Glycoprotein IIb/IIIa Inhibitors			
Abciximab	Adjunctive therapy for PCI including angioplasty, stent placement Unstable angina pending PCI	10–60 min prior to PCI 0.25 mg/kg IV bolus then 0.125 mcg/kg/min IV (max 10 mcg/min) for 18–24 h concluding 1 h after PCI	Fab fragmented of chimeric antibody to GP IIb/IIIa receptor Binds both activated and nonactivated platelets Reverse effects with platelet transfusions
Eptifibatide	Acute coronary syndrome Adjunctive therapy for PCI	Immediately prior to PCI 180 mcg/kg IV bolus × 2 10 min apart, then 2 mcg/kg/min IV for 12–24 h	Binds GP IIb/IIIa receptor of activated platelets only, effects not reversed by platelet transfusion Reduce dose in renal failure Single bolus used in patients with ACS
Tirofiban	Acute coronary syndrome but may be continued through later PCI	Prior to PCI (for acute coronary syndrome) 0.4 mcg/kg/min for 30 min, then 0.1 mcg/kg/min for 12–24 h post-PCI	Similar to eptifibatide Partially metabolized by liver Reduce dose in renal failure

MI, myocardial infarction; PCI, percutaneous coronary interventions; PO, by mouth; TIA, transient ischemic attack

TABLE 8.11. Declotting Catheters—Procedures

Drug	Dosage	Duration	Comments
Thrombolytics			All agents may be effective in occlusions due to fibrin clots Indications include complete catheter occlusion and the inability to withdraw blood Should be administered locally in clotted port or ports of catheter; after indicated dwell time duration, the drug should be aspirated from the catheter with a syringe; assessment of catheter patency should then occur—catheter should not be flushed to avoid systemic administration of the drug
Alteplase	2 mg/ml and instill volume equal to internal volume of the catheter	Allow to stand for 0.5–1 h prn	
Other Agents			
Ethanol 70%	1–2 ml or equal to the internal volume of the catheter	Allow to stand for 20 min prn	Useful for occlusions caused by drugs or fat emulsion
Hydrochloric acid 0.1 N	0.2–1 ml or equal to the internal volume of the catheter	Allow to stand for 0.5–1 h prn	Useful for occlusions caused by drugs or fat emulsion; calcium, phosphorus, and mineral salts
Sodium bicarbonate 8.4%	0.25–3 ml, or equal to the internal volume of the catheter	Allow to stand for 15 min prn	Useful for occlusions caused by phenytoin

TABLE 8.12. Heparin-Induced Thrombocytopenia[a]

Clinical Condition	Platelet Count Monitoring
Therapeutic-dose UFH	qod until day 14 or until UFH stopped
Postoperative antithrombosis prophylaxis with UFH, postoperative cardiac surgery receiving UFH or LMWH	qod between day 4–14 or until UFH stopped
Medical or obstetric patient with prophylactic-dose UFH, postoperative patients receiving prophylactic-dose LMWH, postoperative patients receiving intravascular catheter UFH flushes, medical or obstetric patient receiving LMWH after first receiving UFH	Every 2–3 days from day 4–14 or until heparin stopped
Medical/obstetrical patients receiving LMWH only, medical patients receiving intravascular catheter UFH flushes	No routine platelet monitoring

Diagnosis

HIT antibody (high titer anti-platelet factor 4) formation or washed platelet activation assay and unexplained platelet count fall:

- Usually >50% even if nadir $>150 \times 10^9$/L
- May occur 5–14 days after initiating heparin therapy
- Rapid-onset HIT where counts fall within 24 hours of starting heparin after recent heparin exposure (within past 100 days)

or

Skin lesions at heparin injection sites

or

Acute systemic reaction such as chills, cardiorespiratory distress after IV heparin bolus (obtain platelet count immediately)

or

Venous or arterial thrombosis.

Treatment

Direct thrombin inhibitors

Lepirudin	With or without 0.4 mg/kg IV bolus, infusion rate 0.15 mg/kg/h IV	Treatment of thrombosis complicating HIT Monitor aPTT 1.5–2.0 times baseline Renal excretion
Argatroban	2 μg/kg/min (no bolus) HIT undergoing PCI IV bolus of 350 μg/kg then 25 μg/kg/min IV	Prevent and treat HIT-associated thrombosis Anticoagulation during angioplasty Increases INR Hepatobiliary excretion
Bivalirudin	0.15–0.20 mg/kg/h IV (no bolus)	Anecdotal experience in HIT Anticoagulation during PCI Monitor aPTT 1.5–2.5 times baseline

HIT, heparin-induced thrombocytopenia; INR, International Normalized Ratio; IV, intravenous; LMWH, low molecular weight heparin; PCI, percutaneous coronary intervention; UFH, unfractionated heparin

(*Adapted from the 7th ACCP Conference on Antimicrobial and Thrombolytic Therapy. Chest 2004;126:Supplement.)

Neurologic and Psychiatric Therapeutics

TABLE 9.1. Seizures—Urgent Management

Drug	Dosage	Comment
Thiamine	100 mg IV/IM	To avoid Wernicke's encephalopathy in alcoholics after glucose administration
Dextrose 50%	25–50 ml IV	For hypoglycemic seizures
Diazepam	2.5–10 mg IV, repeat after 5–10 min if needed	May cause respiratory depression and hypotension Seizures may recur because duration of efficacy is short
Phenytoin	10–20 mg/kg IV	Maximum infusion rate 50 mg/min Precipitates if injected into glucose-containing solutions Arrhythmias develop during rapid administration; monitor ECG Can produce hypotension
Fosphenytoin	10–20 PE/kg IV	Fosphenytoin should be prescribed in PE Fosphenytoin 75 mg = phenytoin 50 mg Infusion rate should be 100–150 mg PE/min Continuous monitoring of ECG, BP, and respiration is essential during IV loading Peak phenytoin levels occur approximately 2 h after the end of the loading infusion Fosphenytoin should not be administered IM for the treatment of status epilepticus
Phenobarbital	10–20 mg/kg IV	Maximum infusion rate 50 mg/min Respiratory depression and hypotension should be anticipated
Thiopental	25–100 mg IV	Hypotension and apnea are expected 5 mg/kg induces general anesthesia, but with a variable response
Neuromuscular blocking agents	See Table 2.4	Neuromuscular blocking agents possess no anticonvulsant properties For intractable seizures or life-threatening acidosis or muscle contractions Use of these agents can mask seizure activity; therefore, EEG monitoring is required
General anesthesia		For intractable seizures or life-threatening acidosis or muscle contractions

ECG, electrocardiogram; EEG, electroencephalogram; IV, intravenous; IM, intramuscular; PE, phenytoin sodium equivalent; BP, blood pressure

TABLE 9.2. Seizures—Maintenance Therapy

Drug	Daily Dosage	Optimal Blood Level (μg/ml)	Comment
Carbamazepine	5–25 mg/kg PO divided tid-qid	4–8	Metabolized to active metabolite Side effects: nystagmus, dysarthria, diplopia, ataxia, drowsiness, nausea, blood dyscrasias, hepatotoxicity
Fosphenytoin	Maintenance dose: 4–6 mg/kg PE total daily dose IV/IM divided doses q8h Temporary substitution for oral Dilantin: same as daily oral Dilantin dose in mg	10–20 (measured as phenytoin) Free level 1–2	Fosphenytoin 75 mg = phenytoin 50 mg Maximum infusion rate 150 mg PE/min IV infusion requires continuous ECG, BP, and respiratory monitoring Administer fosphenytoin substitution doses at the same frequency as oral Dilantin Side effects: tingling, paresthesias after IV administration; other side effects similar to phenytoin
Gabapentin	900 mg PO divided tid	—	Side effects: fatigue, somnolence, dizziness, ataxia
Lamotrigine	25 mg PO every other day if on valproic acid + enzyme inducer; 50 mg/d if not on valproic acid, but on enzyme inducer	—	Side effects: rash, abnormal thinking, dizziness, ataxia, nervousness, somnolence, diplopia, nausea, vomiting, weight gain
Phenobarbital	2–5 mg/kg PO/IV qd	10–40	Maximum infusion rate 50 mg/min Side effects: drowsiness, nystagmus, ataxia, skin rash, learning difficulties
Phenytoin	4–8 mg/kg PO/IV qd	Total level:10–20 Free level 1–2	Maximum infusion rate 50 mg/min Side effects: nystagmus, ataxia, dyskinesias, sedation, gingival hyperplasia, hirsutism, blood dyscrasias, rashes, systemic lupus erythematosus, peripheral neuropathy
Primidone	5–20 mg/kg PO divided tid	Primidone: 5–15 Phenobarbital: 15–40	Metabolized to phenobarbital, which contributes to pharmacologic activity Side effects: sedation, nystagmus, ataxia, vertigo, nausea, skin rashes, megaloblastic anemia

(continued)

TABLE 9.2. *(continued)* **Seizures: Maintenance Therapy**

Drug	Daily Dosage	Optimal Blood Level (μg/ml)	Comment
Topiramate	Goal of 200 mg PO bid Starting dose 50 mg PO bid	—	Adequate fluid intake should be maintained to minimize the risk of kidney stone formation Side effects: psychomotor slowing, difficulty in concentrating, speech and language problems, somnolence and fatigue, kidney stone formation
Valproic acid	10–60 mg/kg PO divided tid	50–100	Side effects: nausea, vomiting, diarrhea, drowsiness, alopecia, weight gain, hepatotoxicity, thrombocytopenia, tremor
Valproate sodium injection	10–60 mg/kg IV divided tid-qid IV dose equals the oral dose when used as a temporary substitute for oral therapy		IV product is intended for temporary substitution of oral valproate in same daily dose and dosing interval IV dose should be infused as a 60 min infusion, but not faster than 20 mg/min

BP, blood pressure; ECG, electrocardiogram; IM, intramuscular; IV, intravenous; PE, phenytoin sodium equivalent; PO, by mouth

TABLE 9.3. Increased Intracranial Pressure

Agent	Dosage	Comment
Adjunctive therapy		Airway and hemodynamic management may be indicated Neurosurgical consultation
Mannitol	0.25–1.0 g/kg IV, then 0.25–0.5 g/kg IV q4h	As needed to maintain ICP without exceeding serum osmolality of 320–400 mOsm Adverse effects: transient immediate hypervolemia followed by diuresis and hypovolemia; hyperosmolar state; possible rebound increase in ICP after termination, particularly if mannitol is retained by abnormal tissue; exacerbation of intracranial bleeding
Hypertonic saline 23.4%	Standard dose of 30 ml (120 mEq) over 15–20 min (2ml/min) Maximum dose 60 ml	Must be administered through a central line Administration without a central line is an absolute contraindication This is for acute osmotherapy with the goal of reduced ICP Obtain serum sodium after every dose of 30 ml of 23.4% saline
Hypertonic saline 3%	Mixture 3% saline (50% as acetate 50% as chloride) Or mixture as 3% saline (100% as chloride) Starting dose 40–50 ml/h Titrate to serum sodium goal (140–160 meq) Serum sodium concentration of 160 is the maximum tolerated serum sodium concentration Common bolus volume is 250 cc	Must be administered through a central line Administration without a central line is an absolute contraindication Obtain serum sodium levels every 2–4 h while infusing and immediately after bolusing
Hypertonic saline 2%	Given as an IV bolus or continuous infusion Serum sodium should be monitored every 4 h while in the infusion	No absolute contraindications
Furosemide	10–20 mg IV q4h	Titrated Decreases edema and CSF production Does not produce rapid decreases in ICP
Pentobarbital	3–5 mg/kg IV bolus, over 30 min then 1 mg/kg/h Loading dose: 10mg/kg/h for 3 h then 2mg/kg/h	Monitoring: EEG burst suppression, therapeutic level of 20–50 μg/ml Burst suppression goal 1:10 to 1:30 ratio of complexes to seconds
Lidocaine	0.5–1.5 mg/kg IV or intratracheally	Useful with acute airway manipulations to reduce coughing Can precipitate seizures
Dexamethasone	4–20 mg IV q6h	Decreases brain swelling with vasogenic edema Increases mortality in head trauma

CSF, cerebral spinal fluid; EEG, electroencephalogram; ICP, intracranial pressure; IV, intravenous

TABLE 9.4. Cerebral Vasospasm

Goal	Treatment	Comments
If arterial pressure excessively elevated, lower toward normal range	Trimethaphan or labetalol	Refer to Tables 3.11 and 3.12; vasodilator agents may increase intracranial blood volume and intracranial pressure and are usually avoided in symptomatic vasospasm
Ensure adequate intravascular volume	Colloid and/or crystalloid solutions as appropriate	Fluids maximize cardiac performance and blunt catecholamine release and activation of renin-angiotensin system; if cerebral edema is severe, may need invasive monitoring
Avoid arterial hypotension	If hypotension does not correct with fluids, use phenylephrine	CPP = mean arterial pressure – intracranial pressure Phenylephrine does not constrict cerebral vessels; alternatives are dopamine or norepinephrine, dobutamine
Ensure adequate oxygenation	Supplemental oxygen as needed	Maximize cerebral oxygen delivery
Decrease severity of neurologic deficits	Nimodipine 60 mg PO q4h for 21 d	Calcium channel blocker that affects cerebral vessels preferentially; in subarachnoid hemorrhage protects against calcium-induced ischemic cell damage through unknown mechanisms; no side effects except occasional hypotension
Reversal of neurologic deterioration caused by vasospasm	Expansion of intravascular volume and elevation of systemic arterial pressure	Rapid expansion of intravascular volume with colloid and crystalloid to pulmonary artery wedge pressure of 12–18 mm Hg; raise systemic arterial pressure in increments of 10 mm Hg with dopamine until deficits reverse; hazardous if initiated in the presence of an untreated or unruptured aneurysm

CPP, cerebral perfusion pressure; PO, by mouth

TABLE 9.5. Psychiatric Disorders

Disorder	Treatment	Dosage	Comments
Anxiety and Agitation			Benzodiazepines are the treatment of choice in controlling psychotic agitation and when panic and phobic anxiety account for agitated behavior
Benzodiazepines	Diazepam	PO: 2–10 mg bid-qid	Rapid onset Especially useful for rapid tranquilization
		IV/IM: 2–10 mg q4–6h prn	Available in IV and oral liquid dosage forms Active metabolites accumulate with multiple doses Reduced metabolism in the elderly and patients with liver disease Potential for drug interactions May cause excessive sedation
	Lorazepam	PO: 0.5–3 mg bid-tid IV/IM: 1–2 mg q1–4h prn	Slower onset than diazepam Available in IV and oral liquid dosage forms No active metabolites May cause excessive sedation
	Alprazolam	PO: 0.25–1 mg bid-tid	Useful in patients who have a panic or phobic component to their anxiety Lower doses should be used in elderly patients, patients with liver disease or low albumin
Delirium			Neuroleptic medications are thought to be specific for the treatment of delirium and psychosis, attendant agitation may be controlled more effectively by the use of a benzodiazepine with a neuroleptic agent
Neuroleptics	Haloperidol	(See Table 9.6) Mild agitation: 0.5–2 mg IV Moderate agitation: 2–5 mg IV Severe agitation: 5–10 mg IV Continuous infusion: 2–10 mg/h Less severe symptoms: 0.5–2 mg PO/IV/IM qhs-bid	IV medication required in acute delirium IM administration is not recommended because of the potential for erratic absorption in hemodynamically unstable patients Oral dose has about half of the potency of the IV dose Torsade de pointes is a potential complication Monitor QT interval and electrolytes when using high doses or continuous infusions, or in combination with other drugs that prolong QT interval
Benzodiazepines	Lorazepam	IV/IM: 1–10 mg q1–4h prn	Promotes additional calming when used in combination or alternating with haloperidol May result in decreased doses of haloperidol needed for clinical effect Diazepam or midazolam may be used in place of lorazepam when agitation is explosive and rapid control is desired

(continued)

TABLE 9.5. *(continued)* **Psychiatric Disorders**

Disorder	Treatment	Dosage	Comments
Depression			
Psychostimulants	Methylphenidate	PO: 2.5–20 mg bid	Useful in patients who are lethargic, hard to mobilize, listless, or who show no interest in their care Give the afternoon dose before 3:00 PM so that the ability to fall asleep is not impaired
Conventional antidepressants			Useful if the response to psychostimulants is partial or ineffective Tricyclic antidepressants have a slow onset, have anticholinergic side effects, and can affect the cardiac conduction system The patient's medical record should be reviewed to determine if he or she has previously been treated with antidepressants and to assess his or her response to these agents
	Doxepin	PO: 25 mg qhs	Useful in depressed patients who have difficulty in falling asleep Increase by 25 mg nightly until an adequate sleep dose is achieved
	Nortriptyline	PO: 25 mg qhs	Increase 25 mg weekly up to 75 mg qhs, aiming for a serum concentration between 50–150 ng/ml
Serotonin reuptake inhibitors			Potential adverse effects of this class of antidepressants are overstimulation, agitation, and increased anxiety
	Fluoxetine	PO: 20 mg q AM	Metabolized through the cytochrome P450 system and has the potential for drug interactions
	Paroxetine	PO: 20 mg q AM	Metabolized through the cytochrome P450 system and is a potent inhibitor of this enzyme system; serious potential for many drug interactions
	Sertraline	PO: 50 mg q AM	Least potential for drug interactions
	Nefazodone	PO: 50 mg qhs	Possesses antidepressant and antianxiety properties, so it is useful in patients with an anxiety component to their depression An alternative to doxepin
	Citalopram	20 mg PO qd starting up to 60 mg PO qd maximum	SSRI antidepressant and reduced anxiety

(continued)

TABLE 9.5. *(continued)* **Psychiatric Disorders**

Disorder	Treatment	Dosage	Comments
	Escitalopram	10 mg PO qd starting May increase to 20 mg after 1 wk	SSRI antidepressant and reduced anxiety
	Venlafaxine	75 mg qd total daily dose Immediate release 25 mg PO tid or 37.5 mg bid Sustained release 75 mg PO qd	SSRI antidepressant and reduced anxiety
	Bupropion	100 mg PO bid starting dose Maximum 450 mg PO in bid or sustained release	Side effects are seizures SSRI with decreased depression and anxiety

IM, intramuscular; IV, intravenous; PO, by mouth; SSRI, selective serotonin reuptake inhibitor

TABLE 9.6. Guidelines for Intravenous Haloperidol

Severity of Agitation	Haloperidol Dose
Mild	0.5–2 mg
Moderate	2–5 mg
Severe	5–10 mg

1. Allow 10 to 15 minutes between doses.
2. For continued agitation, double the previous dose.
3. For continued agitation after 3 doses, give lorazepam 0.5–10 mg IV either concurrently or alternating with haloperidol every 30 minutes.
4. Consider a haloperidol continuous infusion (2–10 mg/h) if the agitation is poorly controlled with intermittent IV doses.
5. Once the patient is calm, determine the total dose of haloperidol administered, and give this dose over the next 24 hours. The daily requirement can be divided into 2 doses, with the largest dose administered at bedtime.
6. Give this dose for 24–48 hours; if the patient remains calm, begin reducing the dose by 50% every day.
7. If the patient is stable and able to take oral medications, the tapering doses may be given orally (the oral dose = 2 × the IV dose).
8. Monitor QT interval and decrease dose or discontinue if QT interval prolonged because of risk of serious arrhythmia.

TABLE 9.7. Alcohol Withdrawal—Drug Therapy

Drug	Typical Dosage	Comment
Supportive Care		
Folate	1 mg PO/IV/IM qd	Folate, thiamine, and multivitamins should be given before the administration of dextrose to avoid precipitating Wernicke's syndrome
Thiamine	100 mg IM/PO qd × 3 d	
Multivitamin	1 PO qd	Fluid and electrolytes should be administered to correct fluid and electrolyte disturbances
Magnesium	1–2 g IV/IM qd-tid × 3 d	IV multivitamins—1 vial/day in IV fluid
Benzodiazepines		Although there is no evidence that one benzodiazepine is more effective than another, benzodiazepines with long half-lives and active metabolites may be beneficial in alcohol withdrawal because they may help to smooth a tapering effect Late-onset seizures have been reported in patients being treated with short-acting benzodiazepines
Diazepam	5–10 mg PO tid, tapering over 5–10 d	Active metabolites Long half-life
Lorazepam	1–2 mg IV q4–6h titrated to sedation, tapering over 5–10 d	No active metabolites Intermediate half-life Preferred agent in patients with liver disease
Control of Adrenergic Symptoms		
Atenolol	25–50 mg PO qd	
Metoprolol	5–20 mg IV q4h	
Clonidine	0.1–0.4 mg PO q8–12h	Central acting sympathomimetic that may diminish the use of sedatives; weekly patch (0.1–0.3 mg) may be used but is delayed in onset
Other		
Alcohol	5% solution for IV infusion	Postpones withdrawal, toxic, difficult to titrate, and generally is not recommended
Haloperidol	2.5–150 mg/day in divided doses	May lower the seizure threshold; usually not indicated even when withdrawal hallucinations occur
Phenytoin	15 mg/kg load then 300 mg per day	For treatment of seizures

IM, intramuscular; IV, intravenous; PO, by mouth

Note: The need for prophylaxis in patients undergoing alcohol withdrawal has been questioned recently. Therapy based on symptoms may be equally effective and diminish the need to treat large numbers of patients who may not experience withdrawal.

TABLE 9.8. Treatment of Withdrawal Reactions

Agent	Therapy	Comments
Alcohol		See Table 9.7
Benzodiazepines		
Short, intermediate-acting	Lorazepam 2 mg PO qid-tid, then taper over 5–7 d	
Long-acting	Diazepam 5–10 mg PO qid-tid × 5 d, then taper over 5–7 d	Active metabolites are beneficial in tapering agent after discontinuation
Opiates		
Replacement therapy	Methadone 20 mg PO or 10 mg IM × 1 dose A second dose may be given if significant relief is not obtained 1 h after the 1st dose	Dosing for withdrawal reactions requires less methadone than dosing for methadone maintenance; some patients require 20–40 mg daily to avoid psychological withdrawal
Sympatholytic therapy	Clonidine 6 μg/kg PO loading dose followed by 6–17 μg/kg/d PO divided tid × 7 d, then taper over 3 d	Hypotension may be associated with higher doses May use clonidine topical patches for tapering regimen Dose may be decreased by changing patches every 3 d

IM, intramuscular; PO, by mouth

TABLE 9.9. Myasthenia Gravis

Problem	Management	Comment
Acute diagnosis	Edrophonium 2 mg (0.2 ml) IV initially, if tolerated 8 mg (0.8 ml) IV after 30 s (results in improvement in muscle strength, 5 min duration) Or Neostigmine 1.5 mg IM (duration 2 h)	Assessment of patient with fluctuating weakness of voluntary muscles with symptoms of diplopia, ptosis, difficulty swallowing Atropine sulfate (0.6 mg IV/IM) should be available to reverse muscarinic effects Monitor respiratory function, avoid aminoglycosides
Therapy	*Chronic therapy:* Neostigmine 7.5–30 mg PO qid or pyridostigmine 30–180 mg PO qid Corticosteroids (prednisone 60–100 PO qd) in patients who respond poorly to anticholinergics and have undergone thymectomy. Alternatively azathioprine may be given 2–3 mg/kg/d Plasmapheresis	Conversion to IV dose is 1:60 conversion; with the IV dose being 1/60 of the oral dose of neostigmine and pyridostigmine Thus 60 qid of pyridostigmine bromide equaling 1,240 mg TTL daily dose would equal 4mg/ day of IV neostigmine as an IV infusion given over 24 h

IM, intramuscular; IV, intravenous; PO, by mouth; TTL, total

TABLE 9.10. Acute Spinal Cord Injury

Problem	Management	Comment
Airway	Skilled and experienced operator necessary to prevent secondary injury Neutral traction during placement of airway	Lesions above C_3–C_4 require intubation and mechanical ventilation because of loss of diaphragm (C_3–C_5) Lesions below C_5–C_6 may result in reduced vital capacity and flow and require mechanical ventilation
Hypotension	Fluid resuscitation often with central pressure monitoring Vasopressors (see Table 3.8) after fluid resuscitation	Causes other than spinal shock should be aggressively sought because of associated thoracic and abdominal trauma
Bradydysrhythmias	Atropine 0.5–1 mg IV Pacemaker	If cardiac accelerator nerves (T_1–T_4) are involved, bradycardia and bradydysrhythmias may occur because of loss of sympathetic tone and unopposed vagal activity
Tachydysrhythmias	β-Blockers (see Table 3.6)	Often accompany autonomic hyperreflexia If hypertension present, α-adrenergic blockade required with β-blockers
Loss of neurologic function	Stabilization of spine by traction and surgical fixation Surgical decompression of subdural or epidural hematomas Methylprednisolone 30 mg/kg IV, infused over 15 min; after 45 min, continuous infusion (5.4 mg/kg/h) for 23 h	Methylprednisolone treatment should be initiated as soon as possible (i.e., within 3 h of injury) Recent trials suggest that when therapy is initiated 3–8 h after injury, patients should be maintained on therapy for 48 h
Autonomic hyperreflexia	Minimize episodes of noxious or visceral stimuli (e.g., bladder or bowel distension) Pharmacologic therapy: trimethaphan, phentolamine (see Table 3.12)	Usually when flaccid paralysis or spinal shock occurs, it occurs below level of injury
Abnormal response to depolarizing muscle relaxants	Avoid depolarizing agents 12 h after injury (e.g., succinylcholine) and use nondepolarizing neuromuscular blockade (see Table 2.4)	Massive amounts of K^+ can be released from skeletal muscle to extracellular space following depolarizing muscle relaxant Magnitude of K^+ release is a function of muscle mass affected and may occur before spasticity is apparent

IV, intravenous

TABLE 9.11. Thrombolysis for Acute Ischemic Stroke

Agent	Dosage	Comments
Tissue plasminogen activator	0.9 mg/kg (maximum dose 90 mg) infused over 60 min, with 10% of total dose given as IV bolus over 1 min	Indicated for thrombotic arterial occlusion with no evidence of intracranial hemorrhage on CT scan Treatment should be started within 3 h after onset of symptoms Antithrombotic and antiplatelet drugs should be withheld for 24 h Contraindications—intracranial hemorrhage, or other bleeding risk[a]

CT, computed tomography

[a]Suspicion of subarachnoid hemorrhage or other bleeding, recent intracranial surgery or head trauma, recent major surgery, uncontrolled hypertension, intracranial neoplasm, aneurysm or vascular malformation, recent treatment with heparin or warfarin, or platelet count <100,000/cu mm.

TABLE 9.12. Experimental Therapies for Acute Hemorrhagic and Ischemic Stroke

Agent	Dosing	Comments
Acute Hemorrhagic Stroke		
Recombinant activated factor VIIa (Table 8.2)	20,80 μg/kg dosing in IV push over 2 min Presently in randomized phase III trial 80 μg/kg is the preferred dose for hemorrhage Must administer within 3 h of onset of ICH	Many adverse events including myocardial ischemia, pulmonary embolus, and ischemic stroke have been documented in this setting
Ischemic Stroke		
Tenecteplase	Phase 2-B study of TNK in acute ischemic stroke (TNK-S2B) Dosing: 0.1 mg/kg TNK, 0.25 mg/kg TNK, or 0.4 mg/kg TNK Given as an IV bolus within 3 h of onset	This is an experimental therapy and is currently only used in the clinical research setting with informed consent and IRB approval
Desmoteplase	62.5μg/kg, 90μg/kg, 125μg/kg IV given as a single bolus 3–9 h if patient has a perfusion mismatch on MRI or CT perfusion scans	This is an experimental drug and is currently only used in the clinical research setting with informed consent and IRB approval

CT, computed tomography; ICH, intracranial hemorrhage; IRB, institutional review board; MRI, magnetic resonance imaging

Infectious Diseases

TABLE 10.1. Parenteral Antimicrobial Agents of Choice for Specific Pathogens

(These recommendations for empiric therapy should be modified based on local susceptibility patterns. The susceptibility of clinically important pathogens must be substantiated by laboratory testing for most pathogens.)

Pathogen	First Choices	Alternatives
Acanthamoeba		
Encephalitis	None definitely effective	Pentamidine Trimethoprim-sulfamethoxazole + rifampin
Keratitis	0.1% propamidine (topical) + neomycin/gramicidin/polymyxin (topical)	Polyhexamethylene biguanide 0.02% (topical) Chlorhexidine 0.02% (topical)
Acinetobacter calcoaceticus—baumanni complex	Imipenem or Meropenem or Tobramycin + ciprofloxacin	Tobramycin + piperacillin Colistin Tigecycline Ampicillin-sulbactam
***Actinomyces israeli* and others**	Penicillin G or Ampicillin	Clindamycin Doxycycline Erythromycin Ceftriaxone
Adenovirus	None	Cidofovir
Aeromonas hydrophila		
Bacteremia	Ciprofloxacin	Trimethoprim-sulfamethoxazole Imipenem or Meropenem Cefepime
Diarrhea	Trimethoprim-sulfamethoxazole	Doxycycline Ciprofloxacin
Alcaligenes xylosoxidans	Imipenem or Meropenem or Piperacillin-tazobactam	Trimethoprim-sulfamethoxazole
Ameba	See *Entameba histolytica* or *Naegleria*	
Anaplasma	Doxycycline	Ciprofloxacin
***Aspergillus* species**	Voriconazole	Liposomal amphotericin B (AmBisome) or ABLC Amphotericin B Itraconazole Caspofungin Micafungin
Babesia microti	Atovaquone + azithromycin	Clindamycin + quinine
Bacillus anthracis		
Inhalational or gastrointestinal	Ciprofloxacin + clindamycin + rifampin ± penicillin G	Doxycycline + clindamycin + rifampin
Bacillus anthracis cutaneous	Ciprofloxacin	Doxycycline
***Bacillus cereus* (invasive)**	Vancomycin or Clindamycin	Imipenem or Meropenem Levofloxacin
Bacillus subtilis	Vancomycin or Clindamycin	Imipenem or Meropenem Levofloxacin
Bacteroides fragilis	Metronidazole	Imipenem or Meropenem Piperacillin-tazobactam
Bacteroides melaninogenicus	Metronidazole	Piperacillin-tazobactam Imipenem or Meropenem
***Bartonella* species (Cat scratch fever)**	Erythromycin or Azithromycin	Clarithromycin Doxycycline Ciprofloxacin
Blastomyces dermatitidis	Liposomal amphotericin B (AmBisome) or ABLC	Itraconazole Fluconazole Amphotericin B

(continued)

TABLE 10.1. *(continued)* **Parenteral Antimicrobial Agents of Choice for Specific Pathogens**

Pathogen	First Choices	Alternatives
Bordetella pertussis	Azithromycin	Trimethoprim-sulfamethoxazole Erythromycin Clarithromycin
Borrelia burgdorferi		
Early	Doxycycline	Amoxicillin
Facial nerve palsy	Doxycycline	Amoxicillin
Arthritis	Doxycycline	Ceftriaxone
Carditis	Ceftriaxone	Doxycycline
Meningitis/Encephalitis	Ceftriaxone	Penicillin G
Burkholderia cepacia	Imipenem or Meropenem	Trimethoprim-sulfamethoxazole
Campylobacter fetus	Imipenem or Meropenem	Gentamicin Erythromycin
Campylobacter jejuni	Erythromycin or Azithromycin	Doxycycline Ciprofloxacin
***Candida* species (mucosal—not life-threatening)**	Fluconazole (IV/PO) or Caspofungin	Itraconazole (IV/PO) Amphotericin B Liposomal amphotericin B (AmBisome) or ABLC Micafungin
***Candida* species (invasive)**	Liposomal amphotericin B (AmBisome) or ABLC or Caspofungin	Fluconazole Amphotericin B Micafungin
Capnocytophaga ochracea (DF-1)	Clindamycin	Imipenem or Meropenem Ceftriaxone Ciprofloxacin Doxycycline
Capnocytophaga canimorsus (DF-2)	Ampicillin-sulbactam	Ciprofloxacin Ceftriaxone Imipenem or Meropenem
Cardiobacterium	Ceftriaxone	Ampicillin + gentamicin
Chlamydia pneumoniae	Doxycycline or Azithromycin	Clarithromycin Erythromycin Levofloxacin or Gatifloxacin
Chlamydia psittaci	Doxycycline	Erythromycin Azithromycin
Chlamydia trachomatis		
Pelvic inflammatory disease (PID)	Doxycycline	Azithromycin Ofloxacin
Citrobacter diversus	Imipenem or Meropenem	Ciprofloxacin Gentamicin
Citrobacter freundii	Imipenem or Meropenem	Ceftriaxone Ciprofloxacin
***Clostridium botulinum* (botulism)**	Trivalent equine antitoxin (CDC)[a] (+ penicillin for wound botulism)	Metronidazole + antitoxin
***Clostridium difficile* (diarrhea)**	Metronidazole (PO)	Vancomycin (PO) Bacitracin (PO) Metronidazole (IV)
***Clostridium* species (non-tetanus) (non-botulinum)**	Penicillin G ± Clindamycin	Piperacillin-tazobactam Imipenem or Meropenem Doxycycline
***Clostridium tetani* (tetanus)**	Penicillin G + human tetanus immune globulin (CDC)[a]	Metronidazole Doxycycline Clindamycin Imipenem or Meropenem (all with antitoxin)

(continued)

TABLE 10.1. *(continued)* **Parenteral Antimicrobial Agents of Choice for Specific Pathogens**

Pathogen	First Choices	Alternatives
Coccidioides immitis	Liposomal amphotericin B (AmBisome) or ABLC	Itraconazole (IV/PO) Amphotericin B
Corynebacterium diphtheriae	Penicillin + antitoxin (CDC)[a]	Erythromycin + antitoxin Clindamycin + antitoxin
***Corynebacterium JK* strain**	Vancomycin	Penicillin G + gentamicin Ciprofloxacin
Coxiella burnetii	Doxycycline	Ciprofloxacin
Cryptococcus neoformans	Liposomal amphotericin B (AmBisome) or ABLC ± flucytosine	Fluconazole Amphotericin B
Cysticercosis	Albendazole ± prednisone	Praziquantel ± prednisone
Cytomegalovirus	Ganciclovir ± IV immune globulin (IVIG)	Foscarnet ± IV immune globulin (IVIG) Ganciclovir + foscarnet ± IVIG Cidofovir
DF-1 (Capnocytophaga)	Clindamycin	Imipenem or Meropenem Cefoxitin Ceftriaxone
DF-2 (Capnocytophaga)	Ampicillin-sulbactam	Ciprofloxacin Ceftriaxone Imipenem or Meropenem
Ehrlichia chaffeensis, phagocytophila,* and other *Ehrlichia	Doxycycline	Ciprofloxacin
Eikenella corrodens	Ampicillin or Penicillin G	Cefotaxime Imipenem or Meropenem Ciprofloxacin
Entameba histolytica		
Severe intestinal	Metronidazole (IV) or Tinidazole (PO) followed by Paromomycin (PO)	Dehydroemetine followed by Iodoquinol (PO)
Mild	Metronidazole (IV/PO) or Tinidazole (PO) followed by Iodoquinol (PO)	Paromomycin
Asymptomatic	Paromomycin (PO)	Iodoquinol (PO) Diloxanide (PO)
***Enterobacter* species**	Ciprofloxacin Imipenem or Meropenem	Aztreonam Cefepime Piperacillin-tazobactam
***Enterococcus* (sensitive)**	Ampicillin ± gentamicin	Vancomycin ± gentamicin Daptomycin
***Enterococcus* (Vancomycin-resistant)**	Linezolid Daptomycin	Synercid
Escherichia coli	Ceftriaxone	Gentamicin Imipenem or Meropenem Ciprofloxacin Aztreonam Piperacillin-tazobactam Ampicillin (if sensitive)
Flavobacterium meningosepticum	Vancomycin	Trimethoprim-sulfamethoxazole Erythromycin Clindamycin Imipenem or Meropenem
Francisella tularensis	Streptomycin or Gentamicin	Ciprofloxacin Doxycycline
Fusobacterium	Penicillin G or Metronidazole	Cefoxitin or Imipenem Clindamycin

(continued)

TABLE 10.1. *(continued)* **Parenteral Antimicrobial Agents of Choice for Specific Pathogens**

Pathogen	First Choices	Alternatives
Gardnerella vaginalis	Metronidazole	Clindamycin (topical or PO)
Helicobacter pylori	Amoxicillin + omeprazole (or rabeprazole) + clarithromycin	Bismuth subsalicylate (PO) + metronidazole + tetracycline + omeprazole
Hemophilus influenzae	Cefotaxime or Ceftriaxone	Piperacillin-tazobactam Imipenem or Meropenem Levofloxacin, Gatifloxacin, or Moxifloxacin
Herpes simplex		
Keratoconjunctivitis	Trifluridine (topical) + acyclovir	Idoxuridine (topical) Vidarabine (topical)
Local Mucocutaneous	Acyclovir	Foscarnet
Disseminated	Acyclovir (high dose)	Foscarnet
Encephalitis	Acyclovir (high dose)	Foscarnet
Herpes zoster		
Local	Famciclovir (PO) ± prednisone Valacyclovir (PO) ± prednisone Acyclovir ± prednisone	Foscarnet
Disseminated	Acyclovir (high dose)	Foscarnet
Influenza A (H3N2)	Oseltamivir	Zanamivir (Inhal)
Influenza A Avian (H5N1)	Oseltamivir	Zanamivir (Inhal)
Influenza B	Oseltamivir	Zanamivir (Inhal)
Hantavirus	None	(No documented benefit from ribavirin)
Histoplasma capsulatum	Liposomal amphotericin B (AmBisome) or ABLC	Itraconazole (IV/PO) Amphotericin B
***Klebsiella* species**	Ceftriaxone	Gentamicin Piperacillin Imipenem or Meropenem Piperacillin-tazobactam Aztreonam Ciprofloxacin or Levofloxacin
***Legionella* species**	Ciprofloxacin or Levofloxacin or Azithromycin or Erythromycin ± rifampin	Trimethoprim-sulfamethoxazole + rifampin Moxifloxacin
Leptospira	Penicillin G or Ampicillin	Doxycycline
Lice see *Pediculosis*		
Listeria monocytogenes	Ampicillin ± gentamicin or Penicillin ± gentamicin	Trimethoprim-sulfamethoxazole Erythromycin
Lyme disease	See *Borrelia burgdorferi*	
Malaria	See *Plasmodia*	
Moraxella catarrhalis (Branhamella catarrhalis)	Ceftriaxone	Levofloxacin, Gatifloxacin, Moxifloxacin Telithromycin (PO) Azithromycin Trimethoprim-sulfamethoxazole
***Morganella* species**	Imipenem or Meropenem or Ceftriaxone	Gentamicin Ciprofloxacin or Levofloxacin
Mucormycosis	Liposomal amphotericin B (AmBisome) or ABLC	Amphotericin B Posaconazole (investigational)
***Mycobacterium avium intracellulare* (Non-AIDS)**	Clarithromycin + ethambutol ± rifabutin	Rifabutin (PO) + ciprofloxacin (or moxifloxacin) + amikacin

(continued)

TABLE 10.1. *(continued)* **Parenteral Antimicrobial Agents of Choice for Specific Pathogens**

Pathogen	First Choices	Alternatives
***Mycobacterium avium-intracellulare* (AIDS)**	Clarithromycin (PO) or Azithromycin (PO/IV) + ethambutol (PO)	Rifabutin (PO) + moxifloxacin (or ciprofloxacin) + amikacin
Mycobacterium chelonae	Clarithromycin or Azithromycin + amikacin	Amikacin + cefoxitin
Mycobacterium fortuitum	Amikacin + cefoxitin + probenecid	Clarithromycin (PO) Doxycycline Imipenem
Mycobacterium kansasii	Isoniazid (PO/IV) + rifampin (PO/IV) + ethambutol (PO)	Trimethoprim-sulfamethoxazole Amikacin (IV) Ciprofloxacin (PO/IV) Clarithromycin
Mycobacterium tuberculosis	Isoniazid (PO/IM/IV) + rifampin (PO/IV) + pyrazinamide (PO) + ethambutol (PO)	Cycloserine (PO) Ethionamide (PO) Streptomycin (IM/IV) Amikacin (IV) Linezolid (PO, IV) Moxifloxacin (PO, IV)
Mycoplasma pneumoniae	Clarithromycin Azithromycin	Levofloxacin Gatifloxacin Moxifloxacin Doxycycline
Naegleria fowleri	Amphotericin B intraventricular + liposomal amphotericin (AmBisome) or ABLC	
***Neisseria gonorrhea* (uncomplicated)**	Ceftriaxone (IM) or Ofloxacin (PO/IV) or Doxycycline (PO)	Cefotaxime Ciprofloxacin
***Neisseria gonorrhea* Disseminated**	Ceftriaxone or Cefotaxime	Ciprofloxacin Levofloxacin
Neisseria meningitidis	Penicillin G	Ampicillin Cefotaxime, or Ceftriaxone
Nocardia asteroides	Trimethoprim-sulfamethoxazole ± amikacin	Imipenem + amikacin Ceftriaxone + amikacin
Nocardia brasiliensis	Trimethoprim-sulfamethoxazole ± amikacin	Ampicillin-sulbactam Ceftriaxone + amikacin
Pasteurella multocida	Penicillin G	Cefazolin Piperacillin-tazobactam Doxycycline
***Pediculosis* (lice) Body, Head**	Permethrin 5% (topical) (Elimite) or Ivermectin (PO)	Malathion 0.5% (topical) Lindane 1% (Kwell) (topical) Pyrethrin (RID) (topical)
Peptostreptococcus	Penicillin G or Ampicillin	Clindamycin Metronidazole Imipenem or Meropenem Vancomycin
Plasmodia* species potentially resistant *Falciparum	Quinidine gluconate (PO/IV) or Quinine (PO) + either Doxycycline, Clindamycin, or Fansidar (PO)	Artesunate (PO) + mefloquine (PO)
***Plasmodia* species (not potentially resistant)**	Chloroquine (PO/IM) (followed by primaquine)	Quinine (PO) Quinidine (PO/IV)

(continued)

TABLE 10.1. *(continued)* **Parenteral Antimicrobial Agents of Choice for Specific Pathogens**

Pathogen	First Choices	Alternatives
***Pneumocystis jiroveci* (mild)**	Trimethoprim-sulfamethoxazole	Atovaquone (PO) Clindamycin + primaquine (PO) Pentamidine (IV) Trimetrexate (IV)
***Pneumocystis jiroveci* (severe)**	Trimethoprim-sulfamethoxazole + prednisone	Pentamidine (IV) + prednisone or Trimetrexate + prednisone
Propionibacterium acnes	Penicillin	Clindamycin
Proteus	Ceftriaxone	Gentamicin Piperacillin-tazobactam Aztreonam Imipenem or Meropenem
***Providencia* species**	Ceftriaxone or Ciprofloxacin	Piperacillin-tazobactam Imipenem or Meropenem Aztreonam
Pseudomonas aeruginosa	Imipenem ± Gentamicin or Ciprofloxacin	Piperacillin-tazobactam Cefepime Levofloxacin Ceftazidime Aztreonam
Respiratory Syncytial Virus (RSV)	Ribavirin (aerosol)	Palivizumab
***Rhizopus* species**	Liposomal amphotericin B (AmBisome) or ABLC	Amphotericin B Posaconazole (investigational)
Rhodococcus equi	Vancomycin + ciprofloxacin	Vancomycin + amikacin Imipenem or Meropenem Erythromycin or Azithromycin Ciprofloxacin
***Rickettsia* species**	Doxycycline	Levofloxacin
Salmonella typhi	Ceftriaxone	Trimethoprim-sulfamethoxazole Ciprofloxacin Cefotaxime or Ceftizoxime
***Salmonella* species (non*typhi*)**	Cefotaxime	Piperacillin-tazobactam Trimethoprim-sulfamethoxazole Cefotaxime Ciprofloxacin
Scabies	Permethrin 5% cream (topical)	Ivermectin (PO) Crotamiton 10% (topical)
Serratia marcescens	Ceftriaxone ± gentamicin	Either Gentamicin or Amikacin ± either Piperacillin-tazobactam or Ceftriaxone Cefepime Imipenem or Meropenem Ciprofloxacin Aztreonam
***Shigella* species**	Ciprofloxacin	Trimethoprim-sulfamethoxazole
***Staphylococcus aureus* (methicillin-sensitive)**	Oxacillin ± gentamicin	Vancomycin Cefazolin Imipenem or Meropenem Daptomycin Linezolid
***Staphylococcus aureus* (methicillin-resistant)**	Vancomycin ± either Rifampin or Gentamicin	Linezolid Daptomycin
Staphylococcus epidermidis	Vancomycin ± rifampin	Linezolid Daptomycin

* Primaquine indicated for P. vivax and P. ovale

(continued)

TABLE 10.1. *(continued)* **Parenteral Antimicrobial Agents of Choice for Specific Pathogens**

Pathogen	First Choices	Alternatives
Staphylococcus haemolyticus	Trimethoprim-sulfamethoxazole	Ciprofloxacin
Staphylococcus lugdunensis	Oxacillin	Daptomycin Vancomycin Cefazolin
Staphylococcus saprophyticus	Ampicillin-sulbactam	Cefazolin Levofloxacin Trimethoprim-sulfamethoxazole
Stenotrophomonas maltophilia	Trimethoprim-sulfamethoxazole	Ciprofloxacin
Streptococcus* groups *A, B, C, G; bovis; milleri; viridans	Penicillin G ± gentamicin	Cephazolin Vancomycin Cefepime
***Streptococcus* pneumoniae (penicillin sens.)**	Penicillin G ± gentamicin	Levofloxacin, Moxifloxacin Imipenem or Meropenem Ceftriaxone
***Streptococcus pneumoniae* (moderate penicillin resistance)**	Cefotaxime or Ceftriaxone	Vancomycin Levofloxacin, Moxifloxacin Linezolid
***Streptococcus pneumoniae* (high level penicillin-resistant; MIC > 1.0 μg/ml)**	Levofloxacin	Vancomycin ± rifampin Moxifloxacin Gatifloxacin Linezolid
Strongyloides stercoralis	Ivermectin (PO)	Albendazole (PO)
Toxoplasma gondii	Sulfadiazine (PO) + pyrimethamine (PO) + folinic acid (PO/IV)	Clindamycin (IV) + pyrimethamine (PO) + folinic acid (PO/IV) Trimethoprim-sulfamethoxazole Atovaquone (PO) + pyrimethamine (PO) + folinic acid (PO/IV) Trimethoprim-sulfamethoxazole (IV) + pyrimethamine (PO) or Trimetrexate (IV) + folinic acid (PO/IV)
Treponema pallidum	Penicillin G (Neuro: 12–24M U/d IV) (Late latent, cardiac, or other tertiary: Benzathine 2.4M U IM q7d × 3)	Doxycycline Ceftriaxone
Variola virus	Cidofovir	
Vibrio cholerae	Doxycycline	Trimethoprim-sulfamethoxazole Ciprofloxacin
Vibrio vulnificus	Doxycycline ± ceftazidime	Cefotaxime Ciprofloxacin
Yersinia enterocolitica	Trimethoprim-sulfamethoxazole	Ceftriaxone Ciprofloxacin Tobramycin Amikacin
Yersinia pestis	Streptomycin or Gentamicin ± doxycycline	Doxycycline Ciprofloxacin

IM, intramuscular; IV, intravenous; PO, by mouth
[a]CDC: obtain from Centers for Disease Control (404) 639–2206 (days) or (404) 639–2888 (nights, weekends, holidays)

TABLE 10.2. Empiric Therapy for Common Infectious Syndromes in the ICU

(Initial therapy for likely pathogens pending identification of causative organisms and their specific antimicrobial susceptibilities; pathogen susceptibility may vary at different hospitals.)

Syndrome	Clinical Circumstance	Usual Causative Organism(s)	Empiric Regimens 1° = Primary Alt = Alternate
Bone			
Osteomyelitis	Child	*S. aureus* *Streptococci*	1° = vancomycin Alt = linezolid Alt = daptomycin
	Adult (Hematogenous)	*S. aureus*	1° = vancomycin (add cefepime or ciprofloxacin if gram negative rod suspected) Alt = linezolid Alt = daptomycin
	Postoperative	Mixed aerobic/anaerobic *S. aureus* *Enterobacteriaceae* *Pseudomonas*	1° = vancomycin + ciprofloxacin (or levofloxacin) + piperacillin-tazobactam[a] Alt = vancomycin + cefepime + metronidazole Alt = linezolid + ciprofloxacin + metronidazole
	Decubitus ulcer Diabetes Vascular insufficiency	*S. aureus* *Enterobacteriaceae* *Pseudomonas* Anaerobes	1° = imipenem or meropenem + ciprofloxacin Alt = piperacillin-tazobactam plus ciprofloxacin or gentamicin Alt = vancomycin + ciprofloxacin + metronidazole
Catheter Related—see Vascular			
Central Nervous System			
Brain abscess	Primary, otogenic, or paranasal sinus	Polymicrobial: *Viridans streptococci* Anaerobic *Streptococci* *Bacteroides*	1° = vancomycin + ceftriaxone + metronidazole Alt = penicillin G (high dose) + metronidazole + ceftriaxone ± vancomycin
		Enterobacteriaceae S. aureus	Alt = linezolid + metronidazole + aztreonam
	Postsurgical, posttraumatic	*S. aureus* *Enterobacteriaceae*	1° = vancomycin or linezolid + ceftriaxone ± gentamicin Alt = piperacillin-tazobactam + vancomycin ± gentamicin Alt = vancomycin + meropenem

(continued)

TABLE 10.2. *(continued)* **Empiric Therapy for Common Infectious Syndromes in the ICU**

Syndrome	Clinical Circumstance	Usual Causative Organism(s)	Empiric Regimens 1° = Primary Alt = Alternate
Brain abscess (*continued*)	HIV-1 infected (AIDS)	*Toxoplasma gondii*	1° = sulfadiazine + pyrimethamine + folinic acid Alt = clindamycin + pyrimethamine + folinic acid Alt = trimethoprim-sulfamethoxazole
Meningitis	Age 1 mo–50 y	*S. pneumoniae* *N. meningitides* *H. influenzae*	1° = ceftriaxone + vancomycin (also consider dexamethasone[a]) Alt = meropenem + vancomycin (also consider dexamethasone[a])
	Age >50 yrs or alcohol or debilitating medical illness	*S. pneumoniae* *Listeria* Gram-negative bacilli	1° = ceftriaxone or cefotaxime + vancomycin + ampicillin (consider dexamethasone[a]) Alt = meropenem + vancomycin + trimethoprim-sulfamethoxazole (also consider dexamethasone[a])
	HIV-1 infected (AIDS)	As in 1–50 y range, plus *Cryptococcus* *M. tuberculosis* *T. pallidum* *HIV-1*	1° = cefotaxime or ceftriaxone + vancomycin 1° = if *cryptococcus* identified, use ABLC or AmBisome ± flucytosine
	Postcranial trauma 0–3 d	*S. pneumoniae*	1° = cefotaxime or ceftriaxone + vancomycin Alt = ampicillin-sulbactam + vancomycin
	Postneurosurgical or postcranio/spinal trauma ≥3 d	*S. aureus* *Enterobacteriaceae* *Pseudomonas* *S. pneumoniae*	1° = vancomycin + ceftazidime or cefepime Alt = vancomycin + piperacillin-tazobactam
	Persistent cerebrospinal fluid leak (no prior antibiotics)	*S. pneumonia*	1° = cefepime + vancomycin Alt = vancomycin + meropenem

[a]Dexamethasone 0.15 mg/kg IV q6h × 2–4 d with first dose prior to antibiotics

(continued)

TABLE 10.2. *(continued)* **Empiric Therapy for Common Infectious Syndromes in the ICU**

Syndrome	Clinical Circumstance	Usual Causative Organism(s)	Empiric Regimens 1° = Primary Alt = Alternate
	Neutropenia	*S. aureus* *Streptococci* *Enterobacteriaceae*	1° = vancomycin + cefepime + ampicillin ± gentamicin Alt = vancomycin + aztreonam + trimethoprim-sulfamethoxazole Alt = vancomycin + meropenem + trimethoprim-sulfamethoxazole
	Ventricular shunt	*S. epidermidis* *Diphtheroids* *Enterobacteriaceae*	1° = vancomycin + cefepime ± rifampin
Ear			
Malignant otitis externa		*P. aeruginosa*	1° = ceftazidime or cefepime or meropenem ± gentamicin Alt = ciprofloxacin ± gentamicin
Eye			
Conjunctivitis			
Nonsuppurative		Adenovirus	None
Suppurative	Hospital or community acquired	*H. influenzae* *S. pneumoniae*	1° = gatifloxacin topical 0.3% or levofloxacin topical 0.5% or moxifloxacin topical 0.5% Alt = polymyxin B + trimethoprim topical
Keratitis		Gram-positive cocci	Ophthalmic drops = cefazolin (50 mg/ ml, 1 drop q1h) (must be compounded) Subconjunctival = cefazolin (100 mg in 0.5 ml) Systemic = cefazolin (if severe)
		Gram-negative bacilli	Ophthalmic drops = tobramycin (13.6 mg/ml, 1 drop q30min) or ciprofloxacin 0.3% Subconjunctival = tobramycin (20 mg in 0.5 ml) Systemic = piperacillin-tazobactam or meropenem (if severe)

(continued)

TABLE 10.2. *(continued)* **Empiric Therapy for Common Infectious Syndromes in the ICU**

Syndrome	Clinical Circumstance	Usual Causative Organism(s)	Empiric Regimens 1° = Primary Alt = Alternate
Keratitis (*continued*)		No organisms seen	Ophthalmic drops = cefazolin + tobramycin or sulfacetamide or neomycin-polymyxin-bacitracin Subconjunctival = cefazolin + tobramycin Systemic = piperacillin-tazobactam (if severe)
		Fungi	Ophthalmic drops = pimaricin (natamycin) 5% (1 drop q3–4h) Alt drops = amphotericin B 0.05% to 0.15% Subconjunctival = miconazole (10 mg in 0.5 ml) Systemic = none
		HSV	Ophthalmic drops = trifluridine 1% (1 drop q2h) or vidarabine ointment ± corticosteroids Subconjunctival = none Systemic = acyclovir
Endophthalmitis		*S. aureus* *S. epidermidis* *Pseudomonas* *Diphtheroids* *Candida*	1° = vancomycin + cefepime Alt = vancomycin + piperacillin-tazobactam Intravitreal = vancomycin + ceftazidime ± corticosteroids; add amphotericin B if fungus suspected
Periorbital cellulitis		*Streptococci* *Staphylococci* *H. influenzae* Anaerobes	1° = vancomycin + cefepime ± metronidazole Alt = piperacillin-tazobactam + linezolid
Gallbladder, Biliary Tree, And Pancreas			
Gallbladder and biliary tree	Cholecystitis, cholangitis, biliary sepsis	*Enterobacteriaceae* *Enterococci* *Bacteroides* *Clostridium* species	1° = vancomycin + imipenem or meropenem ± gentamicin Alt = cefepime + ampicillin ± ciprofloxacin Alt = piperacillin-tazobactam ± gentamicin Alt = vancomycin + aztreonam + metronidazole ± gentamicin
	Common duct obstruction	Seldom infected unless manipulated	If infection suspected: per biliary sepsis above
Pancreas	Necrotizing pancreatitis	*Enterobacteriaceae* *Enterococci*	1° = imipenem or meropenem ± ciprofloxacin Alt = piperacillin-tazobactam ± ciprofloxacin

(continued)

TABLE 10.2. *(continued)* **Empiric Therapy for Common Infectious Syndromes in the ICU**

Syndrome	Clinical Circumstance	Usual Causative Organism(s)	Empiric Regimens 1° = Primary Alt = Alternate
	Pancreatic abscess; infected pseudocyst	*Enterobacteriaceae* *Enterococci*	1° = vancomycin + imipenem or meropenem ± ciprofloxacin Alt = piperacillin-tazobactam ± gentamicin
Gastrointestinal			
Diarrhea (severe with fever, hemorrhage, or severe dehydration)	No recent antibiotic use	*Shigella* *Salmonella* *C. jejuni* *E. coli 0157:H7* *C. difficile*	1° = ciprofloxacin or levofloxacin ± metronidazole
	Antibiotic use	*C. difficile* *Salmonella* *Shigella* *Campylobacter*	1° = metronidazole (IV or PO) + ciprofloxacin Alt = vancomycin (PO) + ciprofloxacin Alt = metronidazole (IV or PO) + ciprofloxacin
Diverticulitis		*Enterobacteriaceae* *Bacteroides* *Enterococci*	1° = cefoxitin ± gentamicin Alt = vancomycin+ metronidazole + ciprofloxacin Alt = imipenem or meropenem ± gentamicin
Neutropenic enterocolitis (Typhlitis)	Neutropenia	*Clostridium septicum* *Enterobacteriaceae* *Pseudomonas*	1° = metronidazole + ciprofloxacin + vancomycin Alt = meropenem or imipenem ± levofloxacin
Perirectal abscess	Immunologically normal	*Enterobacteriaceae* *Bacteroides* species *Enterococci*	1° = metronidazole + ciprofloxacin + vancomycin Alt = meropenem or imipenem Alt = piperacillin-tazobactam
	Neutropenia	Same, plus *Pseudomonas*	Refer to "Sepsis, neutropenic"
Genital Tract: Female			
Amnionitis, septic abortion	Early postpartum (initial 48 h)	*Bacteroides* *Streptococci* *Enterobacteriaceae* *C. trachomatis*	1° = doxycycline + meropenem or imipenem Alt = ampicillin-sulbactam + doxycycline Alt = clindamycin + aztreonam + doxycycline or ofloxacin

(continued)

TABLE 10.2. *(continued)* **Empiric Therapy for Common Infectious Syndromes in the ICU**

Syndrome	Clinical Circumstance	Usual Causative Organism(s)	Empiric Regimens 1° = Primary Alt = Alternate
Amnionitis, septic abortion (*continued*)	Late postpartum (48 h to 6 wk)	*C. trachomatis*	1° = doxycycline (avoid if nursing) Alt = ofloxacin or erythromycin
Gonorrhea	Disseminated or endocarditis	*N. gonorrhea*	1° = ceftriaxone + doxycycline Alt = ciprofloxacin + azithromycin
Pelvic inflammatory disease (PID), salpingitis, tuboovarian abscess	Hospitalized	*N. gonorrhea* *Chlamydia* *Enterobacteriaceae* *Streptococci* *Bacteroides*	1° = doxycycline + cefoxitin Alt = clindamycin + gentamicin + doxycycline
Syphilis	Primary, secondary, latent <1 y	*T. pallidum*	1° = benzathine penicillin Alt = doxycycline or erythromycin Alt = ceftriaxone
	latent: >1 y cardiovascular		1° = benzathine penicillin Alt = doxycycline
	Neurosyphilis		1° = penicillin G followed by benzathine penicillin Alt = desensitize to penicillin in penicillin-allergic patients
Vaginitis	Candidiasis	*Candida* species	1° = fluconazole (PO/IV) Alt = miconazole, clotrimazole, butoconazole, or terconazole (all topical) Alt = caspofungin
	Trichomoniasis	*Trichomonas vaginalis*	1° = metronidazole (PO, IV) 1° = tinidazole (PO)
Genital Tract: Male			
Epididymitis/ orchitis	Age <35 y, not recently hospitalized	*N. gonorrhea* *C. trachomatis*	Treat for gonorrhea and chlamydia 1° = ceftriaxone + doxycycline Alt = ofloxacin
	Age >35 y	*Enterobacteriaceae*	1° = ciprofloxacin Alt = trimethoprim-sulfamethoxazole Alt = β-lactam/ piperacillin-tazobactam Alt = imipenem or meropenem or cefepime

(continued)

TABLE 10.2. *(continued)* **Empiric Therapy for Common Infectious Syndromes in the ICU**

Syndrome	Clinical Circumstance	Usual Causative Organism(s)	Empiric Regimens 1° = Primary Alt = Alternate
Gonorrhea	As in female patients		
Prostatitis	Acute, age <35 y	*N. gonorrhea* *C. trachomatis*	Treat for gonorrhea and chlamydia 1° = ceftriaxone + doxycycline Alt = ofloxacin
	Acute, age ≥35 y	*Enterobacteriaceae*	1° = ciprofloxacin Alt = trimethoprim-sulfamethoxazole
	Chronic bacterial	*Enterobacteriaceae* *Enterococci* *P. aeruginosa*	1° = ciprofloxacin Alt = trimethoprim-sulfamethoxazole
Syphilis	As in female patients		
Urethritis nongonococcal		*C. trachomatis* *Ureaplasma* *Mycoplasma*	1° = doxycycline Alt = azithromycin Alt = ofloxacin
Heart			
Infective endocarditis (native valve)	Initial empiric therapy	*S. aureus* *Enterococci* *S. pneumoniae* Group A *streptococci* (In IV drug abusers, also *Pseudomonas*) and Group D *streptococci*	1° = vancomycin + penicillin G + gentamicin Alt = daptomycin + gentamicin Alt = imipenem + gentamicin
	Streptococcal	*Viridans streptococci* (MIC ≤0.1 μg/ml) *S. bovis*	1° = penicillin G + gentamicin Alt = ceftriaxone or vancomycin Alt = penicillin G
		Enterococci *Viridans streptococci* (MIC >0.1 μg/ml)	1° = penicillin G + gentamicin Alt = vancomycin + gentamicin
	Staphylococcal	*S. aureus (sensitivity unknown or ORSA)*	1° = vancomycin + gentamicin Alt = daptomycin
		S. aureus oxacillin sensitive	1° = oxacillin + gentamicin Alt = cefazolin + gentamicin
Infective endocarditis (prosthetic valve)	Early (<2 mo post operative) Organism unknown initially	*S. aureus* *Enterobacteriaceae* *S. epidermidis* *Diphtheroids* (also *Candida and Aspergillus*)	1° = vancomycin + gentamicin + rifampin Alt = daptomycin + gentamicin + rifampin (Antifungal therapy only if fungus documented)

(continued)

TABLE 10.2. *(continued)* **Empiric Therapy for Common Infectious Syndromes in the ICU**

Syndrome	Clinical Circumstance	Usual Causative Organism(s)	Empiric Regimens 1° = Primary Alt = Alternate
Infective endocarditis (prosthetic valve) (*continued*)	Late (>2 mo postoperative) Organism unknown initially	*Viridans streptococci* *Enterococci* *S. aureus* *S. epidermidis* *Enterobacteriaceae*	1° = vancomycin + gentamicin + rifampin Alt = oxacillin + gentamicin
Purulent pericarditis		*S. aureus* *S. pneumoniae* Group A *streptococci* *Enterobacteriaceae*	1° = vancomycin + gentamicin Alt = oxacillin + gentamicin Alt = linezolid + gentamicin
Joint			
Septic arthritis	Children >6 y and adults	*S. aureus* Group A *streptococci* *Enterobacteriaceae*	1° = vancomycin + cefepime Alt = daptomycin + ciprofloxacin Alt = linezolid + aztreonam
	Adult with probable sexual transmission	*N. gonorrhea*	1° = ceftriaxone Alt = ciprofloxacin
	Prosthetic joint, postoperative, or postintraarticular injection	*S. epidermidis* *S. aureus* *Enterobacteriaceae* *Pseudomonas*	1° = vancomycin + cefepime + rifampin Alt = vancomycin + rifampin + either aztreonam, ciprofloxacin, or gentamicin Alt = linezolid + rifampin + imipenem or meropenem
Septic bursitis		*S. aureus*	1° = vancomycin Alt = linezolid Alt = daptomycin
Kidney			
Acute pyelonephritis	Hospitalized not septic	*Enterobacteriaceae* *Enterococci*	1° = ciprofloxacin Alt = piperacillin-tazobactam Alt = vancomycin + gentamicin
	Hospitalized + septic	*Enterobacteriaceae* *Enterococci*	1° = ceftriaxone + ampicillin + ciprofloxacin Alt = piperacillin-tazobactam + gentamicin
	Perinephric abscess	*S. aureus* *Enterobacteriaceae*	1° = ciprofloxacin + vancomycin 1° = vancomycin + levofloxacin Alt = linezolid + aztreonam or ciprofloxacin

(continued)

TABLE 10.2. *(continued)* **Empiric Therapy for Common Infectious Syndromes in the ICU**

Syndrome	Clinical Circumstance	Usual Causative Organism(s)	Empiric Regimens 1° = Primary Alt = Alternate
Line Infection/Line Sepsis See Vascular			
Liver			
Liver abscess	Amebic	*E. histolytica*	1° = metronidazole (IV) followed by iodoquinol (PO) Alt = dehydroemetine followed by paromomycin (PO)
	Bacterial	*Enterobacteriaceae* *Bacteroides* *Enterococci*	1° = ciprofloxacin + vancomycin + metronidazole Alt = linezolid + piperacillin-tazobactam Alt = imipenem or meropenem + vancomycin
Lung			
Pneumonia	Adults and children (age >5 y), without underlying disease, community acquired	Viral *Mycoplasma pneumoniae* *Chlamydia* pneumoniae *S. pneumoniae* *Legionella* species *H. influenzae*	1° = levofloxacin + vancomycin Alt = imipenem or meropenem or cefepime + azithromycin + linezolid Alt = piperacillin-tazobactam + azithromycin + vancomycin
	Chronic debilitating diseases (e.g., alcoholism, diabetes, heart failure), community acquired	All of above, plus *Klebsiella and Enterobacteriaceae*	1° = vancomycin + levofloxacin + cefepime Alt = linezolid + ceftriaxone or cefepime + azithromycin or ciprofloxacin Alt = vancomycin + piperacillin-tazobactam
	Aspiration-prone	*S. pneumoniae,* oral anaerobes, including *Bacteroides* species, *Klebsiella,* and other *Enterobacteriaceae*	1° = imipenem or meropenem + vancomycin + ciprofloxacin Alt = azithromycin or linezolid + cefoxitin Alt = vancomycin + metronidazole + azithromycin + gentamicin

(continued)

TABLE 10.2. *(continued)* **Empiric Therapy for Common Infectious Syndromes in the ICU**

Syndrome	Clinical Circumstance	Usual Causative Organism(s)	Empiric Regimens 1° = Primary Alt = Alternate
Pneumonia (*continued*)	Hospital associated ± mechanically ventilated; not neutropenic	*Enterobacteriaceae* *Pseudomonas* *S. aureus* *Legionella* species *Acinetobacter*	1° = vancomycin + meropenem or imipenem + ciprofloxacin Alt = linezolid + piperacillin-tazobactam + gentamicin + azithromycin Alt = vancomycin + metronidazole + gentamicin+ ciprofloxacin
Pneumonia	Neutropenic (<500/cu mm) and/or severely immune suppressed (non-HIV)	All of above, plus *Rhizopus* species (mucormycosis) and *Aspergillus* ± PCP	1° = vancomycin + ciprofloxacin + trimethoprim-sulfamethoxazole Alt = linezolid + cefepime + levofloxacin + trimethoprim-sulfamethoxazole Alt = linezolid + piperacillin-tazobactam + moxifloxacin + pentamidine (Empiric antifungal therapy indicated in some clinical situations)
	Postinfluenza	*S. aureus* *S. pneumoniae* *H. influenza*	1° = levofloxacin or gatifloxacin or moxifloxacin + vancomycin Alt = ceftriaxone or cefotaxime + linezolid Alt = piperacillin-tazobactam[a] + vancomycin
	HIV-1 infected with CD4 count >200/cu mm	*S. pneumoniae* *S. aureus* *H. influenzae* Viral (Rule out tuberculosis)	1° = azithromycin + ceftriaxone + vancomycin Alt = levofloxacin + linezolid Alt = levofloxacin or gatifloxacin or moxifloxacin + linezolid
	HIV-1 infected with CD4 count <200/cu mm^3, or clinical AIDS	*Pneumocystis jiroveci* *S. pneumoniae* *S. aureus*	1° = trimethoprim-sulfamethoxazole + levofloxacin or gatifloxacin + vancomycin

(continued)

TABLE 10.2. *(continued)* **Empiric Therapy for Common Infectious Syndromes in the ICU**

Syndrome	Clinical Circumstance	Usual Causative Organism(s)	Empiric Regimens 1° = Primary Alt = Alternate
		H. influenzae (rule out tuberculosis)	Alt = pentamidine + vancomycin or linezolid + azithromycin (Add prednisone if PCP suspected while awaiting diagnosis and PO_2 is <70% on room air)
Cystic fibrosis	Acute exacerbation of pulmonary symptoms	*P. aeruginosa* (often resistant) *B. cepacia*	1° = gentamicin + ciprofloxacin + trimethoprim-sulfamethoxazole Alt = piperacillin-tazobactam + trimethoprim-sulfamethoxazole
Empyema		*S. pneumoniae* *S. aureus (MRSA)* Group A *streptococci*	1° = vancomycin + cefepime Alt = linezolid + ciprofloxacin
Peritoneum			
Peritonitis	Primary (spontaneous bacterial peritonitis)	*S. pneumoniae* Group A *streptococci* *Enterobacteriaceae*	1° = piperacillin-tazobactam + vancomycin Alt = cefepime + linezolid Alt = vancomycin + imipenem or meropenem
	Secondary (bowel perforation)	*Enterobacteriaceae* *Bacteroides* *Pseudomonas* *Enterococci*	1° = imipenem or meropenem + gentamicin + vancomycin Alt = vancomycin + metronidazole + ciprofloxacin
	Associated with chronic ambulatory peritoneal dialysis (CAPD), mild	*S. epidermidis* *S. aureus* *Streptococci* *Enterobacteriaceae* *Candida* species	1° = vancomycin (500–1,000 mg/L in 1st bag then 15–25 mg/L) + aminoglycoside (gentamicin or tobramycin 35–70 mg/L in 1st bag then 4–8 mg/L) in dialysate only
	CAPD, severe	Same	1° = vancomycin IV + gentamicin IV + vancomycin in dialysate + gentamicin in dialysate per above

(continued)

TABLE 10.2. *(continued)* **Empiric Therapy for Common Infectious Syndromes in the ICU**

Syndrome	Clinical Circumstance	Usual Causative Organism(s)	Empiric Regimens 1° = Primary Alt = Alternate
Pharynx			
Epiglottitis	Adults	*H. influenzae* *S. pneumoniae* Group A *streptococci*	1° = levofloxacin + vancomycin Alt = piperacillin-tazobactam + linezolid Alt = cefepime + vancomycin
Pulmonary—see Lung			
Sinuses			
Sinusitis, acute	Healthy adults	*S. pneumoniae* *H. influenzae* *M. catarrhalis* Group A *streptococci* Anaerobes Viruses	1° = piperacillin-tazobactam Alt = imipenem or meropenem Alt = ceftriaxone
	Diabetes mellitus; neutropenia	Above, plus *Rhizopus* species (*Mucormycosis*) *Aspergillus*	As above (Antifungal therapy only after definitive diagnosis)
	Patient with nasotracheal or nasogastric tube; nosocomial; postsinus surgery	Above, plus *S. aureus* *Enterobacteriaceae* *Pseudomonas*	1° = vancomycin + imipenem or meropenem ± gentamicin 1° = linezolid + piperacillin-tazobactam ± gentamicin Alt = daptomycin + ceftriaxone ± gentamicin Alt = clindamycin + aztreonam
Sinusitis, chronic	Adults (often after various antibiotics)	Anaerobes *S. aureus* *S. pneumonia* *H. influenza* *Enterobacteriaceae*	1° = vancomycin + imipenem or meropenem Alt = vancomycin + clindamycin + ceftriaxone Alt = vancomycin + clindamycin + aztreonam Alt = levofloxacin + metronidazole or clindamycin
Skin/Soft Tissue			
Bites:			
Dog and cat		*S. aureus* Anaerobes *P. multocida* *C. canimorsus* (DF2)	1° = ampicillin-sulbactam Alt = levofloxacin or ciprofloxacin + metronidazole

(continued)

TABLE 10.2. *(continued)* **Empiric Therapy for Common Infectious Syndromes in the ICU**

Syndrome	Clinical Circumstance	Usual Causative Organism(s)	Empiric Regimens 1° = Primary Alt = Alternate
Monkey		*Herpes B (simiae)*	1° = valacyclovir (prophylaxis) 1° = ganciclovir (therapy)
Rat		*Streptobacillus*	1° = ampicillin-sulbactam Alt = doxycycline
Human		*S. aureus* *Streptococci* Anaerobes	1° = ampicillin-sulbactam ± vancomycin Alt = clindamycin + ciprofloxacin
Cellulitis, erysipelas	Extremities, not associated with venous catheter	Group A *streptococci* *S. aureus*	1° = vancomycin Alt = linezolid Alt = daptomycin
	Facial, adult	Group A *streptococci* *S. aureus*	1° = vancomycin Alt = linezolid Alt = daptomycin
	Diabetes mellitus	Polymicrobial: Group A *streptococci, S. aureus, Enterobacteriaceae,* anaerobes, *enterococci*	1° = piperacillin-tazobactam + vancomycin Alt = imipenem or meropenem + linezolid Alt = vancomycin + clindamycin + aztreonam or ciprofloxacin or levofloxacin
	Hemorrhagic bullous lesions or shock with history of sea water exposure or raw seafood ingestion	*Vibrio vulnificus*	1° = ceftazidime or cefotaxime Alt = doxycycline Alt = ciprofloxacin
Decubitus ulcer	Sepsis likely	Polymicrobial: aerobic + anaerobic *streptococci* *Enterobacteriaceae* *Pseudomonas* *Bacteroides* species *S. aureus*	1° = imipenem or meropenem + vancomycin + ciprofloxacin or levofloxacin Alt = piperacillin-tazobactam + linezolid + aztreonam Alt = vancomycin + metronidazole + ciprofloxacin or levofloxacin
Infected wound, post-operative	Sepsis likely	*S. aureus* Group A *streptococci* *Enterobacteriaceae* *Pseudomonas*	1° = imipenem or meropenem + ciprofloxacin + vancomycin Alt = linezolid + ceftriaxone ± gentamicin Alt = daptomycin + ciprofloxacin or aztreonam ± gentamicin

(continued)

TABLE 10.2. *(continued)* **Empiric Therapy for Common Infectious Syndromes in the ICU**

Syndrome	Clinical Circumstance	Usual Causative Organism(s)	Empiric Regimens 1° = Primary Alt = Alternate
Crepitant cellulitis/ myonecrosis	With possible perirectal, GI, or GU involvement	*Bacteroides* species *Clostridia* Other anaerobes *Enterococci* Group B and C *streptococci* *Enterobacteriaceae*	1° = vancomycin + imipenem or meropenem + ciprofloxacin Alt = vancomycin + metronidazole + gentamicin Alt = piperacillin-tazobactam + linezolid + aztreonam
Infected wound	Hemodynamically stable	*S. aureus* *Streptococci*	1° = vancomycin ± meropenem Alt = piperacillin-tazobactam + linezolid Alt = vancomycin Alt = daptomycin
Sepsis	Adult; nonimmunocompromised; community acquired	*S. aureus* *S. pneumoniae* *H. influenzae* *N. meningitidis* *Enterobacteriaceae*	1° = vancomycin + piperacillin-tazobactam + ciprofloxacin Alt = linezolid + imipenem or meropenem + gentamicin Alt = daptomycin + metronidazole + ciprofloxacin
	Adult; nonimmunocompromised; hospital acquired	Gram-positive cocci Aerobic gram-negative bacilli Anaerobes *Candida*	1° = vancomycin + ceftriaxone + ciprofloxacin 1° = linezolid + imipenem or meropenem + gentamicin 1° = daptomycin + piperacillin-tazobactam + ciprofloxacin 1° = vancomycin + ciprofloxacin + metronidazole + gentamicin (Antifungal therapy only if fungus documented or very high risk)
	IV drug abuser	*S. aureus*	1° = vancomycin + ciprofloxacin Alt = linezolid + ciprofloxacin Alt = vancomycin + imipenem or meropenem
	Asplenic	*S. pneumoniae* *H. influenzae* *N. meningitidis*	1° = cefotaxime, ceftriaxone, or cefuroxime + vancomycin Alt = linezolid + levofloxacin

(continued)

TABLE 10.2. *(continued)* **Empiric Therapy for Common Infectious Syndromes in the ICU**

Syndrome	Clinical Circumstance	Usual Causative Organism(s)	Empiric Regimens 1° = Primary Alt = Alternate
	Neutropenia (<500/cu mm)	*Enterobacteriaceae* *Pseudomonas* *S. aureus* *S. epidermidis* *Viridans streptococci* *Corynebacterium JK*	1° = imipenem or meropenem + ciprofloxacin + vancomycin Alt = linezolid + metronidazole + aztreonam or ciprofloxacin Alt = daptomycin + piperacillin-tazobactam + gentamicin
	Toxic shock syndrome	*Streptococci*	1° = oxacillin ± penicillin + clindamycin Alt = vancomycin + clindamycin
		S. aureus	1° = oxacillin + clindamycin Alt = linezolid + clindamycin
Vascular or Catheter Related			
Intravascular catheter infections (nonseptic)	Immunocompetent	*S. aureus* *S. epidermidis*	1° = vancomycin 1° = linezolid 1° = daptomycin Alt = imipenem or meropenem + vancomycin
	Neutropenia	*S. aureus* *S. epidermidis* *Enterobacteriaceae* *Pseudomonas*-like organisms	1° = vancomycin + imipenem or meropenem + gentamicin Alt = linezolid + piperacillin-tazobactam or ticarcillin-clavulanic acid + ciprofloxacin Alt = daptomycin + ciprofloxacin + gentamicin
Intravascular catheter-related sepsis	Immunocompetent	*S. aureus* *S. epidermidis* *Enterobacteriaceae* *Pseudomonas* species	1° = vancomycin + ciprofloxacin Alt = imipenem or meropenem or cefepime + ciprofloxacin + daptomycin Alt = linezolid + ciprofloxacin + piperacillin-tazobactam

(continued)

TABLE 10.2. *(continued)* **Empiric Therapy for Common Infectious Syndromes in the ICU**

Syndrome	Clinical Circumstance	Usual Causative Organism(s)	Empiric Regimens 1° = Primary Alt = Alternate
Intravascular catheter-related sepsis (*continued*)	Neutropenia	*S. aureus* *S. epidermidis* *Enterobacteriaceae* *Pseudomonas* species	1° = vancomycin + either piperacillin-tazobactam + ciprofloxacin Alt = linezolid + imipenem or meropenem + gentamicin Alt = ceftriaxone + ciprofloxacin + daptomycin (Add AmBisome or caspofungin if *Candida* suspected)
Septic thrombophlebitis	Immunocompetent	*S. epidermidis* *S. aureus* *Candida* species	1° = vancomycin + either ceftriaxone or meropenem or imipenem + ciprofloxacin Alt = linezolid + gentamicin Antifungal therapy only if fungus documented Consider heparin
	Neutropenia (<500/cu mm)	As above, plus *Pseudomonas* *Enterobacteriaceae* *Corynebacterium JK* *Aspergillus* *Rhizopus*	1° = imipenem or meropenem + gentamicin + vancomycin 1° = either piperacillin-tazobactam or ticarcillin-clavulanic acid + ciprofloxacin + linezolid 1° = daptomycin + ciprofloxacin + gentamicin Consider heparin
Septic pelvic vein thrombophlebitis	Postpartum, post-abortion, or post-pelvic surgery	*Streptococci* *Bacteroides* *Enterobacteriaceae*	1° = imipenem or meropenem + vancomycin + gentamicin 1° = linezolid + either piperacillin-tazobactam or + ciprofloxacin Alt = vancomycin + ciprofloxacin + gentamicin Consider heparin

(continued)

TABLE 10.2. *(continued)* **Empiric Therapy for Common Infectious Syndromes in the ICU**

Syndrome	Clinical Circumstance	Usual Causative Organism(s)	Empiric Regimens 1° = Primary Alt = Alternate
Cavernous sinus thrombosis		*S. aureus* Group A *streptococci* *H. influenzae* *Aspergillus* *Rhizopus/ mucormycosis*	1° = cefepime + vancomycin ± gentamicin Alt = vancomycin + either aztreonam or ceftriaxone ± gentamicin Antifungal therapy only if fungus documented

GI, gastrointestinal; GU, genitourinary

TABLE 10.3. Antimicrobial Drugs—Doses, Toxicities

Agent	Usual Adult Dosage	Adverse Effects/ Comments
Penicillins		
β-Lactamase Susceptible, Nonantipseudomonal Penicillins		
Penicillin G	IV low dose: 600,000–1,200,000 U/d IV high dose: 4M U load, then 1M U q1h	Hypersensitivity: drug fever, rash Anaphylactic reactions (approximately 1 in 10,000) Blood: positive Coombs, hemolytic anemia, cytopenia, nephrotoxicity, seizures, phlebitis at IV site Use pump for infusion to avoid inadvertent bolus 2 mEq Na^+/MU of penicillin G sodium
Benzathine penicillin	IM: 600,000–1,200,000 U qd	As with penicillin G, plus local reactions at injection site; not for IV administration
Ampicillin	IV: 1–3 g q4–6h	Rash Urticarial rash, often not true penicillin allergy: especially patients with infectious mononucleosis, lymphocytic leukemia, or those on allopurinol Fever, low WBC, high SGOT (rare), anaphylactic reactions; convulsions (with excessively rapid infusions) Interstitial nephritis 2.9 mEq Na^+/g
β-Lactamase Susceptible, Antipseudomonal Penicillins		
Piperacillin	IV: 2–4 g q4–6h Urinary tract: IV: 2 g q6h	Similar to other penicillins 1.85 mEq Na^+/g
Combination β-Lactamase Inhibitors and β-Lactam Agents		
Ticarcillin-clavulanic acid	IV: 3.1 g q4–6h	Similar to ticarcillin alone 4.75 mEq Na^+/g
Ampicillin-sulbactam	IV: 1.5–3 g q6h	Similar to ampicillin alone 5 mEq Na^+/1.5g
Piperacillin-tazobactam	IV: 3.375 g q4–6h	Similar to piperacillin alone 2.35 mEq Na^+/g piperacillin For pseudomonas; use q4h regimen
β-Lactamase Resistant Penicillins		
Nafcillin	Moderate infection: IV/IM: 1 g q4h Severe infection: IV: 2 g q4h	Phlebitis, rash, drug fever, eosinophilia, hemolytic anemia, neutropenia, interstitial nephritis, elevated SGOT, nausea, diarrhea 2.9 mEq Na^+/g

(continued)

TABLE 10.3. *(continued)* **Antimicrobial Drugs—Doses, Toxicities**

Agent	Usual Adult Dosage	Adverse Effects/ Comments
Oxacillin	Moderate infection: IV/IM: 1 g q4h Severe infection: IV: 2 g q4h	Similar to nafcillin (neutropenia less frequent) 2.5 mEq Na^+/g
Cephalosporins/Cephamycins/Carbacephem		
Parenteral		
Cefazolin	IV/IM: 0.5–3 g q6–8h	Rash, elevated SGOT, elevated alkaline phosphatase, phlebitis (less than with cephalothin), positive Coombs 2 mEq Na^+/g
Cefepime	IV/IM: 2 g q12h	Rash Cefepime is sodium free
Cefotaxime	Moderate infection: IV/IM: 1 g q8–12h Life-threatening infection: IV/IM: 2 g q4h	Phlebitis, rash, eosinophilia, positive Coombs, neutropenia Elevated SGOT, diarrhea 2.2 mEq Na^+/g
Cefoxitin	IV/IM: 1–2 g q4–6h	Phlebitis, pruritus, rash, fever, eosinophilia, positive Coombs (without hemolysis), leukopenia, mildly elevated BUN Falsely elevated serum creatinine Transiently elevated SGOT, SGPT, LDH, alkaline phosphatase 2.3 mEq Na^+/g
Ceftazidime	IV/IM: 0.5–2 g q8–12h	Phlebitis Hypersensitivity: rash, eosinophilia, fever Positive Coombs, neutropenia, thrombocytosis Elevated SGOT Diarrhea, elevated BUN 2.3 mEq Na^+/g
Ceftriaxone	IV/IM: 0.5–2 g q12–24h	Phlebitis Hypersensitivity: rash, eosinophilia, fever Neutropenia, thrombocytosis Elevated SGOT “Pseudocholelithiasis” secondary to sludge in gallbladder 3.6 mEq Na^+/g
Cefuroxime	IV/IM: 0.75–1.5 g q8h	Phlebitis, rash, positive Coombs, lowered hematocrit, eosinophilia, neutropenia Elevated SGOT, alkaline phosphatase, LDH, bilirubin Diarrhea, nausea 2.4 mEq Na^+/g

(continued)

Agent	Usual Adult Dosage	Adverse Effects/ Comments
Carbapenems		
Ertapenem	IV: 1 g q24h	Similar to meropenem, imipenem 6.0 mEq Na^+/g
Imipenem-cilastatin	IV: 0.5–1 g q6–8h	Phlebitis Hypersensitivity: rash, pruritus, eosinophilia Positive Coombs, neutropenia Oliguria Elevated SGOT, SGPT, alkaline phosphatase Confusion, seizures, myoclonus Nausea, vomiting (especially with too rapid IV infusion), diarrhea, pseudomembranous colitis In elderly patients with poor renal function, cerebrovascular disease, or seizure disorders, consider avoiding this agent because of high risk of neurological side effects 1.6 mEq Na^+/500 mg
Meropenem	IV: 1–2 g q8h	Similar to imipenem but less contraindicated for patients with renal, cerebrovascular, or seizure disorders 3.92 mEq Na^+/500 mg
Monobactams		
Aztreonam	Moderately severe infection: IV: 1 g q8h Life-threatening infection: IV: 2 g q6h	Phlebitis Hypersensitivity, rash (no cross-reactivity with penicillin G), eosinophilia Elevated SGOT Diarrhea, nausea, vomiting Seizures Aztreonam is sodium-free
Aminoglycosides and Related Antibiotics (See Table 10.4)		
Amikacin	IV: 15 mg/kg/d divided q8h IV: for extended interval (i.e., q24h) see Table 10.4	Nephrotoxicity (proteinuria, elevated BUN), ototoxicity Eosinophilia, arthralgia, fever, skin rash, probable neuromuscular blockade q24h regimen not as well studied, but can be given at high doses at extended intervals, i.e., 20–32 mg/kg q24h if renal function is normal (see Table 10.4)
Gentamicin	IV: For extended interval (i.e., q24h) see Table 10.4 IV: 3–5 mg/kg/d divided q8h or given q24h Intrathecal: 4 mg q12h (Preservative free)	Nephrotoxicity (proteinuria, elevated BUN), ototoxicity (especially vestibular), fever, rash, neuromuscular blockade q24h regimen not well studied for life-threatening disease; but can be given as high doses at extended intervals, i.e., 5–8 mg/kg q24h (see Table 10.4)

(continued)

TABLE 10.3. *(continued)* Antimicrobial Drugs—Doses, Toxicities

Agent	Usual Adult Dosage	Adverse Effects/ Comments
Neomycin sulfate	Hepatic coma: PO 4–12 g/d Enteropathogenic *E. coli*: PO 100 mg/kg/d	Nausea, vomiting, diarrhea, "malabsorption" Ototoxicity, nephrotoxicity, neuromuscular blockade if sufficiently absorbed
Streptomycin	IM/IV: 0.5–2 g/d	Ototoxicity (vestibular, auditory) nephrotoxicity, drug fever, neuromuscular blockade, rash, circumoral paresthesias Often in short supply
Tobramycin	IV: 3–5 mg/kg/d divided q8h	Nephrotoxicity, ototoxicity, (dizziness, hearing loss) neuromuscular blockade, rash
Macrolides, Cloramphenicol Glycopeptides, and Others		
Azithromycin	IV: 500 mg qd × 1–2 d	Diarrhea, nausea, abdominal pain, pain at infusion site If unable to convert to PO therapy, reduce IV dose to 100 mg IV qd; provides approximately same systemic expose as 250 mg PO daily, with oral bioavailability equal to 37%
Chloramphenicol	IV: 50 mg/kg/d	Rarely used except in unusual circumstances because of risk of aplasia or litigation or both Decreased RBC in approximately one-third of patients; aplastic anemia incidence of 1 of 21,000 courses Fever, skin rash, anaphylactoid reactions, optic atrophy or neuropathy, digital paresthesias, minor disulfiramlike reactions 2.3 mEq Na^{+}/g
Clindamycin	IV: 150–900 mg q8h	Diarrhea, pseudomembranous colitis with toxic megacolon Rash, neutropenia, eosinophilia Occasional elevated SGOT and alkaline phosphatase Neuromuscular blockade
Erythromycin	IV: 500 mg–1 g q6h	Nausea, vomiting, abdominal cramps (both PO and IV), diarrhea, phlebitis at infusion site

(continued)

TABLE 10.3. *(continued)* **Antimicrobial Drugs—Doses, Toxicities**

Agent	Usual Adult Dosage	Adverse Effects/ Comments
Erythromycin (*continued*)		Rare rash, elevated SGOT, cholestatic jaundice (especially with erythromycin estolate; rare with erythromycin ethyl succinate) Reversible deafness (high dose), PVCs, torsade de pointes For legionellosis, 1g IV q6h is preferred over lower doses
Spectinomycin	IM: 2 g once	Rash, drug fever, local pain on injection Anaphylaxis
Synercid (Quinupristin-Dalfopristin)	IV: 7.5 mg/kg q8–12h	Myalgias
Vancomycin	IV: 1 g q12h PO: 125–500 mg q6h Intrathecal: 5–10 mg q48–72h	Phlebitis, fever, rash, nausea, ototoxicity Neutropenia, eosinophilia, anaphylactoid reactions "Red man syndrome" (flushing over upper chest)—rate dependent Hypotension with rapid IV push Oral doses not absorbed systemically; oral therapy limited to treatment of antibiotic associated diarrhea due to *C. difficile*
Tetracyclines		
Doxycycline	IV: 100 mg q12h on 1st day then 100–200 mg/d	Hepatotoxicity, negative nitrogen balance, pseudotumor cerebri; phlebitis (central line preferred)
Tigecycline	IV: 100 mg × 1 then 50 mg q12h	Nausea, vomiting Avoid in pregnancy
Fluoroquinolones		
Ciprofloxacin	IV: 400 mg q8–12h	Nausea, diarrhea, vomiting, abdominal pain Headache, insomnia, nightmares, toxic psychosis, confusion, seizures Rash, angioedema Elevated SGOT, alkaline phosphatase, WBC, creatinine
Gatifloxacin	IV: 200–400 mg qd	Similar to ciprofloxacin

(continued)

TABLE 10.3. *(continued)* **Antimicrobial Drugs—Doses, Toxicities**

Agent	Usual Adult Dosage	Adverse Effects/ Comments
Levofloxacin	IV: 500–750 mg qd	Similar to ciprofloxacin Use higher dose for most ICU settings
Moxifloxacin	IV: 400 mg qd	Similar to ciprofloxacin
Ofloxacin	IV: 200–400 mg q12h	Similar to ciprofloxacin
Miscellaneous Antibacterial Agents		
Colistin	IV: 1.25–2.5 mg/kg q12h	Nephrotoxicity, abnormal vision, paresthesias, confusion
Daptomycin	IV: 4–6 mg/kg qd	Myalgias
Linezolid	IV/PO: 600 mg q12h	Thrombocytopenia Neuropathies (prolonged use) Serotonin syndrome
Metronidazole	IV: 500 mg q6h	Nausea, vomiting, diarrhea, metallic taste, headache, rare paresthesias, ataxia, seizures, urticaria, phlebitis at injection site 14 mEq Na^+/500 mg
Tinidazole	PO: 2 g once or qd	Similar to metronidazole
Trimethoprim (TMP)-sulfamethoxazole (SMX)	IV: TMP 320 mg/SMX 1,600 mg q8h	Urticaria, maculopapular and morbilliform rashes, nausea, vomiting, diarrhea Glossitis, rare jaundice Headache, depression, rare hallucinations, pseudotumor cerebri Renal: falsely elevated creatinine, renal failure, hyperkalemia Neutropenia, thrombocytopenia, agranulocytosis May trigger asthma in sulfite-sensitive individuals
Antifungals		
Amphotericin B	IV: 0.5–1.5 mg/kg qd	Premeds: diphenhydramine 50 mg IV, meperidine 50 mg IV, acetaminophen 650 mg PO Hydration: ≥500 ml 0.9% NaCl pre- and postinfusion Administer in D5W, not in electrolyte solutions Administer over 1–4 h (1 h may be as well tolerated as 4 h) Hydrocortisone: 25–100 mg IV if fever, chills not controlled by other premeds Toxicity: renal (dose related elevation of creatinine), renal tubular wasting, lowered K, lowered Mg, fever, chills, nausea, vomiting, phlebitis, anemia, headache

(continued)

TABLE 10.3. *(continued)* **Antimicrobial Drugs—Doses, Toxicities**

Agent	Usual Adult Dosage	Adverse Effects/ Comments
Amphotericin B (*continued*)		Initiating doses in stepwise fashion (1 mg, 5 mg, 10 mg, etc.) is probably unnecessary
	Bladder irrigation: 50 mg/ 1,000 cc sterile water	
ABLC (Abelcet)	IV: 5 mg/kg qd	Same as amphotericin B but less frequent ABLC (amphotericin B lipid complex)
Liposomal ampho B (AmBisome)	IV: 5–7.5 mg/kg qd	Same as amphotericin B but less common Higher doses have been used
Anidulafungin	IV: 35 mg qd	Minimal to date
Caspofungin	IV: 70 mg × 1 d then 50 mg qd	Elevated transaminase Histamine release
Fluconazole	IV/PO: 400 mg q24h	Nausea, vomiting, diarrhea Elevated ALT/AST, confusion, rash, eosinophilia
Flucytosine	PO: 37.5 mg/kg q6h	Nausea, vomiting, diarrhea, leukopenia, thrombocytopenia Elevated ALT/AST Rash Falsely elevated creatinine if EKTACHEM analysis used
Itraconazole	PO: 200 mg bid IV: 200 mg PO bid × 4 doses then 200 mg qd	Nausea, abdominal pain, rash, edema, hypokalemia, hepatitis Administer capsule with meals, administer oral solution on an empty stomach
Micafungin	IV: 150 mg qd (acute therapy)	Leukopenia Histamine release
Posaconazole (Investigational)	PO: 400 mg q12h	Elevated ALT/AST
Voriconazole	IV: 6 mg/kg q12h × 24 h then 4 mg/kg q12h PO: 400 mg q12h × 1 d then 200 mg q12h (if >40 kg body weight)	Elevated transaminase Visual disturbances Rash Thrombocytopenia
Antiretroviral		Should discontinue all antiretrovirals if adherence or gastrointestinal absorption not ensured No intravenous preparations are available
Anti-HIV nucleosides/ nucleotides		All drugs in this class can cause hepatic steatosis and lactic acidosis
Abacavir	PO: 300 mg bid/600 mg qd	Rash, myalgia, fever: never rechallenge after stopping for rash, fever, or myalgias
Didanosine (ddI)	PO: 400 mg qd	Pancreatitis, peripheral neuropathy

(continued)

TABLE 10.3. *(continued)* **Antimicrobial Drugs—Doses, Toxicities**

Agent	Usual Adult Dosage	Adverse Effects/ Comments
Emtricitabine (FTC)	PO: 200 mg qd	Few
Lamivudine (3TC)	PO: 150 mg bid	Toxicities are rare
Stavudine (d4T)	PO: 30–40 mg bid	Pancreatitis, peripheral neuropathy
Tenofovir	PO: 300 mg qd	Renal tubular dysfunction If stopped, beware hepatitis B flare
Anti-HIV Nonnucleosides		
Efavirenz	PO: 600 mg qd	CNS effects (e.g., insomnia, vivid dreams), rash, drug interactions
Anti-HIV Proteases		Drug interactions with agents metabolized by cytochrome P450 system can be significant
Lopinavir-Ritonavir	PO: 3 capsules bid or 2 tablets bid or 6 capsules qd or 4 tablets qd	Diarrhea, nausea, hypertriglyceridemia, elevated transaminase
Antivirals (Nonantiretrovirals)		
Acyclovir	PO (HSV): 200 mg 5 doses/day PO (VZV): 800 mg 5 doses/day IV (most HSV): 5 mg/kg q8h IV (HSV encephalitis or disseminated VZV): 10–12 mg/kg IV q8h	Phlebitis (IV) Lethargy Tremors/seizures Confusion Crystalluria Elevated ALT/AST 4.2 mEq Na^+/g
Adefovir	PO: 10 mg PO qd	Few
Cidofovir	IV: 5 mg/kg qw × 2, then qow	Nephrotoxicity, neutropenia, hypotony Given with oral probenecid 2 g at 2 h predose infusion, and administer 1 g orally at 2 and 8 h postinfusion Given with 1 liter 0.9% NaCl preinfusion
Foscarnet	IV: 60 mg/kg q8h or 90 mg/kg q12h (acute) 90–120 mg/kg q24h (chronic)	Infuse over 2 h after 1 L 0.9% NaCl load Nephrotoxicity Nausea, vomiting Headache, seizures Leukopenia, anemia Elevated SGOT Penile ulcers
Ganciclovir	IV: 5 mg/kg q12h (acute) 5 mg/kg q24h (chronic)	Leukopenia Thrombocytopenia Fever Rash Elevated ALT/AST 46 mEq Na^+/500 mg vial
Palivizumab	IV: 15 mg/kg IM (pediatric)	Elevated ALT/AST Allergic response to Ig
Ribavirin	Aerosol: 6g over 12–18 h per day IV: Investigational	Bronchospasm, environmental hazard precautions Hemolytic anemia Concentration 20 mg/ml (6 g in 300 ml sterile H_2O without preservatives)

(continued)

TABLE 10.3. *(continued)* **Antimicrobial Drugs—Doses, Toxicities**

Agent	Usual Adult Dosage	Adverse Effects/ Comments
Trifluridine topical	1 drop of 1% q2h (max 9 drops/d)	Burning, edema, hypersensitivity
Interferon alpha	SC/IM (hepatitis B): 5M U qd SC/IM (hepatitis C): 3M U qd	Fever Myalgia, fatigue Headache Anorexia Rash Leukopenia, thrombocytopenia
Antiparasitics		
Chloroquine	PO: 600 mg base at T = 0, then 300 mg base at 6 h, 24 h, 48 h for malaria	Nausea, vomiting, pruritus, rash, hemolytic anemia, leukopenia, thrombocytopenia
Ivermectin	PO: 12 mg PO qd × 2 d	Headache, fever, abdominal pain
Pentamidine	IV: 4 mg/kg q24h	Infuse over 1 h Nephrotoxicity Hyperglycemia followed by hypoglycemia Torsades de pointes Can be given IM but causes sterile abscesses
Pyrimethamine	PO: 100 mg/d × 1 then 25–100 mg qd	Leukopenia, rash, ataxia, tremors, seizures
Quinine	PO: 600 mg tid	Tinnitus, headache, nausea, hemolysis
Quinidine	IV: 10 mg/kg load (maximum 600 mg) in 0.9% NaCl over 1 h followed by 0.02 mg/kg/min × 72 h, then oral quinine 600 mg tid to complete 7 d for malaria	More available than quinine IV: hypotension
Sulfadiazine	PO: 1–2 g PO q6h IV: none (consider using TMP/SMX)	Rash, fever, nephritis, nausea, hemolysis
Antimycobacterials		
Isoniazid	PO/IM/IV: 300 mg qd	Administer with pyridoxine Hepatitis, neuropathy, rash, fever, headache, psychosis, seizures
Rifabutin	PO: 300 mg qd	Myalgias, arthralgias, leukopenia, neuritis
Rifampin	PO/IV: 600 mg qd	Orange urine and secretions, hepatitis, fever, nausea
Ethambutol	PO: 15–25 mg/kg qd	Rash, optic neuritis, confusion, gout
Pyrazinamide	PO: 15–30 mg/kg qd	GI intolerance, rash, arthralgia, hepatotoxicity, hyperuricemia
Streptomycin	IM/IV: 15 mg/kg (adult <40 y), qd 10 mg/kg (>40 y) qd	Ototoxicity, nephrotoxicity Call (800) 254–4445 to obtain from Pfizer

ALT, aminotransferase; AST, aspartate aminotransferase; BUN, blood urea nitrogen; CNS, central nervous system; ICU, intensive care unit; IM, intramuscular; IV, intravenous; HSV, herpes simplex virus; LDH, lactate dehydrogenase; PO, by mouth; PVC, premature ventricular contractions; RBC, red blood cells; SGOT, serum glutamic-oxaloacetic transaminase; SGPT, serum glutamic-pyruvic transaminase; VZV, varicella zoster virus; WBC, white blood cells

TABLE 10.4. Aminoglycoside Dosing Protocols

I. Multiple Daily Dosage Regimen

Aminoglycoside	Condition	Dosage	Comments
A. Loading Doses—To be given once initially—See Section C for determining when to use actual body weight (ABW) and lean body weight (LBW)			
Gentamicin/ Tobramycin	Non–head injured	2.5–3 mg/kg ABW	Expected peak concentrations: 6–8 mg/L
	Head injured	2–2.5 mg/kg ABW	
	Uncomplicated urinary tract infection	2 mg/kg LBW	
Amikacin	Non–head injured	10–12 mg/kg ABW	Expected peak concentration: 25–35 mg/L
	Head injured	8–10 mg/kg ABW	
	Uncomplicated urinary tract infection	8 mg/kg LBW	
B. Maintenance Doses—See Section C for determining when to use actual body weight (ABW) and lean body weight (LBW) and how to determine dosing interval			
Gentamicin/ Tobramycin	Non–head injured	1.8–2 mg/kg ABW at selected interval	Expected peak concentrations: 6–8 mg/L
	Head injured	1.5–1.8 mg/kg ABW at selected interval	
	Uncomplicated urinary tract infection	1 mg/kg LBW at selected interval	Due to the high concentrations of drug excreted into the urine, allowing lower dose therapy, routine monitoring of serum concentrations in uncomplicated urinary tract infections may not be required
Amikacin	Non–head injured	7.5–8 mg/kg ABW at selected interval	Expected peak concentration: 25–35 mg/L
	Head injured	6–7.5 mg/kg ABW at selected interval	
	Uncomplicated urinary tract infection	4 mg/kg LBW at selected interval	Due to the high concentration of drug excreted into the urine, routine monitoring of serum concentrations in uncomplicated urinary tract infections may not be required

C. Determining Aminoglycoside Dosing Weights and Dosing Intervals

Calculating Aminoglycoside Dose

1. Use actual body weight to determine the dose for infections in critically ill patients.
2. Use lean body weight to determine the dose for treating urinary tract infections.

Calculating Lean Body Weight (kg)

Males: 50 kg + [(2.3 kg) × (inches >5 feet)]
Females: 45.5 kg + [(2.3 kg) × (inches >5 feet)]

(continued)

TABLE 10.4. *(continued)* **Aminoglycoside Dosing Protocols**

C. Determining Aminoglycoside Dosing Weights and Dosing Intervals (*continued*)

Calculating Dosing Interval

1. Determine or estimate creatinine clearance (CrCl).
2. Measured creatinine clearance can be determined from 4-, 12-, or 24-hour urine collections.
3. Estimating creatinine clearance (ml/min) using the Cockcroft and Gault formula (note: the Cockcroft and Gault formula as well as other formulas used to estimate creatinine clearance tend to overestimate creatinine clearance in critically ill patients):

Males: $\frac{(140\text{-age})\ \text{LBW}}{72 \times \text{SCr}}$ Females: $0.85 \times$ male CrCl

Selecting Appropriate Dosing Interval for Multiple Daily Dose Regimen

Intervals for Maintenance Doses

Creatinine Clearance (ml/min)	Dosing Interval
>160	q8h
100–159	q8–12h
60–99	q12–18h
40–59	q18–24h
<40	q24–48h

II. Single Daily Dose or High Dose Extended Interval Regimens

Some clinicians prefer to give larger gentamicin doses once daily to patients with normal renal function on the presumption that these regimens are equally effective, less toxic, and less expensive. Peak gentamicin level measurements are usually unnecessary but trough levels should be drawn and should be undetectable at the end of the selected dosing interval in order to take advantage of the postantibiotic effect and minimize toxicity. Appropriateness in ICU of this approach is controversial.

For critically ill patients with reduced creatinine clearances, the dosing interval may have to be adjusted to greater than 24 hours with the help of trough serum concentration monitoring.

Drug	Dosage	Comments
Gentamicin	5–8 mg/kg ABW	Infuse over 60 min Expected peak concentration: 20–25 mg/L Desired trough level before next dose: 0 mg/L
Amikacin	20–32 mg/kg ABW	Infuse over 60 min Expected peak concentration: 80–100 mg/L Desired trough level before next dose: 0 mg/L

Selecting Appropriate Dosing Interval for High Dose Extended Interval Regimen

Intervals for Maintenance Doses

Creatinine Clearance (ml/min)	Dosing Interval
>110	q24h
81–110	q36h
60–80	q48h
<60	per levels

TABLE 10.5. Cardiac Lesions That Warrant Antibiotic Prophylaxis Against Endocarditis

Prophylaxis should be administered only if the patient has appropriate cardiac pathology *and* a procedure warranting prophylaxis.

Prophylaxis Recommended	Prophylaxis *Not* Recommended
High-risk category	**Negligible-risk category (no greater risk than the general population)**
Prosthetic cardiac valves (including bioprosthetic and homograft valves)	Isolated secundum atrial septal defect
Previous bacterial endocarditis	Surgical repair of atrial septal defect, ventricular septal defect, or patent ductus arteriosus (without residua, beyond 6 mo)
Complex cyanotic congenital heart disease (i.e., single ventricle states, transposition of the great arteries, tetralogy of Fallot)	Previous coronary artery bypass graft surgery
Surgically constructed systemic pulmonary shunts or conduits	Mitral valve prolapse without valvular regurgitation
Moderate-risk category	Physiologic, functional, or innocent heart murmurs
Most other congenital cardiac malformations (other than above and below)	Previous Kawasaki disease without valvular dysfunction
Acquired valvular dysfunction (i.e., rheumatic heart disease)	Previous rheumatic fever without valvular dysfunction
Hypertrophic cardiomyopathy	Cardiac pacemakers (intravascular and epicardial) and implanted defibrillators
Mitral valve prolapse with valvular regurgitation and/or thickened leaflets	

(Adapted from Dajani AS, et al. Prevention of bacterial endocarditis; recommendations by the American Heart Association. JAMA 1997;277;1794–1801.)

TABLE 10.6. Bacterial Endocarditis—Procedures that Require Prophylaxis

Prophylaxis should be administered only if the patient has appropriate cardiac pathology *and* a procedure warranting prophylaxis.

Procedures that Warrant Prophylaxis*	Procedures that Do *Not* Warrant Prophylaxis
Dental extractions	Restorative dentistry† (operative and prosthodontic) with or without retraction cord††
Periodontal procedures including surgery, scaling and root planning, probing, and recall maintenance	Local anesthetic injections (nonintraligamentary)
Dental implant placement and reimplantation of avulsed teeth	Intracanal endodontic treatment; postplacement and buildup
Endodontic (root canal) instrumentation or surgery only beyond the apex	Placement of rubber dams
Subgingival placement of antibiotic fibers or strips	Postoperative suture removal
Initial placement of orthodontic bands but not brackets	Placement of removable prosthodontic or orthodontic appliances
Intraligamentary local anesthetic injections	Taking of oral impressions
Prophylactic cleaning of teeth or implants where bleeding is anticipated	Fluoride treatments
	Taking of oral radiographs
	Orthodontic appliance adjustment
	Shedding of primary teeth
Respiratory Tract	**Respiratory Tract**
Tonsillectomy and/or a adenoidectomy	Endotracheal intubation
Surgical operations that involve respiratory mucosa	Bronchoscopy with a flexible bronchoscope, with or without biopsy†††
Bronchoscopy with a rigid bronchoscope	Tympanostomy tube insertion
Gastrointestinal Tract**	**Gastrointestinal Tract**
Sclerotherapy for esophageal varices	Transesophageal echocardiography†††
Esophageal stricture dilatation	Endoscopy with or without gastrointestinal biopsy†††
Endoscopic retrograde cholangiography with biliary obstruction	
Biliary tract surgery	
Surgical operations that involve intestinal mucosa	
Genitourinary Tract	**Genitourinary Tract**
Prostatic surgery	Vaginal hysterectomy†††
Cystoscopy	Vaginal delivery†††
Urethral dilation	Caesarean section
	In uninfected tissue: Urethral catheterization; Uterine dilatation and curettage; Therapeutic abortion; Sterilization procedures
	Insertion or removal of intrauterine devices
	Other
	Cardiac catheterization, including balloon angioplasty
	Implanted cardiac pacemakers, implanted defibrillators, and coronary stents
	Incision or biopsy of surgically scrubbed skin
	Circumcision

*Prophylaxis is recommended for patients with high- and moderate-risk cardiac conditions.
**Prophylaxis is recommended for high-risk patients; optional for medium-risk patients.
†This includes restoration of decayed teeth (filling cavities) and replacement of missing teeth.
††Clinical judgment may indicate antibiotic use in selected circumstances that may create significant bleeding.
†††Prophylaxis is optional for high-risk patients.
(Adapted from Dajani AS, et al. Prevention of bacterial endocarditis; recommendations by the American Heart Association. JAMA 1997;277:1794–1801.)

TABLE 10.7. Bacterial Endocarditis Prophylaxis—Drugs of Choice

Patient Category	Drug/Dosage	Time in Relation to Procedure
Dental/Oral/Respiratory Tract or Esophageal Procedures		
Oral		
Penicillin tolerant	Amoxicillin 2 g PO	1 h preprocedure
Penicillin allergic	Azithromycin or Clarithromycin 500 mg PO or	1 h preprocedure
	Clindamycin 600 mg PO or	1 h preprocedure
	Cephalexin or Cefadroxil 2.0 g	1 h preprocedure
Parenteral		
Penicillin tolerant	Ampicillin 2.0 g IV/IM	Within 30 min preprocedure
Penicillin allergic	Vancomycin 1.0 g or	Slowly over 1 h starting preprocedure
	Clindamycin 600 mg IV or	Within 30 min preprocedure
	Cefazolin 1.0 g	Within 30 min preprocedure
Genitourinary or Gastrointestinal (Excluding Esophageal) Procedures		
Parenteral High Risk[a]		
Penicillin tolerant	Ampicillin 2 g IV/IM + gentamicin 1.5 mg/kg IV/IM (not to exceed 120 mg) followed 6 h later by Ampicillin 1 g IV/IM or Amoxicillin 1 g PO	Within 30 min preprocedure and follow-up 6 h post 1st dose
Penicillin allergic	Vancomycin 1 g IV over 1–2 h + gentamicin 1.5 mg/kg IV (not to exceed 120 mg)—complete infusions within 30 min of starting procedure	Complete within 30 min preprocedure
Parenteral Moderate Risk		
Penicillin tolerant	Ampicillin 2 g IV/IM	Within 30 min preprocedure
Penicillin allergic	Vancomycin 1 g IV over 1–2 h	Within 30 min preprocedure
Oral Moderate Risk	Amoxicillin 2 g PO	1 h preprocedure

IM, intramuscular, IV, intravenous; PO, by mouth

[a] High risk: prosthetic valve, history of endocarditis, surgically constructed systemic/pulmonary shunts or conduits

(Adapted from Dajani AS et al. Prevention of bacterial endocarditis: recommendations by the American Heart Association. JAMA 1997;277:1794–1801.)

TABLE 10.8. Antimicrobial Prophylaxis in Surgery

Procedure	Prophylactic Drug(s)	Drug Regimen (Usually Given During Hour Prior to Surgery;[a] One Dose Preoperative is Adequate in Most Situations; Vancomycin Should be Substituted for Cephalosporin to Cover MRSA)
Cardiothoracic		
Median sternotomy	Cefazolin or	1–2 g IV preoperatively (± q4–8h × 1–3 d)
	Cefuroxime or	1.5 g IV preoperatively (± q8h × 1–3 d)
	Vancomycin	1 g IV preoperatively (q12h × 1–3 d)
Pacemaker insertion	None or Cefazolin or Vancomycin	1–2 g IV preoperatively (± q8h × 24 h)
Pneumonectomy or lobectomy	Cefazolin or	1–2 g IV preoperatively (± q8h × 24 h postoperatively)
	Vancomycin	1 g IV preoperatively (± q12h × 24 h postoperatively)
Peripheral vascular	Cefazolin or	1–2 g IV preoperatively (± q8h × 24 h postoperatively)
	Vancomycin	1 g IV preoperatively (± q12h postoperatively)
General Surgery		
Cholecystectomy	None or	
	Cefazolin or	1–2 g IV preoperatively ± q12h × 1–3 d
	Clindamycin +	600 mg IV preoperatively (± q8h × 24 h)
	gentamicin	1.5 mg/kg IV preoperatively (± q8h × 24 h)
Cholangitis		Treat for infection per Table 10.2
Herniorrhaphy	None	
Colon surgery	*Oral (alone or with IV)*	
	Neomycin + erythromycin + laxative	1 g PO of each antibiotic at 1 PM, 2 PM, 11 PM preoperatively; 4L polyethylene glycol electrolyte solution PO over 2h at 10 AM preoperatively
	IV	
	Cefoxitin or	1–2 g IV preoperatively (± q4h × 3)
	Cefazolin +	1–2 g IV preoperatively plus
	metronidazole	0.5–1.0 g IV
	Clindamycin +	600 mg IV × 1
	gentamicin or	1.5 mg/kg IV × 1
	Ciprofloxacin	400 mg IV × 1
Gastrectomy	Cefazolin or	1 g IV preoperatively if high risk
	Gentamicin +	120 mg IV preoperatively
	clindamycin or	600 mg IV preoperatively
	Ciprofloxacin	400 mg IV preoperatively
Appendectomy	Cefoxitin or	2 g IV preoperatively (± q6h × 3 doses if nonperforated) and for 3–5 d if perforated
	Cefazolin +	1–2 g IV and q8h × 3 doses if nonperforated, and for 3–5 d if perforated
	metronidazole	500 mg IV preoperatively once if nonperforated or preoperatively and q8h IV × 3–5 d if perforated
	Alternative:	
	Ciprofloxacin +	400 mg preoperatively q6h × 3 doses if nonperforated, or for 3–5 d if perforated
	clindamycin	900 mg IV preoperatively once if nonperforated or preoperatively and q8h IV if perforated

(continued)

TABLE 10.8. *(continued)* **Antimicrobial Prophylaxis in Surgery**

Procedure	Prophylactic Drug(s)	Drug Regimen (Usually Given During Hour Prior to Surgery;[a] One Dose Preoperative is Adequate in Most Situations; Vancomycin Should be Substituted for Cephalosporin to Cover MRSA)
Mastectomy	None	
Penetrating abdominal trauma	Cefoxitin	2 g IV upon hospital admission, and 2 g IV q6h × 2–5 d if GI perforation found
Ruptured viscus	Cefoxitin + gentamicin or	2 g IV pre-op 1 g IV q8h × ≥5 d 1.5 mg/kg IV q8h × ≥5 d
	Clindamycin + gentamicin	900 mg IV q8h × ≥5 d 1.5 mg/kg IV q8h × ≥5 d
Gynecologic		
Caesarean section (esp high risk)	Cefazolin or	1–2 g IV after clamping cord (± 6 and 12 h later)
	Cefoxitin or	2 g IV after clamping cord
	Metronidazole or	500 mg IV after clamping cord
	Clindamycin + gentamicin or levofloxacin	600 mg IV after clamping cord 1.5 mg/kg IV 750 mg IV
Dilatation and curettage	None	
Instillation abortion, 2nd trimester	Cefazolin or	1–2 g IV preprocedure and 6 and 12 h postprocedure
	Metronidazole	500 mg PO preprocedure (± q4h for 2 doses postprocedure)
Induced abortion, 1st trimester	Penicillin or	2 MU IV before (± 3 h postprocedure)
	Doxycycline	100 mg PO pre- and 200 mg 30 min postprocedure
Hysterectomy, abdominal or vaginal	Cefazolin or	1 g preoperatively and 6 and 12 h later
	Cefoxitin or	2 g IV preoperatively
	Metronidazole or	500 mg IV
	Clindamycin + gentamicin or levofloxacin	600 mg preoperatively 1.5 mg/kg preoperatively or 750 mg IV
Head and Neck		
Tonsillectomy	None	
Radical resection	Cefazolin or	2 g IV preoperatively (± q8h × 2 doses)
	Clindamycin + gentamicin	600 mg IV preoperatively (± q8h × 2 doses) 1.5 mg/kg IV preoperatively (± q8h × 2 doses)
Neurosurgical		
CSF Shunts	None or	
	Cefazolin or	1–2 g IV preoperatively
	Vancomycin	1 g IV preoperatively
Craniotomy	Clindamycin or	600 mg IV preoperatively (± 4 h × 1–3 d postoperatively if high risk)
	Vancomycin + gentamicin	500 mg IV preoperatively 1.5 mg/kg IV preoperatively

(continued)

TABLE 10.8. *(continued)* **Antimicrobial Prophylaxis in Surgery**

Procedure	Prophylactic Drug(s)	Drug Regimen (Usually Given During Hour Prior to Surgery;[a] One Dose Preoperative is Adequate in Most Situations; Vancomycin Should be Substituted for Cephalosporin to Cover MRSA)
Orthopedic		
Arthroplasty and replacement	Cefazolin or	1–2 g IV preoperatively (± q8h × 3–4 doses)
	Vancomycin or	1 g IV preoperatively (± q12h × 3–6 doses)
	Clindamycin	600 mg IV preoperatively (± q6h × 3–4 doses
Open reduction of closed fracture	Cefazolin or	1–2 g IV preoperatively (± q8h × 3 doses)
	Vancomycin	1g IV ± 1 g IV q12h × 2 doses
Reduction of open fracture	Cefazolin or	1–2 g upon admission (± q8h × 10 d)
	Vancomycin	1 g IV ± 1 g IV q12h × doses
Laminectomy or spinal fusion	None or	
	Cefazolin or	1–2 g IV preoperatively (± q8h × 3 d)
	Vancomycin	1 g IV preoperatively (± q12h × 3 d)
Urology		
Prostatectomy	None	
	Ciprofloxacin	400 mg IV if documented organism

GI, gastrointestinal; IV, intravenous; MRSA, methicillin resistant staphylococcus aureus; PO, by mouth

Antimicrobial prophylaxis for surgery: (An advisory statement from the National Surgical Infections Prevention Project, Clinical Infectious Diseases 2004;38:1706–15.)

[a]Prophylactic drugs should ideally be given during the 1 hour period prior to surgery. (Vancomycin or quinolones can be given 2 hours prior to surgery.) For prolonged procedures or when blood loss is extensive, subsequent doses may be necessary at intervals 1–2 times the half-life of the drug. Postoperative antibiotics are rarely documented to be necessary, although two or more postoperative doses are FDA approved for many regimens. Thus many experts try to avoid continuing antibiotic prophylaxis postoperatively unless the surgical field is contaminated, e.g., a perforated viscus. The one exception is cardiothoracic surgery: continuation for 72 hours postoperatively is recommended.

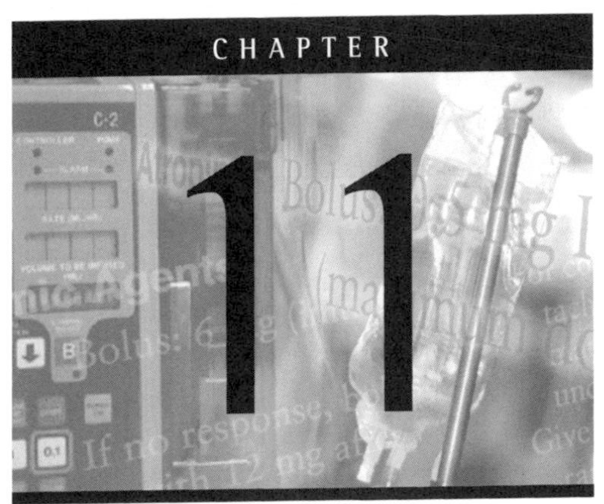

Allergy

TABLE 11.1. Anaphylaxis and Contrast Dye Reactions[a]—Prophylaxis

Agent	Dosage	Time Prior to Exposure
Prednisone or	50 mg PO	13 h, 7 h, and 1 h prior to exposure
Hydrocortisone	100 mg IV	
Diphenhydramine	50 mg PO or IV	13 h, 7 h, and 1 h prior to exposure
H_2-blocker[b]	See below	13 h and 1 h prior to exposure
Ephedrine (optional)	25 mg PO	1 h prior to exposure

IV, intravenous; PO, by mouth

Note: Consider for patients with prior history of dye reaction; may also consider use of nonionic contrast material

[a]This regimen also appropriate for other prophylactic situations.

[b]Ranitidine: 150 mg PO or 50 mg IV

Famotidine: 20 mg PO/IV

Cimetidine: 300 mg PO/IV

TABLE 11.2. Anaphylaxis—Therapy

Situation	Intervention	Comments
Systemic anaphylaxis	Epinephrine 1:1,000, 0.3 cc SC, repeat at 5–10 min intervals Diphenhydramine 25–100 mg IV H_2-blocker[a] Hydrocortisone 100–250 mg IV q6h	Repeat doses of diphenhydramine may be required for symptom relief
Special Problems		
Upper airway obstruction	Nebulized racemic epinephrine, 0.3 ml diluted in 3 ml 0.9% NaCl	Administer oxygen; consider tracheal intubation and mechanical ventilation
Bronchospasm	Epinephrine 1:1,000, 0.3–0.5 ml SC, may repeat at 5–10 min intervals, or Albuterol, 1–2 puffs metered dose inhaler or 2.5–5 mg nebulized in 2–3 ml 0.9% NaCl, or Aminophylline, 6 mg/kg IV initially (see Table 4.4)	With severe bronchospasm or hypotension, consider epinephrine, 1:10,000, 0.5–1.0 ml IV (rather than SC)
Shock	Volume resuscitation with 0.9% NaCl ≥500 ml rapidly, with or without vasopressors Dopamine 5–20 μg/kg/min, titrated to blood pressure, or Norepinephrine, 2 μg/min, titrated to blood pressure Patients on β-blockers who are hypotensive may also be treated with glucagon, 1 mg IV	

IV, intravenous; SC, subcutaneous
[a]Ranitidine: 50 mg IV
Famotidine: 20 mg IV
Cimetidine: 300 mg IV

TABLE 11.3. Desensitization Procedure for Beta-lactam and Other Antibiotics

For patients with severe or life-threatening infections and a history of previous significant allergic reactions to an essential antibiotic (e.g., a history of wheezing, hypotension, angioedema, or other symptoms and signs of systemic anaphylaxis on exposure to the antibiotic or class). This may be documented with skin testing to penicillin if reagents are available. For other classes of antibiotics, the decision to desensitize is based on the clinical history.

1. The procedure should be carried out in a monitored setting with a physician available.
2. A secure IV line should be established.
3. Epinephrine, diphenhydramine, parenteral glucocorticosteroids should be immediately available for acute anaphylactic reactions (see Table 11.2).
4. Six serial 10-fold dilutions of the desired antibiotic dose should be prepared each in 20 ml bags or syringes.
5. Each dose from the most dilute to the least dilute should be administered intravenously over 20 minutes (1 ml/min).
6. A physician should examine the patient prior to each dose.

Example: Ceftriaxone

2 mcg/20 ml over 20 minutes
20 mcg/20 ml over 20 minutes
200 mcg/20 ml over 20 minutes
2 mg/20 ml over 20 minutes
20 mg/20 ml over 20 minutes
200 mg/20 ml over 20 minutes
2 gm/20 ml (full dose) over 20 minutes

- In the absence of an allergic reaction, the standard dose of the antibiotic may be administered after approximately 2 hours.
- If a mild to moderate reaction such as flushing, wheezing, or chest tightness occurs, the infusion should be stopped and the subject treated with antihistamines, epinephrine, or both.
- When the patient's symptoms/signs have resolved, the infusion may be repeated or resumed at 0.5 ml/min.
- If a severe reaction occurs, the infusion should be stopped and the line aspirated to remove any residual antibiotic. The subject should be treated as described in the anaphylaxis therapy protocol (Table 11.2) and the desensitization effort discontinued.
- When there is a need to provide immediate antibiotic coverage because of severe infection, an alternative antibiotic should be administered for at least one dose prior to the desensitization procedure.
- The desensitization procedure should limit or prevent acute allergic reactions to the antibiotic during the initiation of the antibiotic but will need to be reimplemented if a time period greater than 48 hours elapses between doses of therapy.

CHAPTER 12

Poisonings

TABLE 12.1. General, Supportive, and Emergency Measures in Drug Overdose or Poisoning*

For poisoning emergency call 1-800-222-1222. The call is routed to the local poison control center serving the caller based on area code and exchange of the caller. The number is functional 24 hours/day in all 50 states, the District of Columbia, the U.S. Virgin Islands, and Puerto Rico.

Condition	Measures	Comments
Arrhythmias (see Tables 3.9 and 3.10)	Evaluate underlying causes (e.g., hypoxia, electrolytes, etc.)	
	Ventricular arrhythmias:	
	lidocaine	May cause seizures with cocaine
	phenytoin	May increase risk of ventricular tachycardia with antidepressant overdose
	Tachyarrhythmias:	
	β-blockade	May lead to unopposed α-adrenergic effects and coronary vasoconstriction in cocaine overdose May increase risk of ventricular tachycardia in cyclic antidepressant overdose Wide QRS tachycardia (if tricyclic antidepressant suspected or cocaine overdose): $NaHCO_3$ 50–100 mEq IV
Coma	Airway, ventilation, oxygenation, IV access	
	Dextrose 50%, 50–100 mL IV	
	Thiamine 100 mg IV (especially if history of alcoholism)	
	Naloxone (IV/IM, or via endotracheal tube) 0.2–0.4 mg IV; in patients with suspected narcotic addiction 2 mg q 2–3 min until 10 mg total given	May precipitate withdrawal Synthetic opioids, such as fentanyl, may require larger doses
	Flumazenil 0.2 mg q 30–60 sec, total dose 3–5 mg IV if sedative-hypnotic overdose suspected	Contraindicated in patients with epilepsy receiving long-term benzodiazepine therapy and in severe mixed overdose with benzodiazepine and a proconvulsant drug (i.e., aminophylline, amitriptyline, or chloroquine)
Gastrointestinal decontamination	(See specific poisoning for indications)	
	Ipecac syrup: 30 mL followed by 8 oz water, may repeat after 30 min; nausea and vomiting may delay the use of activated charcoal for up to 6 h	Contraindicated if drowsy, unconscious, convulsing, hydrocarbon ingestion, corrosive poisoning, or rapidly acting convulsants (strychnine, camphor, tricyclic antidepressants)
	Gastric lavage: stomach tube; 37–40F, usually most effective within first 4 h after overdose; lavage with 100–200 ml aliquots of 0.9% NaCl or water, usually 1–2 L sufficient to clear contents	Contraindicated in stuporous or comatose patient with absent gag unless intubated with endotracheal tube

(continued)

TABLE 12.1. *(continued)* **General, Supportive, and Emergency Measures in Drug Overdose or Poisoning***

Condition	Measures	Comments
	Activated charcoal: 1–2 g/kg oral aqueous slurry with sorbitol cathartic with first dose and then q 2nd or 3rd dose; repeat dose 20–30 g q2–4h; may hasten drug elimination but cathartics should not be used with each dose	Contraindicated in stuporous, comatose, or convulsing patient unless airway protected by endotracheal tube and gastric tube in place
	Catharsis: Magnesium sulfate 10%, 2–3 mL/kg PO or sorbitol 70%, 1–2 mL/kg PO	Contraindications: magnesium-based cathartics may accumulate in renal failure, oil-based cathartics carry risk of aspiration, sodium-based cathartics may exacerbate hypertension or heart failure
	Whole bowel irrigation: polyethylene glycol, electrolyte solution (COLYTE, GoLYTELY) 1–2 L/h via gastric tube until rectal effluent clear to push tablets through GI tract (especially iron ingestion, sustained release and enteric coated tablets)	
	Pharmacobezoars may form from sustained-release products and result in continual drug absorption after gastrointestinal decontamination	May require endoscopic identification and removal or surgical removal if intestinal obstruction
Hypertension (see Tables 3.11 and 3.12)	Nitroprusside 0.25–10 μg/kg/min or Phentolamine 2–5 mg IV; add β-blocker as needed	β-blockade may lead to unopposed α-adrenergic effects and coronary vasoconstriction in cocaine overdose
Hyperthermia (>40°C)	Rapid cooling measures and benzodiazepines to decrease heat production if agitated or seizing If ineffective and extreme muscle rigidity present, then neuromuscular blockade (see Tables 2.4 and 2.5) If malignant hyperthermia, dantrolene 2.5 mg/kg IV (see Table 2.14) If neuroleptic malignant syndrome, bromocriptine 2.5–7.5 mg PO qd or dantrolene 2.5 mg/kg IV (maximum total dose 10 mg/kg)	

(continued)

TABLE 12.1. *(continued)* **General, Supportive, and Emergency Measures in Drug Overdose or Poisoning***

Condition	Measures	Comments
Hypotension	Fluid resuscitation Vasopressor (e.g., dopamine) If suspected/documented overdose is: tricyclic antidepressant: $NaHCO_3$ IV 1–2 mEq/kg β-blocker: glucagon 5–10 mg IV calcium antagonist: calcium chloride 10% 10–15 ml IV	
Renal excretion	Forced diuresis and urinary pH manipulation: limited utility of alkaline diuresis, 50–100 mEq of $NaHCO_3$ in 1 L of 0.2% NaCl or D5W to urinary pH of 7–8 to prevent tubular reabsorption of acidic drugs, such as phenobarbital, salicylates, and isoniazid	Monitor for hypokalemia, metabolic alkalosis, hypernatremia
	Dialysis indicated if lethal amounts of dialyzable drug present	Hemodialysis: acetaminophen, arsenic, bromide, chloral hydrate, ethanol, ethylene glycol, lithium, mercuric chloride, methanol, salicylates Hemoperfusion cartridges with activated charcoal: amobarbital, butabarbital, carbamazepine, digitoxin, ethchlorvynol, methotrexate, paraquat, pentobarbital, phenobarbital, phenytoin, secobarbital, theophylline
Seizure (see Table 9.1)	Diazepam 2.5–10 mg IV Lorazepam 2–3 mg IV Midazolam 5–10 mg IV or IM Phenobarbital 10–20 mg/kg IV (over 30 min) Phenytoin 10–20 mg/kg (infusion should not exceed 50 mg/min)	

GI, gastrointestinal; IM, intramuscular; IV, intravenous; PO, by mouth

*Fifty percent of all adult overdoses and 90% of all opioid overdoses are mixed ingestions. Most frequently abused: alcohol in combination with drugs, cocaine, heroin or morphine, acetaminophen, aspirin, marijuana, alprazolam, ibuprofen, diazepam, amitriptyline.

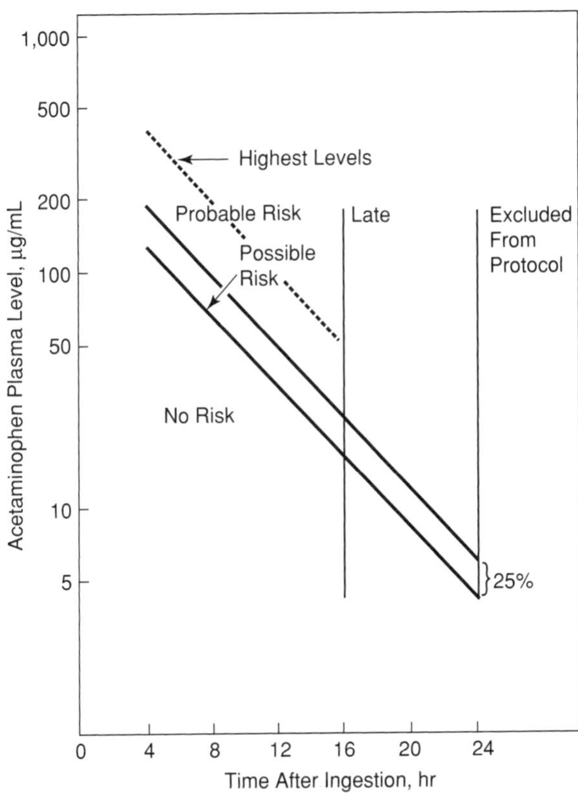

FIGURE 12.1. Acetaminophen Overdose: N-acetylcysteine Dosing Nomogram

Acetaminophen treatment protocol. (Adapted from Rumack BH, Peterson RC, Koch GG, et al. Acetaminophen overdose. 662 cases with evaluation or oral acetylcysteine treatment. Arch Intern Med 1981;141:382. Used with permission.)

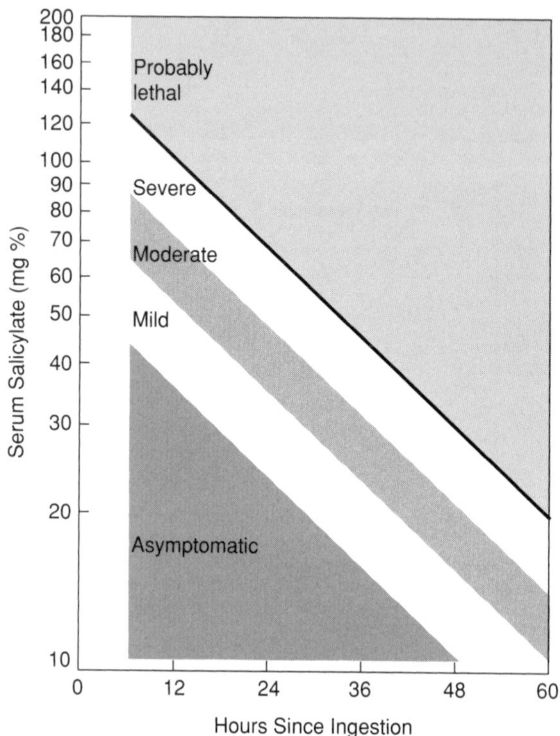

FIGURE 12.2. Salicylate Overdose Nomogram

Nomogram relating serum salicylate level to severity of intoxication.
Mild toxicity: mild to moderate hyperpnea without acidosis, lethargy, and vomiting.
Moderate toxicity: severe hyperpnea with acidosis, marked lethargy or excitability but no coma or convulsions, and marked gastrointestinal distress.
Severe toxicity: severe hyperpnea, severe neurologic impairment that may include coma or convulsions and marked acidosis.
(Adapted from Done AK. Aspirin overdose: incidence, diagnosis and management. Pediatrics 1978;62(suppl):895. Reproduced with permission.)

TABLE 12.2. Specific Therapy for Poisonings and Overdoses

Agent Ingested	Emergency/Supportive Care	Specific Therapy	Comments
Acetaminophen	Empty stomach (emesis or lavage) Activated charcoal	Acetylcysteine Oral solution; load 140 mg/kg then 70 mg/kg q4h × 17 doses IV solution; load 150 mg/kg IV over 15 min, then 50 mg/kg infuse over 4 h, then 100 mg/kg infuse over 16 h	Refer to nomogram (Figure 12.1) to predict risk of toxicity Serum acetaminophen levels should be obtained (see Table 12.4). Levels 0–4 h after ingestion uninterpretable; NAC administration has priority over charcoal if levels are toxic Best if given within 8–10 h of overdose Narcotics and anticholinergics may interfere with oral absorption IV formulation may cause anaphylactoid reaction; interrupt infusion until allergic symptoms treated
Acid corrosives (pool, toilet bowl cleaners)	Do not induce emesis Dilute by drinking 8 oz milk or water Do not give bicarbonate Immediate lavage if possible	Surgical intervention for perforation, peritonitis, bleeding	UGI endoscopy to assess extent of tissue damage, do not pass beyond site of injury
Alkalis (lye, oven cleaners, Clinitest tablets, drain cleaners, disk batteries)	Do not induce emesis Dilute by drinking milk or water Immediate lavage if possible	Endoscopic removal of batteries Surgical intervention for perforation, peritonitis, bleeding	UGI endoscopy to assess extent of tissue damage, do not pass beyond site of injury
Amphetamines (dextroamphetamine, methylphenidate propylhexedrine, ephedrine, d-methamphetamine)	Airway, assisted ventilation Do not induce emesis (seizure risk) Gastric lavage Activated charcoal	Agitation or psychosis; diazepam 5–10 mg IV or midazolam 0.1–0.2 mg/kg IV/IM, lorazepam 1–2 mg IV Hypertension: labetalol 10–20 mg IV, or phentolamine 1–5 mg IV, or nifedipine 10–20 mg PO Tachyarrhythmias: esmolol 50–300 μg/kg/min IV	β-adrenergic blocker alone can worsen hypertension due to unopposed α adrenergic effects

(continued)

TABLE 12.2. *(continued)* **Specific Therapy for Poisonings and Overdoses**

Agent Ingested	Emergency/Supportive Care	Specific Therapy	Comments
Antiarrhythmics (class IA: quinidine, procainamide, disopyramide; class IC: flecainide)	Activated charcoal and cathartic	Atrioventricular block, hypotension, QRS interval widening: sodium bicarbonate 50–100 mEq IV Torsade de pointes: magnesium sulfate 1–2 g IV or isoproterenol 1–5 μg/min or overdrive pacing	
Anticoagulants (warfarin, rodenticides)	Emesis or gastric lavage Activated charcoal	If prothrombin time elevated, give phytonadione (vitamin K) 5–10 mg IV If serious bleeding, give fresh frozen plasma to correct coagulopathy Recombinant activated factor VII (off label use) 15–30 μg/kg IV q12h life threatening bleeding may use 90–120 μg/kg IV bolus q2h	
Antidepressants (tricyclic or tetracyclic, amitriptyline, maprotiline)	Airway, assisted ventilation Do not induce emesis (seizure risk) Gastric lavage Activated charcoal	Cardiotoxic effects: (supraventricular and ventricular tachycardias) sodium bicarbonate 50–100 mEq IV and specific therapy, alkalinize blood pH to 7.5 Seizures: diazepam 5–10 mg IV q1–2h prn Hyperthermia: sedate and paralyze Hypotension: volume resuscitation and then dopamine 5–20 μg/kg/min or norepinephrine 5–100 μg/min or epinephrine 1–20 μg/min	QRS widening >0.10 correlates with increased risk of seizure, >0.16 increased risk of seizure and arrhythmias Class 1A (quinidine, disopyramide, procainamide), and class 1C (e.g., flecainide) contraindicated Phenytoin may worsen risk of ventricular tachycardia β-blockade may worsen cardiac depression and hypotension Physostigmine, a cholinergic agonist, may cause seizures, ventricular fibrillation, and asystole Flumazenil contraindicated; may aggravate seizures and cardiotoxicity

nontricyclic (amoxapine)	Airway, assisted ventilation, supplemental oxygen, gastric lavage, activated charcoal	Seizures/status epilepticus: diazepam 5–10 mg IV q1–2h prn phenytoin 15 mg/kg IV load, infusion not to exceed 50 mg/min, then 100 mg IV q8h	Cardiovascular side effects less common than with tricyclic antidepressants
selective serotonin reuptake inhibitors (SSRI) (fluvoxamine, fluoxetine, paroxetine, sertraline)	Airway, assisted ventilation, supplemental oxygen, gastric lavage, activated charcoal	Agitation or mania, diazepam 2–5 mg IV or midazolam 3–5 mg IV	Low incidence of cardiac toxicity and seizures but if they occur are managed in same manner as tricyclic antidepressant overdose
Antihypertensives sympatholytics (clonidine, prazosin, methyldopa)	Airway, assisted ventilation Emesis or gastric lavage Activated charcoal Cathartic	Supportive therapy with fluids and vasopressor support (e.g., dopamine, Table 3.8)	
Arsenic	Emesis or gastric lavage Activated charcoal Supportive care with IV fluids	Antidote for massive overdose; dimercaprol injection (BAL), 10% solution in oil, 2–3 mg/kg IM q4h × 48 h, q6h × 24, then q12h for 10 d, pretreat with diphenhydramine 25–50 mg PO Follow with dimercaptosuccinic acid (succimer) 10 mg/kg/dose PO q8h × 5d, then q12h × 14 d	
Atropine (anticholinergics)	No emesis if antidepressants with anticholinergic effects ingested, due to seizure risk, otherwise: Emesis or gastric lavage Activated charcoal	If pure atropine overdose, administer physostigmine salicylate 0.5–1 mg IV over 5 min, with ECG monitoring	Sedation and cooling measures (tepid baths, cooling blanket for increased temperature)
β-adrenergic blockers	Airway, assisted ventilation Do not induce emesis (seizure risk) Empty stomach by gastric lavage Activated charcoal	Bradycardia or AVB: atropine 0.5–2 mg IV, isoproterenol 2–20 μg/min IV, or pacemaker (transvenous or transcutaneous) If above fail, glucagon 5 mg IV followed by infusion 1–5 mg/h	Catecholamine infusion alone may lead to arrhythmias or hypotension. Use in conjunction with IV calcium chloride 1 gm of a 10% solution (10mL) via central line slow infusion, max 3 g and/or insulin 0.1 units/kg/h with glucose 1 gm/kg/h (continued next page)

(continued)

TABLE 12.2. *(continued)* **Specific Therapy for Poisonings and Overdoses**

Agent Ingested	Emergency/Supportive Care	Specific Therapy	Comments
β-adrenergic blockers (*continued*)			Monitor glucose levels q30–60 min for first 4 h
Benzodiazepines	See Sedative-hypnotics		
Calcium channel blockers	Airway, assisted ventilation Do not induce emesis (seizure risk) Gastric lavage Activated charcoal	Bradycardia, AV block: atropine 0.5–2 mg IV, isoproterenol 2–20 μg/min IV, or pacemaker (transvenous or transcutaneous) Negative inotropic effects: calcium chloride 10% 5–10 ml IV or calcium gluconate 10% 10–15 ml IV Epinephrine infusion 1–4 μg/min Glucagon 5 mg IV followed by infusion 1–5 mg/h Insulin 0.1 unit/kg/h with glucose 1 gm/kg/h Monitor glucose levels q30–60 min for first 4 h	
Carbon monoxide (CO)	Airway, assisted ventilation	100% O_2 via tight fitting mask or endotracheal tube Hyperbaric O_2 may be useful for patients with coma, seizure, pregnancy	Half life of CO is 4–5 h breathing room air but is reduced by high FiO_2
Chlorinated insecticides (DDT, chlordane, lindane, toxaphene)	Do not induce emesis (seizure risk) Gastric lavage Activated charcoal	Diazepam 5–10 mg IV for seizures	
Cocaine	Airway, supplemental oxygen	Anxiety, agitation, seizures: IV diazepam, or lorazepam Hyperthermia: rapid cooling, benzodiazepine	Excess sympathetic tone (centrally mediated) contributes to agitation, seizures, hypertension, tachyarrhythmias and is treated with benzodiazepines

		Hypertension: benzodiazepine IV, nitroprusside or phentolamine Arrhythmias (QRS prolongation): $NaHCO_3$ 1–2 mEq/kg IV Myocardial ischemia: aspirin, nitroglycerin or calcium-channel blocker (see Table 3.1)	β-blockade may lead to unopposed α-adrenergic effects and worsen coronary vasoconstriction Associated with rhabdomyolysis
Cyanide	Airway and assisted ventilation For ingestion: emesis or gastric lavage and activated charcoal	Cyanide antidotes: (a) amyl nitrate inhalant 0.3 ml q3min × 2 (b) sodium nitrite 6 mg/kg IV over 3–5 min (c) sodium thiosulfate 250 mg/kg IV (usually 50 ml or 12.5 g of a 25% solution) Decrease or discontinue nitroprusside infusion	Elevated venous oxygen saturation (>90%) Nitrites induce methemoglobinemia which binds free cyanide (may induce hypotension); thiosulfate promotes conversion of cyanide to thiocyanate (see Table 12.4)
Digitalis, cardiac glycosides	Airway and assisted ventilation Do not induce emesis (enhanced vagotonia) Gastric lavage Activated charcoal	Monitor potassium Ventricular arrhythmias: lidocaine (1–3 mg/kg IV) or phenytoin (10–15 mg/kg IV over 30 min) Bradycardia (atropine 0.5–2 mg IV), isoproterenol 2–20 μg/min or pacemaker transvenous or transcutaneous)	Digoxin specific antibodies (see Table 12.3)
Ethanol	IV hydration	None	Identify and correct hypovolemia, hypoglycemia, respiratory monitoring and IV thiamine (100 mg) in patients at risk for Wernicke's encephalopathy Severe metabolic acidosis with increased anion gap may indicate cointoxication with other alcohols (methanol, ethylene glycol) (continued next page)

(continued)

TABLE 12.2. *(continued)* **Specific Therapy for Poisonings and Overdoses**

Agent Ingested	Emergency/Supportive Care	Specific Therapy	Comments
Ethanol (*continued*)			Increased levels of ketones or acetones may indicate isopropyl alcohol ingestion
Ethylene glycol or methanol	Airway and assisted ventilation Emesis or gastric lavage Activated charcoal (limited effectiveness)	Fomepizole as soon as possible; loading dose 15 mg/kg IV in 100 mL D5W over 30 min, followed by 10 mg/kg IV q12h or 48 h, then 15 mg/kg q12h until ethylene glycol levels reduced (<20 mg/dL) or methanol levels reduced (<50 mg/dL), pH is normal, and patient is asymptomatic Dialysis should be considered in addition to fomepizole if renal failure present, worsening acidosis, or if elevated levels (>20 mg/dL ethylene glycol or >50 mg/dL methanol) Metabolic acidosis: sodium bicarbonate 50–100 mEg IV Ethanol: (alternative therapy if fomepizole unavailable) loading dose 750 mg/kg PO or IV (as 5% to 10% solution), maintenance 100–150 mg/kg/h (increase to 175–250 mg/kg/h during hemodialysis)	Fomepizole rapidly competitively inhibits alcohol dehydrogenase. It prolongs half-life of ethanol and simultaneous use not recommended Fomepizole is dialyzable and dose frequency should be increased to q4h during dialysis Adjunctive therapy for ethylene glycol poisoning; pyridoxine 50 mg IV/IM q6h and thiamine 100 mg IV/IM q6h and consideration of forced diuresis with fluids and mannitol to prevent oxalate crystal injury to renal tubules Methanol poisoning; folate 50–70 mg IV q4h × 24 h Maintain serum ethanol concentration 100–130 mg/dl (See Table 12.4)
Hallucinogens			
(LSD, mescaline, 3, 4 methylene-dioxymethamphetamine; "ecstasy" or MDMA, methylenedioxy-amphetamine or MDA		Hypersuggestible state managed with calm, supportive environment	Large doses of MDMA or MDA may produce amphetaminelike effects; hyperthermia, rhabdomyolysis, hyponatremia, cerebral infarction

Iron	Airway, assisted ventilation Emesis or lavage Activated charcoal not effective	Fluid resuscitation for vomiting, diarrhea, and corrosive effects on GI tract Endoscopy, surgery, or whole bowel irrigation for large tablet bolus visible on abdominal x-ray Deferoxamine (if levels >500 μg/dl) 10–15 mg/kg/h IV, or 40–50 mg/kg/h for massive overdose, continue until serum iron <350 μg/dl	Toxic serum iron level is 350–500 μg/dl; toxicity associated with serum iron levels >1,000 μg/dl severe Do not exceed 6 g of deferoxamine in 24 h
Isoniazid	Airway, assisted ventilation Do not induce emesis (seizure risk) Gastric lavage and activated charcoal	Pyridoxine 5 g IV over 1–2 min for each isoniazid gram equivalent Seizures: diazepam 5–50 mg IV Hemodialysis or hemoperfusion may be considered, especially in patients with renal failure	
Lead	Airway, ventilatory assistance Activated charcoal and cathartic for acute ingestion	Severe poisoning: dimercaprol 4–5 mg/kg IM q4h × 5 d and edetate calcium disodium 50 mg/kg/d in 4–6 divided doses or continuous IV Less severe: edetate calcium disodium as above, or dimercaptosuccinic acid (succimer) 10 mg/kg/dose every 8 h × 5d, then q12h for 14 d Lead-containing object may need to be removed by endoscopy, surgery, or whole bowel irrigation	Severe poisoning 70–100 μg/dl
Lithium	Airway, assisted ventilation, gastric lavage	Whole bowel irrigation Hemodialysis for life-threatening toxicity	Serum levels >3.5 mmol/l are life-threatening Not absorbed by charcoal

(continued)

TABLE 12.2. *(continued)* **Specific Therapy for Poisonings and Overdoses**

Agent Ingested	Emergency/Supportive Care	Specific Therapy	Comments
Marine Toxins			
Ciguatera	IV saline infusion	None	Toxins from dinoflagellates concentrate in tissue of fish Vomiting, diarrhea, abdominal cramp, bradycardia, heart block, hypotension
Scambroid	IV hydration	Antihistamines (H_1 and H_2), epinephrine or β-agonists if bronchospasm or angioedema present	Bacterial overgrowth in improperly stored fish produce high levels of histamine result in IgE-like allergic reaction
Paralytic shellfish poisoning	Mechanical ventilation for severe neurologic sequelae	None	Toxins from dinoflagellates taken up by bivalve mollusks (mussels, clams, oysters) Mild to severe neurologic symptoms including paralysis and respiratory failure
Neurotoxic shellfish poisoning	IV hydration Supportive therapy	None	Toxins from dinoflagellates (hemolytic and neurotoxins) taken up by shellfish and aerosolized during algae blooms Results in either GI distress, neurologic symptoms or rhinorrhea with bronchospasm
Pufferfish poisoning (tetrodotoxin)	Supportive care and intestinal decontamination with gut lavage/charcoal	None	Neurotoxin associated with pufferfish upon ingestion results in paresthesias, nausea, loss of reflexes, or in severe cases hypotension and general paralysis
Mercury	Emesis or lavage Activated charcoal and cathartic	Dimercaprol 4–5 mg/kg IM q4h × 5 d or penicillamine 100 mg/kg PO in divided doses or dimercaptosuccinic acid (succimer) 10 mg/kg PO q8h × 5 d	No specific therapy for mercury vapor pneumonitis

Methanol	See Ethylene glycol above		
Methemoglobinemia inducing agents (dapsone, nitrites, nitric oxide, pyridium)	Airway, assisted ventilation Emesis or gastric lavage Activated charcoal	Methylene blue 1–2 mg/kg or 0.1–0.2 ml of 1% solution IV, may repeat × 1 after 20 min	Severe poisoning methemoglobin fraction >40%, at 20% cyanotic appearance with normal pO_2, inaccurate pulse oximetry Dapsone has long half-life requiring repeat doses of methylene blue
Monoamine oxidase inhibitors	Gastric lavage Activated charcoal and cathartic	Severe hypertension: nitroprusside, phentolamine, or labetalol (see Table 3.12) Hyperthermia: aggressive cooling Muscle rigidity, myoclonus, trismus, rhabdomyolysis: similar to neuroleptic malignant syndrome treated with dantrolene 2.5 mg/kg IV q5–10 min until improvement or 1 mg/kg maximum total dose	Hypertension may occur following tyramine-containing foods, sympathomimetic drug use Arrhythmias should not be treated with bretylium because of norepinephrine release Fatal hyperthermia associated with meperidine, fluoxetine, or serotonin-enhancing drugs
Mushrooms	Emesis (usually useless after symptoms occur) Activated charcoal and cathartic	Amatoxin-type cyclopeptides (Amanita): fluid resuscitation, supportive care for hepatic failure Gyromitrin type: pyridoxine 25 mg/kg IV Muscarinic type: atropine 0.01 mg/kg IV, repeat prn Anticholinergic type: physostigmine 0.5–1 mg IV Gastrointestinal irritant: hydration Disulfiram type: avoid alcohol Hallucinogenic type: diazepam 5–10 mg IV or haloperidol 1–2 mg IV q1–2h prn Cortinarius: hemodialysis for renal failure	Liver transplant for severely ill (amatoxin-type cyclopeptides)

(continued)

TABLE 12.2. *(continued)* **Specific Therapy for Poisonings and Overdoses**

Agent Ingested	Emergency/Supportive Care	Specific Therapy	Comments
Nerve "gas" poisoning (GA-tabun, GB-sarin, GD-soman, GF, VX) (see Table 12.6)	Protective gear for health workers Decontaminate skin with hypochlorite (bleach diluted 10:1) or soap and water; rinse eyes with plain water	Atropine for bronchoconstriction and secretions: 2 mg IM/IV for mild dyspnea to 6 mg for severe dyspnea or multisystem signs; may require repeat dose q5min (15–20 mg total within first 3 h) Pralidoxime chloride used with atropine: 1 g IV over 20 min, repeat q1h × 1–2 Brain damage prophylaxis and seizures: diazepam 5–10 mg IV	Volatile liquids not gases, absorbed through skin or inhaled resulting in muscarinic-nicotinic hyperactivity, CNS stimulation-depression, paralysis Pralidoxime ineffective against GF and GD becomes refractory within minutes Pyridostigmine bromide used as pretreatment against GA or GD (30 mg PO q8h), enhances effectiveness of atropine or pralidoxime
Opioids (heroin, methadone, L-alpha-acetyl-methadol or LAAM, propoxyphene, meperidine, pentazocine, fentanyl, others)	Airway, assisted ventilation Emesis or gastric lavage for ingestion Activated charcoal	Naloxone 0.4–2 mg IV/IM, or endotracheal route, repeat as needed Large doses have been used (10–20 mg for fentanyl, codeine, or propoxyphene) Nalmefene 0.25 μg/kg IV/IM/SC q2–5min, total dose 1 μg/kg for postoperative respiratory depression. In nonopioid-dependent adult, initial dose of 0.5 mg/70 kg, followed by 1 mg/70 kg 2–5 min later; no added benefit of doses higher than 1.5 mg/70 kg; if opioid dependency suspected, a challenge dose of 0.1 mg/70 kg is recommended, followed by a 2 min wait for signs or symptoms of opioid withdrawal; if none appear, recommended doses may be given	Duration of naloxone effect 2–3 h (see Table 12.4), nalmefene effect ~11 h Naloxone or nalmefene may precipitate withdrawal in opioid-dependent patients and may be more prolonged with nalmefene Acute opioid withdrawal: anxiety, piloerection, yawning, sneezing, rhinorrhea, nausea, vomiting, diarrhea, abdominal or muscle cramps Usually not life-threatening Symptoms lessened with clonidine

Paraquat	Immediate emesis Gastric lavage Activated charcoal or clay (bentonite or Fuller's earth) repeat q2h × 3–4	Charcoal hemoperfusion reported anecdotally to be lifesaving	Lethal levels: 2 mg/L at 6 h, 0.2 mg/L at 24 h
Pesticides, cholinesterase inhibitors (organophosphates)	Emesis or gastric lavage Activated charcoal	Atropine 2 mg IV (reverses muscarinic stimulation) Pralidoxime (2-PAM) specific antidote for reversing organophosphate binding to cholinesterase enzyme 1–2 g IV q3–4h prn or a continuous IV infusion 200–400 mg/h	Serum and red cell cholinesterase activity <50% below baseline in severe intoxications
Petroleum distillates (kerosene, gasoline, paint thinner)	Emesis or lavage controversial, usually only if agent has known systemic toxicity If lavaged, intubate to prevent aspiration		Risk of systemic toxicity high with camphor, phenol, chlorinated insecticides, benzene, toluene, or other aromatic hydrocarbons; variable risk with turpentine or pine oil
Phencyclidine	Maintain in quiet atmosphere If awake, activated charcoal Obtunded: gastric lavage with protected airway	Agitated patient: diazepam 5–10 mg IV or midazolam 0.1 mg/kg IM/IV or haloperidol 0.1 mg/kg IM (titrated small aliquots of IV anxiolytics may be used) Hyperthermia: cooling measures Muscle rigidity: paralysis with neuromuscular blockade or dantrolene 2.5 mg/kg IV q5–10min as needed	
Salicylates	Airway or assisted ventilation Emesis or gastric lavage Activated charcoal	Hemodialysis may be lifesaving in severe poisoning Urine alkalinization: 100 mEq $NaHCO_3$ in 1 L D5/0.20% NaCl at 200 ml/h with 20 mEq KCL	Acute severe poisoning: >100 mg/dl Chronic poisoning: 60–70 mg/dl Associated hypoglycemia, water, and electrolyte losses (see Figure 12.2)

(continued)

TABLE 12.2. *(continued)* **Specific Therapy for Poisonings and Overdoses**

Agent Ingested	Emergency/Supportive Care	Specific Therapy	Comments
Sedative/hypnotic agents (ethanol, barbiturates, benzodiazepines)	Airway, assisted ventilation Emesis or gastric lavage Activated charcoal	Flumazenil (benzodiazepine antagonist) 0.2 mg IV over 30 s up to total dose 3–5 mg Hemoperfusion for severe phenobarbital intoxication	Coma usually with ethanol levels >300 mg/dl or 65 mmol/L, phenobarbital >80–100 mg/L (see Table 12.4) Flumazenil contraindicated in patients with epilepsy receiving long-term benzodiazepines, and in severe mixed overdose with a benzodiazepine and a proconvulsant drug, such as aminophylline or amitriptyline; may also predispose to catecholamine surge upon awakening resulting in hypertension or, rarely, arrhythmias
Theophylline	Airway, assisted ventilation Emesis or gastric lavage Activated charcoal with catharsis	Hemoperfusion is effective for severe overdose (e.g., status epilepticus) Hypertension and tachycardia: β-blockers (e.g., esmolol 50–300 μg/kg/min IV or propranolol 0.5–1 mg IV)	Acute severe poisoning: >80–90 mg/L Chronic poisoning: >60 mg/L Hypokalemia common
Tranquilizers, phenothiazines	Emesis or gastric lavage Activated charcoal and cathartic	Hypotension and arrhythmias: sodium bicarbonate (50–100 mEq IV, maintain pH 7.4–7.5) Extrapyramidal signs: diphenhydramine 0.5–1 mg/kg IV or benztropine mesylate 1–2 mg IM Neuroleptic malignant syndrome: bromocriptine 2.5–7.5 mg PO qd	Monitor QT interval
Tricyclic antidepressants	See Antidepressants above		
Volatile inhalants (nitrous oxide, gasoline, propane, freons, trichlorethylene, perchloroethylene, toluene)	Airway, assisted ventilation, supplemental oxygen	Supportive therapy	Sudden death presumably due to cardiac arrhythmias Arrhythmogenic drugs such as sympathomimetics should be avoided if possible
Warfarin	See Anticoagulants above		

TABLE 12.3. Digoxin Fab Antibody Therapy

Digibind (Ovine digoxin immune Fab antibody fragments)

Each vial of digibind contains 38 mg of purified digoxin-specific Fab fragments which will bind approximately 0.5 mg of digoxin or digitoxin.

Dosage calculation:

(1) From a known digoxin ingestion:

Dose (# of vials) = Body load (mg) ÷ 0.5 (mg/vial)

Number of Digoxin Tablets or Capsules Ingested*	Digibind Dose	
	mg	Number of Vials
25	340	10
50	680	20
75	1,000	30
100	1,360	40
150	2,000	60
200	2,680	80

*0.25 mg tablets with 80% bioavailability, or 0.2 mg Lanoxicaps.

(2) From a measured serum digoxin concentration:

Dose (# of vials) = serum digoxin concentration (ng/ml) × body weight (kg) ÷ 100

		Serum digoxin concentration (ng/ml)						
		1	2	4	8	12	16	20
Patient	40	0.5	1	2	3	5	7	8
Weight	60	0.5	1	3	5	7	10	12
(kg)	70	1	2	3	6	9	11	14
	80	1	2	3	7	10	13	16
	100	1	2	4	8	12	16	20

(3) From a measured serum digitoxin concentration:

Dose (# of vials) = serum digitoxin concentration (ng/ml) × body weight (kg) ÷ 1000

Administration:

Digibind is administered IV through a 0.22 mm filter over 30 minutes. If cardiac arrest is imminent, a bolus dose can be administered. If, after several hours, overdose has not been reversed adequately or appears to recur, readministration of digibind at a dose guided by clinical judgement may be required. If neither a serum digoxin concentration nor an estimate of amount ingested is available, 20 vials (680 mg) of digibind should be administered.

Monitoring:

Patients should have close monitoring of temperature, blood pressure, and ECG during and after administration of digibind. Potassium concentrations should be monitored carefully. Severe digitalis intoxication can cause life-threatening elevation in potassium concentration, which can lead to increased renal excretion of potassium. After administration of digibind, patients should be monitored for hypokalemia as the effect of digitalis on potassium is neutralized. Digibind is not removed from the systemic circulation by hemodialysis or continuous arteriovenous hemofiltration. Patients with normal renal function rapidly eliminate Fab and digoxin bound to Fab. Patients with end-stage renal disease eliminate Fab and digoxin very slowly (half-life of total digoxin 46–330 hours). They will need free digoxin level monitored if digoxin therapy is going to be reinitiated soon after giving the Fab.

Interference with laboratory tests:

Total serum digoxin concentrations may rise precipitously after the administration of digibind. Immunoassays will not give an accurate measure of the serum digoxin concentration after the administration of digibind and should not be used as a measure of therapeutic success. Digibind will interfere with immunoassay measurements until the digibind/digoxin complex is eliminated from the body, which may take a week or longer, depending on renal function. Free digoxin concentration may be a useful monitoring tool, and levels correlate with recurrences of digoxin toxicity, the need for supplemental Fab doses, and the efficacy of digoxin therapy initiated during Fab therapy.

TABLE 12.4. Poisonings—Antidotes

Indication	Antidote	Initial Dosage	Maintenance Dosage
Benzodiazepines			
Reversal of conscious sedation	Flumazenil	0.2 mg IV over 15 sec	After waiting an additional 45 s, 0.2 mg q1min up to 4 additional times, to a maximum of 1 mg
Reversal of recurrent sedation			Repeat doses at 20-min intervals as needed No more than 1 mg (given as 0.2 mg/min) should be administered at any one time, and no more than 3 mg in any 1 h
Benzodiazepine Overdose			
Initial	Flumazenil	0.2 mg IV over 30 s	After waiting an additional 30 s, 0.3 mg IV over 30 s Repeat doses of 0.5 mg can be administered over 30 s at 1 min intervals up to a cumulative dose of 3 mg
Partial response			With a partial response after 3 mg, additional doses up to a total dose of 5 mg may be administered
Repeat treatment			No more than 1 mg (given as 0.2 mg/min) should be administered at any one time, and no more than 3 mg in any 1 h
Continuous infusion		0.1–0.5 mg/h	Useful for reversal of long-acting benzodiazepines or massive overdoses
Narcotics			
Postoperative narcotic depression	Naloxone	Bolus: 0.1–0.2 mg IV at 2–3 min intervals	Repeat doses may be indicated within 1–2 h depending on amount, type, and time interval since administration of narcotic
	Nalmefene	0.25 μg/kg IV, IM/SC q 2–5 min, total dose 1 μg/kg	Duration of effect ~11 h
Narcotic overdose	Naloxone	Bolus: 0.4–2 mg IV/IM or endotracheal route, repeat as needed	0.4–2 mg may be repeated at 2–3 min intervals If no response is obtained after 10 mg have been administered, the diagnosis of narcotic toxicity or overdose should be questioned Naloxone is preferred for emergency department treatment of opioid overdose because it produces a less prolonged period of withdrawal in opioid-dependent patients than nalmefene
		Infusion: 0.4 mg/h or 0.002 mg/kg/h	Dilute 2 mg in 500 ml of compatible fluid; final concentration of 0.004 mg/ml

(continued)

TABLE 12.4. *(continued)* **Poisonings—Antidotes**

Indication	Antidote	Initial Dosage	Maintenance Dosage
Narcotic overdose (*continued*)	Nalmefene	Nonopioid dependent adult initial dose of 0.5 mg/70 kg, followed by 1 mg/70 kg 2–5 min later; no added benefit of dose greater than 1.5 mg/70 kg; if opioid dependency suspected, a challenge dose of 0.1 mg/70 kg is recommended, followed by a 2 min wait for signs or symptoms of opioid withdrawal; if none appear, then recommended doses may be given	
Narcotic-induced pruritus	Naloxone	Infusion: 5 μg/kg/hr	Useful in patients experiencing pruritis while receiving epidural narcotic infusions
Acetaminophen	N-acetylcysteine	PO: 140 mg/kg diluted 1:3 in cola, juice, soda, or plain water	Additional 17 doses 70 mg/kg PO q4h; refer to nomogram to predict risk of toxicity (Figure 12.1) Administration of activated charcoal is not recommended because it may interfere with the absorption of N-acetylcysteine If administered within 8–16 h of ingestion, N-acetylcysteine minimizes hepatotoxicity, but treatment is still indicated as late as 24 h
		IV solution load 150 mg over 15 min, then infuse 50 mg/kg over 4 h, then 100 mg/kg infused over 16 h	IV formulation may cause anaphylactoid reaction Interrupt infusion until allergic symptoms treated

(continued)

TABLE 12.4. *(continued)* **Poisonings—Antidotes**

Indication	Antidote	Initial Dosage	Maintenance Dosage
Methanol and ethylene glycol	Ethanol	Fomepizole as soon as possible; loading dose 15 mg/kg IV in 100 mL D5W over 30 min, followed by 10 mg/kg IV q12h or 48 h, then 15 mg/kg q12h until ethylene glycol levels reduced (<20 mg/dL) or methanol levels reduced (<50 mg/dL) pH is normal and patient is asymptomatic Dialysis should be considered in addition to fomepizole if renal failure present, worsening acidosis or if elevated levels (>20 mg/dL ethylene glycol or >50 mg/dL methanal) Metabolic acidosis: sodium bicarbonate 50–100 mEg IV	Fomepizole rapidly competitively inhibits alcohol dehydrogenase; it prolongs half-life of ethanol and simultaneous use not recommended Fomepizole is dialyzable and dose frequency should be increased to q4h during dialysis Adjunctive therapy for ethylene glycol poisoning; pyridoxine 50 mg IV/IM q6h and thiamine 100 mg IV/IM q6h and consideration of forced diuresis with fluids and mannitol to prevent oxalate crystal injury to renal tubules Methanol poisoning; folate 50–70 mg IV q4h × 24 h
		Ethanol: (alternative therapy if fomepizole unavailable) loading dose 750 mg/kg PO or IV (as 5% to 10% solution), maintenance 100–150 mg/kg/h (increase to 175–250 mg/kg/h during hemodialysis) 0.75 g/kg (approximately 1 ml/kg) of 10% solution infused over 15 min	Maintain serum ethanol concentration 100–130 mg/dl (see Table 12.4) 130 mg/kg/h (approximately 0.16 ml/kg/h) of a 10% solution titrated to maintain an ethanol level between 100–150 mg/dl Infusion should continue for 2–3 d
Cyanide	Sodium nitrate	10 ml of a 3% solution IV over 3–5 min	If signs of poisoning persist, readminister both sodium nitrate and sodium thiosulfate
	Sodium thiosulfate	50 ml of a 25% solution IV	Note: amyl nitrate may be crushed and inhaled q15–30s until IV access is established

ECG, electrocardiogram; IM, intramuscular; IV, intravenous, PO, by mouth

TABLE 12.5. Antivenin for Snake and Spider Bites

Agent	Indications	Dose	Comments
Antivenin (Crotalidae) Polyvalent (Equine)	Neutralizes absorbed venom of North and South American crotalids or pit vipers (e.g., rattlesnake, copperhead, cottonmouth or water moccasin, tropical moccasins, fer-de-lance, bushmaster, tropical and Asiatic crotalids); prevents or minimizes the effects of poison	Minimal envenomation: 20–40 ml (2–4 vials) Moderate envenomation: 50–90 ml (5–9 vials) Severe envenomation: 100–150 ml (10–15 vials) or more	IV preferred to IM, especially if severe envenomation or shock present The initial 5–10 ml of diluted antivenim[a] should be infused over 3–5 min observing for systemic anaphylaxis reaction; if no signs, then infusion continued at maximal rate Equine derived[a]; entire initial dose should be given ASAP, ideally within 4 h of bite; less effective beyond 12 h but should be given even if 24 h have elapsed Additional doses based on clinical response if swelling progresses, signs or symptoms of envenomation increase, hypotension or a decrease in hematocrit then an additional 10–50 ml (1–5 vials) should be given IV Immobilize bitten extremity Contact Poison Control Center Not for use with coral snake bites
Antivenin (Crotalidae) polyvalent immune Fab (Ovine)	Neutralizes absorbed venom of North and South American crotalidae or pit vipers (e.g. rattlesnake, copperhead, cottonmouth or water moccasins, tropical moccasins, fer-de-lance, bushmaster)	Initial dose; 4–6 vials infused within 6 h after snake bite, infuse over 60 min (20–50 mL/h) for first 10 min, if no allergic reaction seen increase rate to 250 mL/h Repeat (4–6 vials) if control not achieved with initial dose (i.e., local signs of injury continue or if systemic signs and coagulation tests not improved) Maintenance infusion 2 vials q6h × 3 additional doses	Immunoglobin fragments from sheep Side effects include rash, urticaria, pruritus, and rare serum sickness Drug availability 1-800-231-0206

(continued)

TABLE 12.5. *(continued)* **Antivenin for Snake and Spider Bites**

Agent	Indications	Dose	Comments
Antivenin (Micrurus fulvius)	Neutralizes venom of North American coral snake	IV, 30–50 ml (3–5 vials) 50–60 ml (5–6 vials) if pain or neurologic symptoms 80–100 ml (8–10 vials) if bulbar signs present	Equine derived[a] Infuse ASAP even if signs of envenomation are not yet present Additional doses based on clinical response, usually 10–50 ml (1–5 vials)
Antivenin (Latrodectus mactans)	Neutralizes venom of black widow spider or related species	2.5 ml (1 vial) IM or slow IV infusion after skin or conjunctival sensitivity testing[b]	IV infusion preferred for severe cases May be repeated Equine derived[a] Contact Poison Control Center Adjunctive case includes warm baths, 10 ml of 10% calcium gluconate IV to control muscle pain; therapy with antivenin can be deferred and treatment with a skeletal muscle relaxant considered

IM, intramuscular; IV, intravenous

[a]Risk of immediate sensitivity reactions (shock, anaphylaxis in patients with atopic sensitivity to horses) occurs within 30 minutes of administration. Prior to initiating therapy, intradermal sensitivity test should be performed using 0.02–0.03 ml of a 1:10 dilution of normal equine serum or antivenin in 0.9% NaCl. After 5–30 minutes, positive test = urticarial wheal and erythema. Desensitization consists of 0.1, 0.2, and 0.5 ml 1:100 SC injection at 15-minute intervals, then 1:10 dilution, and then undiluted serum. Alternatives to desensitization in critically ill patients include slow IV diluted antivenin with IV antihistamine (e.g., 50–100 mg of diphenhydramine HCl) or IV epinephrine. Serum sickness may occur 5–24 days after administration.

[b]Prior to initializing therapy, 0.02 ml of 1:10 dilution of normal equine serum in 0.9% NaCl is administered intradermally. A positive skin test consists of an urticarial wheal surrounded by erythema. If skin test is negative, the antivenin can be administered. If skin test is positive, a conjunctival test made by placing 1 drop of 1:10 diluted normal equine serum on the conjunctiva and noting results after 10 minutes. A positive conjunctival test reaction consists of vessel congestion, lacrimation, and itching. If both the skin and conjunctival tests are positive, then the antivenin should be avoided. If life-threatening situation, then desensitization should be attempted as in previous footnote.

TABLE 12.6. Chemical Terrorism

Protection of Health Care Workers

- First responders to chemical agent exposure must be equipped with appropriate protective clothing and equipment (boots, gloves, coveralls, masks, and breathing apparatus).
- Reactive skin decontamination lotion (RSDL):
  (a) Neutralizes toxicity of nerve and blister agents (especially nerve agent VX, mustard, lewisite).
  (b) Apply within 3 minutes of contamination, wash away residue at later time.
- Decontamination of patient and health care workers:
  (a) Removal of clothing avoiding contact of skin to residues.
  (b) Copious water showers.
- Key agencies:
  (a) Emergency Federal hotline (U.S. Government Response Center) 1-800-424-8802
  (b) Centers for Disease Control (www.bt.cdc.gov) 1-404-639-3311
  (c) Food and Drug Administrative Counter-Terrorism Office 1-301-827-7777

Category/Example	Action/Syndromes	Medical Management
Biotoxins		
Ricin	Inhibition of protein synthesis Clinical manifestations depend on route of exposure: Ingestion—profuse vomiting, diarrhea, multiorgan failure, and death 36–72 h Inhalation—respiratory distress, fever, cough, pulmonary edema, hypotension, and death within 36–72 h	Supportive care with fluids, mechanical ventilation, oxygen No specific antidote exists
Blister Agents/Vesicants		
Sulfur mustard gas **Nitrogen mustard** **Lewisite**	DNA synthesis inhibition Eye injury and skin burns with vesicle formation Respiratory irritation (wheezing, laryngeal edema, acute lung injury) Garlic smell/onions Radiomimetic effects including leukopenia, pulmonary and GI mucosal damage	No specific therapy for mustard gas effects on skin, eyes, and lungs Supportive treatment, respiratory support, pain relief RSDL neutralizes toxicity of blister agents applied topically Dimercaprol (topical antidote for lewisite)
Toxic Asphyxiants		
Cyanide (hydrocyanic acid) **Arsine (arsenic trihydride)**	Mitochondrial cytochrome oxidase inhibition, inhibit cell respiration, lactic acidosis, cytotoxic hypoxia in cardiovascular and central nervous system Colorless liquid or gas Almond smell (cyanide), garlic smell (arsine) Therapy based on administration of nitrites that form methemoglobin, which combines with cyanide to form cyanomethemoglobin and frees cytochrome oxidase to resume aerobic metabolism	Cyanide poisoning: • 100% O_2 • Sodium nitrite 300 mg IV infused over 5–15 min, may repeat after 30 min with 150 mg IV • Amyl nitrite ampules (0.3 mL) if IV route unavailable; inhale vapors for 30 sec/min × 3 per ampule; repeat up to 5 ampules • Sodium thiosulfate to form thiocyanate complex; after nitrite treatment, 12.5 g IV slow push (50 mL); may repeat in 30 min at one-half the dose • Hydroxocobalamin 10 mL of 40% solution (4g) IV over 20 min • No specific antidote for arsine

(continued)

TABLE 12.6. *(continued)* **Chemical Terrorism**

Category/Example	Action/Syndromes	Medical Management
Arsine (arsenic trihydride) (*continued*)		Supportive treatment for hemolysis (exchange transfusion) and renal failure diuresis with mannitol, alkaline diuresis
Caustics		
Hydrofluoric acid/hydrogen fluoride	Found in refrigerants, herbicides, high-octane gasoline, etching glass/metal Rapidly absorbed through skin into tissues Skin contact—severe burns with ulceration, inhalation; lung injury with pulmonary edema, irritation of eyes and nose Splashes of hydrogen fluoride on skin can be fatal; swallowing small amounts of hydrogen fluoride may be fatal	Remove clothing, wash from skin with large amounts of water, dispose of clothes If hydrogen fluoride is swallowed do not induce vomiting, do not give activated charcoal Calcium or magnesium containing antacids with 1–2 glasses of water if alert Calcium gluconate gel applied to skin to prevent absorption
Pulmonary Irritants		
Chlorine **Phosgene** **Ammonia**	Burn and irritate skin and eyes Direct lung tissue injury, pulmonary edema Smell of new-mown hay (phosgene) Pungent smell (chlorine) Cleaning agent (ammonia)	No antidote exists for any of the pulmonary irritants Remove clothing, rapidly wash body with soap and water Supportive care for acute respiratory distress; Bronchodilators Corticosteroids Mechanical ventilation Oxygen therapy Mydriatic for eyes and topical antibiotic
Nerve Agents		
GX, sarin, tabun, VX	Cholinesterase inhibitors, acetylcholine excess syndrome, severe secretions, smooth muscle stimulation, skeletal muscle neural inhibition, respiratory failure	Atropine IV or IM 2–4 mg then 2 mg IV/IM q5–10min until muscarine symptoms resolve; doses of 200 mg may be required every 24 h Pralidoxime 1–2 g IV with 5 min of presentation, repeat in 20–60 min if weakness unchanged; alternative IM route; 600 mg in large muscle Maintain airway, ventilator assistance, supplementary oxygen Avoid succinylcholine to prevent excess acetylcholine release Seizure—diazepam 5–10 mg IV/IM, repeat after 10–20 min (max 30 mg q8) RSDL applied topically neutralizes nerve agent VX

(continued)

TABLE 12.6. *(continued)* **Chemical Terrorism**

Category/Example	Action/Syndromes	Medical Management
Riot Control Gas		
"Tear gas" **Mace** **Chloroacetophenone (CN)** **Chlorobenzylidene-malononitrile (CS)** **Chloropicrin (PS)** **Bromobenzylcyanide (CA)** **Dibenzoxazepine (CR)**	Irritation of eyes, skin, upper respiratory tract, lower respiratory tract Excessive tearing, blurred vision, runny nose, difficulty swallowing, chest tightens, burns or skin rash, nausea, and vomiting Long-lasting exposure (closed setting) may lead to blindness, immediate death due to chemical burns to throat and lungs, respiratory failure	No specific antidote exists for riot control agents Remove clothing and wash off agent from skin with soap and water. Rinse eyes Supportive care: Bronchodilators Oxygen therapy Corticosteroids

GI, gastrointestinal; IM, intramuscular; IV, intravenous; RSDL, reactive skin decontamination lotion

TABLE 12.7. Radiation Exposure Emergencies[a]

General Principles	Medical Management Principles
Exposure to radiation source (x-rays, gamma rays, neutrons, protons—high dose over short period—minutes) can cause tissue injury. Patients do not become radioactive. *External contamination*: loose particles of radioactive material are deposited on surfaces, skin, clothing *Internal contamination*: radioactive material is inhaled, ingested, or lodged within wound. Contaminated patients should be decontaminated as soon as possible	• Establish triage area for contamination containment and decontamination • Remove contaminated outer garments of patients and staff and double bag using radioactive waste guidelines • Body survey staff and patient with radiation meter • Wash wounds and skin with saline/soap and water • Resurvey and repeat washing until radiation level no more than twice background or unchanged

Additional Resources

Armed Forces Radiobiology Research Institute Medical Radiobiology Team
1-301-295-0530
www.afrri.usuhs.mil

Centers for Disease Control and Prevention
1-800-CDC-INFO
www.bt.cdc.gov/radiation

Radiation Emergency Assistance Center/Training Site (REAC/TS)
1-865-576-3131 (M–F day)
1-865-576-1005 (After hours)
www.orau.gov/reacts

Acute Radiation Syndromes	Dose Exposure	Signs, Symptoms, Outcome
Bone marrow syndrome	>0.7 Gy[b] (70 rads) mild symptoms with 0.3 Gy[a] (30 rads)	• Anorexia, nausea, vomiting • May have latent period of appearing well • Primary cause of death is infection and hemorrhage
Gastrointestinal syndrome	>100 Gy[b] (1,000 rads) same symptoms with 6 Gy (600 rads)	• Anorexia, nausea, vomiting, cramps, diarrhea • May have latent period of appearing well • Death due to infection, dehydration, electrolyte abnormalities • 100% lethality ≈10 Gy
Cardiovascular/central nervous system syndrome	>50 Gy[b] (5,000 rads), some symptoms with 20 Gy (2,000 rads)	• Nervousness, confusion, nausea, vomiting, diarrhea, loss of consciousness, burning sensation of skin • May have partial return of function for hours • Death within 3 days of this level of exposure

(continued)

TABLE 12.7. *(continued)* **Radiation Exposure Emergencies**

If Radiation Exposure Suspected:

Triage	Diagnosis of acute radiation syndrome	Initial treatment and diagnostic evaluation
• Airway, ventilatory, and circulatory support • Physiologic monitoring • Treat major trauma, burns, and respiratory injury	• Diagnosis is difficult and depending on dose, signs and symptoms may occur within hours or days or be in a latent stage	• Treat vomiting • Record clinical symptoms including nausea, vomiting, diarrhea, and itching, reddening, or blistering of skin with time of onset (see Table 12.8)
• Obtain blood samples for complete blood count with differential (attention to lymphocytes) and HLA typing prior to transfusion	• If exposure occurred within 8–12 h, repeat complete blood count with attention to lymphocyte count q2–3h for first 8–12 hrs after exposure and then q4–6h for the following 2–3 d (see Andrews nomogram Table 12.8)	• Consider tissue, blood typing, and initiating viral prophylaxis • Consultation with radiotherapy and hematology experts regarding dosimetry, prognosis, and treatment options • Prophylaxis and treatment of infections • Use of hematopoietic growth factors and/or stem cell transfusions • Chromosome aberration cytogenic bioassay best method of dose assessment

[a] Adapted from www.bt.cdc.gov/radiation.

[b] Exposure of entire body to high dose (>0.7 Gray (Gy) or >70 rads) radiation (i.e., x-rays, gamma rays, neutrons) for short periods of time (usually minutes) resulting in immediate tissue injury and depletion of immature parenchymal stem cells. Symptoms can be immediate or delayed, mild, or severe, depending on radiation dose. Nausea and vomiting may occur minutes to days after the exposure. The time of onset of vomiting is a major sign to assist in diagnosis and dose exposure estimation (Table 12.8).

TABLE 12.8. Estimation of External Radiation Dose Related to Onset of Vomiting and Changes in Absolute Lymphocyte Counts

Vomiting Post Incident	Estimated Dose[a]	Degree of ARS[b]
<10 min	>8 Gy	Lethal
10–30 min	6–8 Gy	Very severe
<1 h	4–6 Gy	Severe
1–2 h	2–4 Gy	Moderate
>2 h after	<2 Gy	Mild

[a]For acute external exposures only. Gray (Gy) is the SI unit of measurement for radiation absorbed dose.
[b]ARS, acute radiation syndrome.
(Adapted from: Berger ME, Leonard RB, Ricks RC, Wiley AL, Lowry PC. Hospital triage in the first 24 hours after a nuclear or radiological disaster, REAC/TS [Radiation Emergency Assistance Center/Training Site];http://www.orau.gov/reacts:2004.)

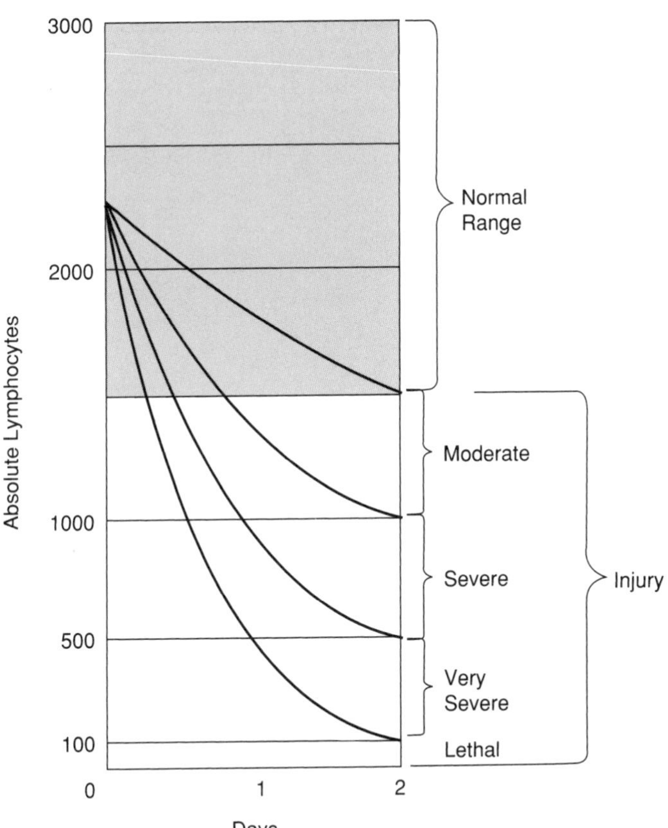

FIGURE 12.3. Andrews Lymphocyte Nomogram

From Andrews GA, Auxier JA, Lushbaugh CC. The importance of dosimetry to the medical management of persons exposed to high levels of radiation. In Personal dosimetry for radiation accidents. Vienna: International Atomic Energy Agency;1965.
Source: http://www.bt.cdc.gov/radiation/arsphysiciantactsheet.asp. Accessed March 21, 2006.

Drug Monitoring

TABLE 13.1. Serum Drug Concentrations—Therapeutic Ranges

Drug	Usual Therapeutic Range	Time to Steady-State with Normal Organ Function	Usual Time Sampling
Antibiotics			
Amikacin	Multiple daily dose: Peak: 20–40 mg/L Trough: <10 mg/L High dose extended interval: Peak: not recommended Trough: 0 mg/L	5–35 h	Peak: 30–60 minutes after a 30-min infusion Trough: Just before next dose Trough: Just before next dose
Chloramphenicol	Peak: 10–25 mg/L Trough: 5–10 mg/L	12–24 h	Peak: 30–90 min after a 30-min infusion Trough: Just before next dose
Gentamicin	Multiple daily dose: Peak: 4–10 mg/L Trough: <2 mg/L High dose extended interval: Peak: not recommended Trough: 0 mg/L	5–35 h	Peak: 30–60 min after a 30-min infusion Trough: Just before next dose Trough: Just before next dose
Streptomycin	Peak: 40–50 mg/L Trough: <5 mg/L	10–500 h	Peak: 30–60 min after a 30-min infusion Trough: Just before next dose
Sulfonamides (sulfamethoxazole, sulfadiazine, co-trimoxazole)	Peak: <150 mg/L	24–48 h	Peak: 2 h after 1-h infusion Trough: Not applicable
Tobramycin	Multiple daily dose: Peak: 4–10 mg/L Trough: <2 mg/L	5–35 h	Peak: 30–60 min after a 30-min infusion Trough: Just before next dose
Vancomycin	Peak: 20–40 mg/L Trough: <10 mg/L	24–36 h	Peak: 1 h after 1-h infusion Trough: Just before next dose
Antiarrhythmics			
Amiodarone	0.5–2 mg/L	Weeks to months	Trough: Just before next dose
Digoxin	0.5–2 ng/ml	7–10 d	Peak: 8–12 h after dose Trough: Just before next dose
Digitoxin	20–35 ng/ml	25–70 d	Peak: 4–12 h after dose Trough: Just before next dose
Disopyramide	2–5 mg/L	24–48 h	Trough: Just before next dose
Flecainide	0.2–1.0 mg/L	70–100 h	Trough: Just before next dose

(continued)

TABLE 13.1. *(continued)* **Serum Drug Concentrations—Therapeutic Ranges**

Drug	Usual Therapeutic Range	Time to Steady-State with Normal Organ Function	Usual Time Sampling
Lidocaine	1.5–5 mg/L	30–90 min after loading dose, 5–10 h without loading dose	Anytime during a continuous infusion
Mexiletine	0.5–2 mg/L	48–72 h	Trough: Just before next dose
Procainamide/ NAPA	Procainamide: 4–10 mg/L NAPA: 10–20 mg/L	Procainamide: 12–24 h NAPA: 24–48 h	IV: 30 min after IV loading dose or anytime during continuous infusion PO: Trough: Just before next dose
Quinidine	2.5–5 mg/L	30–36 h	Trough: Just before next dose
Anticonvulsants			
Carbamazepine	4–12 mg/L	>14 d	Trough: Just before next dose
Fosphenytoin	Total: 10–20 mg/L (measured as phenytoin) Free: 1–2 mg/L	8–50 d Variable depending on daily dose	Peak: IV: 2 h after dose IM: 4 h after dose Trough: just before next dose
Pentobarbital	20–50 mg/L	75–110 h	IV: Peak: Immediately after loading dose or anytime during a continuous infusion
Phenobarbital	15–40 mg/L	10–25 d	Trough: Just before next dose
Phenytoin	Total: 10–20 mg/L Free: 1–2 mg/L	8–50 d Variable depending on daily dose	IV: 2–4 h after dose PO: 3–9 h after administration of phenytoin capsules
Primidone	Primidone: 5–12 mg/L Phenobarbital: 15–40 mg/L	Primidone: 72–170 h Phenobarbital: 10–25 d	Trough: Just before next dose Specimens should be assayed for primidone and phenobarbital
Valproic acid	50–100 mg/L	48–72 h	Trough: Just before next dose
Bronchodilators			
Theophylline	10–20 mg/L	48 h	IV: Prior to IV bolus dose, 30 min after end of bolus dose or anytime during continuous infusion PO: Peak: 2 h after rapid release product, 4 h after sustained release product Trough: Just before next dose

(continued)

TABLE 13.1. *(continued)* **Serum Drug Concentrations—Therapeutic Ranges**

Drug	Usual Therapeutic Range	Time to Steady-State with Normal Organ Function	Usual Time Sampling
Immunosuppressants			
Cyclosporine	*Kidney:* <3 mo: Whole blood: HPLC, M-RIA, M-FPIA: 150–250 ng/ml >3 mo: Whole blood: HPLC, M-RIA, M-FPIA: 100–200 ng/ml *Liver:* Whole blood: HPLC, M-RIA, P-FPIA: 200–300 ng/ml *Heart:* Whole blood: HPLC, M-RIA: 150–300 ng/ml *Bone marrow:* Serum/plasma: HPLC, M-RIA, P-FPIA: 150–300 ng/ml	36–170 h	IV/PO: Trough: Just before next dose
Tacrolimus	Plasma: 0.1–5 μg/L Whole blood: 5–20 μg/L	60–190 h	IV: Anytime during infusion PO: Trough: Just before next dose Preferred assay is MEIA

HPLC, high performance liquid chromatography; IM, intramuscular; IV, intravenous; MEIA, microparticulate enzyme immunoassay; M-FPIA, monoclonal fluorescence polarization immunoassay; M-RIA, monoclonal radioimmunoassay; P-FPIA, polyclonal fluorescence polarization immunoassay; PO, by mouth; NAPA, N-acetylprocainamide

TABLE 13.2. Selected Drug Interactions

Primary Drug	Interacting Drug/Mechanism	Effect	Management
Adenosine	Theophylline/Inhibits the hemodynamic effects of adenosine	Decreases the antiarrhythmic effectiveness of adenosine	May require increased adenosine doses to control arrhythmia
	Dipyridamole/Decreased adenosine metabolism	Potentiates the pharmacologic effect of adenosine	Reduce the dose of adenosine for the treatment of arrhythmias or for diagnostic tests
	Nicotine/Increases the hemodynamic and AV nodal blocking effects of adenosine	Potentiates the pharmacologic effect of adenosine	Cigarette smokers or users of nicotine gum or patches should be monitored for a greater hemodynamic response to adenosine. Reduced adenosine doses may be required in these patients
Aminoglycosides	Neuromuscular blocking agents/Prevent release of acetylcholine at neuromuscular junction	Prolonged paralysis	Monitor neuromuscular function with train-of-four stimulation
	Antipseudomonal penicillins/ Inactivate aminoglycosides in vitro and in vivo	Reduced aminoglycoside levels	Send specimens for aminoglycoside level determination to lab for immediate assay Inactivate aminoglycosides in vivo in patients with severe renal dysfunction
Amiodarone	Cholestyramine/Increased amiodarone elimination	Decreased amiodarone level	Monitor amiodarone level, adjust amiodarone dose accordingly
	Cimetidine/Decreased amiodarone metabolism	Increased amiodarone level	Monitor amiodarone level, adjust amiodarone dose accordingly
	Cyclosporine/Decreased cyclosporine metabolism	Increased cyclosporine level	Monitor cyclosporine level, adjust cyclosporine dose accordingly
	Digoxin/Decreased digoxin clearance	Increased digoxin level	Monitor digoxin level, adjust digoxin dose accordingly
	Phenytoin/Decreased phenytoin metabolism Increased amiodarone metabolism	Increased phenytoin level Decreased amiodarone level	Monitor phenytoin and amiodarone levels, adjust doses accordingly
	Warfarin/Altered protein binding and decreased metabolism	Increased anticoagulant effect	Monitor PT/INR, adjust warfarin dose accordingly

(continued)

TABLE 13.2. *(continued)* **Selected Drug Interactions**

Primary Drug	Interacting Drug/Mechanism	Effect	Management
Anticoagulants	Amiodarone/Altered warfarin protein binding and decreased warfarin metabolism	Increased anticoagulant effect	Monitor PT/INR, adjust warfarin dose accordingly
	Barbiturates/Increased warfarin metabolism	Decreased anticoagulant effect	Monitor PT/INR, adjust warfarin dose accordingly
	Cholestyramine/Decreased warfarin absorption	Decreased anticoagulant effect	Separate doses
	Erythromycins (clarithro-, erythro-)/Decreased warfarin metabolism	Increased anticoagulant effect	Monitor PT/INR, adjust warfarin dose accordingly Consider alternative antibiotic
	Cimetidine/Decreased warfarin clearance	Increased anticoagulant effect	Monitor PT/INR, adjust warfarin dose accordingly
	Ciprofloxacin/Decreased warfarin metabolism	Increased anticoagulant effect	Monitor PT/INR, adjust warfarin dose accordingly Consider alternative antibiotic
	Fluconazole, itraconazole, ketoconazole/Decreased warfarin metabolism	Increased anticoagulant effect	Monitor PT/INR, adjust warfarin dose accordingly
	NSAIDS/Decreased platelet aggregation	Increased bleeding	Monitor for signs and symptoms of bleeding
	Metronidazole/Decreased warfarin metabolism	Increased anticoagulant effect	Monitor PT/INR, adjust warfarin dose accordingly Consider alternative antibiotic
	Propafenone/Decreased warfarin metabolism	Increased anticoagulant effect	Monitor PT/INR, adjust warfarin dose accordingly
	Rifampin/increased warfarin metabolism	Decreased anticoagulant effect	Monitor PT/INR, adjust warfarin dose accordingly
	Salicylates/Decreased platelet aggregation	Increased bleeding	Monitor for signs and symptoms of bleeding
	Sulfonamides/Altered warfarin protein binding	Increased anticoagulant effect	Monitor PT/INR, adjust warfarin dose accordingly Consider alternative antibiotic
Proton Pump Inhibitors	Warfarin	Increased anticoagulant effect	Monitor PT/INR, adjust warfarin dose accordingly
	Phenytoin	Increased phenytoin level	Monitor phenytoin level, adjust phenytoin dose accordingly
Linezolid	Adrenergic agents (i.e., dopamine, epinephrine)	Increased adrenergic response	Reduce and titrate adrenergic dose as needed to achieve desired response
	Serotonergic agents (i.e., fluoxetine, paroxetine, sertraline, etc.)	Increased risk for developing serotonin syndrome	Avoid combination; use alternative antibiotic if possible

Ciprofloxacin	Foscarnet/Decreased seizure threshold	Increased risk of seizures	Monitor for seizure activity Adjust dose of each agent for degree of renal insufficiency
	Mexiletine/Decreased mexiletine metabolism	Increased mexiletine level	Monitor mexiletine level, adjust mexiletine dose accordingly
	Phenytoin/Decreased phenytoin metabolism	Increased phenytoin level	Monitor phenytoin level, adjust phenytoin dose accordingly
	Theophylline/Decreased theophylline metabolism	Increased theophylline level	Monitor theophylline level, adjust theophylline dose accordingly
	Warfarin/Decreased warfarin metabolism	Increased anticoagulant effect	Monitor PT/INR, adjust warfarin dose accordingly Consider alternative antibiotic
Levofloxacin	Warfarin/Decreased warfarin metabolism	Increased anticoagulant effect	Monitor PT/INR, adjust warfarin dose accordingly Consider alternative antibiotic
Cyclosporine	Anticonvulsants (phenytoin, phenobarbital, carbamazepine)/Increased cyclosporine metabolism	Decreased cyclosporine level	Monitor cyclosporine level, adjust cyclosporine dose accordingly
	Diltiazem/Decreased cyclosporine metabolism	Increased cyclosporine level	Monitor cyclosporine level, adjust cyclosporine dose accordingly Consider an alternative calcium channel blocker
	Rifampin/Increased cyclosporine metabolism	Decreased cyclosporine level	Monitor cyclosporine level, adjust cyclosporine dose accordingly
	Ketoconazole, fluconazole, itraconazole/Decreased cyclosporine metabolism	Increased cyclosporine level	Monitor cyclosporine level, adjust cyclosporine dose accordingly
	Erythromycin, clarithromycin/ Decreased cyclosporine metabolism	Increased cyclosporine level	Monitor cyclosporine level, adjust cyclosporine dose accordingly
	Aminoglycosides/ Increased nephrotoxicity	Decreased renal function	Monitor renal function
	Amphotericin B/Increased nephrotoxicity	Decreased renal function	Monitor renal function
	Metoclopramide, cisapride/Increased cyclosporine absorption	Increased cyclosporine level	Monitor cyclosporine level, adjust cyclosporine dose accordingly
	Octreotide/Decreased cyclosporine absorption	Decreased cyclosporine level	Monitor cyclosporine level, adjust cyclosporine dose accordingly

(continued)

TABLE 13.2. *(continued)* **Selected Drug Interactions**

Primary Drug	Interacting Drug/Mechanism	Effect	Management
Cyclosporine (*continued*)	Cimetidine, famotidine, omeprazole/Decreased cyclosporine metabolism	Increased cyclosporine level	Monitor cyclosporine level, adjust cyclosporine dose accordingly
Digoxin	Amiodarone/Decreased elimination	Increased digoxin level	Monitor digoxin level, adjust digoxin dose accordingly
	Diuretics/Increased potassium excretion	Increased potential for digoxin toxicity	Monitor potassium level Consider the need for potassium supplements or potassium sparing diuretics
	Propafenone/Decreased volume of distribution and nonrenal clearance	Increased digoxin level	Monitor digoxin level, adjust digoxin dose accordingly
	Quinidine/Decreased binding and elimination	Increased digoxin level	Monitor digoxin level, adjust digoxin dose accordingly
	Verapamil/Decreased digoxin elimination	Increased digoxin level	Monitor digoxin level, adjust digoxin dose accordingly
Heparin	Nitroglycerin/Altered heparin clearance	Decreased anticoagulant effect	Monitor PTT, adjust heparin infusion accordingly
Meperidine	Monoamine oxidase inhibitors (phenelzine, tranylcypromine)/ Block the reuptake of serotonin	Increased agitation, blood pressure, heart rate, temperature, development of seizures	Avoid drug combination Consider an alternative analgesic
Phenytoin	Cimetidine/Decreased phenytoin metabolism	Increased phenytoin level	Monitor phenytoin level, adjust phenytoin dose accordingly
	Fluconazole/Decreased phenytoin metabolism	Increased phenytoin level	Monitor phenytoin level, adjust phenytoin dose accordingly
Potassium-sparing diuretics/ (amiloride, spironolactone, triamterene)	Potassium supplements/Increased potassium intake	Increased potassium level	Monitor potassium level Review medication profile
	Angiotensin converting enzyme inhibitors/Decrease potassium elimination	Increased potassium level	Monitor potassium level Review medication profile
	Salt substitutes/Increase potassium intake	Increased potassium level	Monitor potassium level Review medication profile
	Theophylline/Increased theophylline metabolism	Decreased theophylline level	Monitor theophylline level, adjust theophylline dose accordingly

Tacrolimus	Aluminum hydroxide/Impaired tacrolimus absorption	Decreased tacrolimus level	Monitor tacrolimus level, adjust tacrolimus dose accordingly
	Dexamethasone/ Increased tacrolimus metabolism	Decreased tacrolimus level	Monitor tacrolimus level, adjust tacrolimus dose accordingly
	Erythromycin/Decreased tacrolimus metabolism	Increased tacrolimus level	Monitor tacrolimus level, adjust tacrolimus dose accordingly
	Fluconazole, itraconazole, ketoconazole/ Decreased tacrolimus metabolism	Increased tacrolimus level	Monitor tacrolimus level, adjust tacrolimus dose accordingly
	Magnesium oxide/pH mediated tacrolimus degradation	Decreased tacrolimus level	Monitor tacrolimus level, adjust tacrolimus dose accordingly
	Rifampin/Increased tacrolimus metabolism	Decreased tacrolimus level	Monitor tacrolimus level, adjust tacrolimus dose accordingly
	Sodium bicarbonate/pH mediated tacrolimus degradation	Decreased tacrolimus level	Monitor tacrolimus level, adjust tacrolimus dose accordingly
Theophylline	See Table 4.6		

AV, atrioventricular; INR, international normalized ratio; NSAIDS, nonsteroid anti-inflammatory drug; PT, prothrombin time; PTT, partial prothrombin time
For a complete review of HIV/AIDS drug interactions (see: Piscitelli SC, Flexner C, Minor JR, et al. Drug interactions in patients infected with human immunodeficiency virus. Clin Inf Dis 1996;23:685–93.)

TABLE 13.3. Dosage Adjustments in Renal and Hepatic Failure

Agent	Adjustment in Renal Failure (CrCl: ml/min/1.73 M^2)		Adjustment in Hepatic Failure	Comments
	CrCl	Dosage		
Acebutolol	>50	100% of daily dose	No change	
	25–49	Reduce daily dose by 50%		
	<25	Reduce daily dose by 75%		
Acyclovir (intravenous)	>50	5 mg/kg q8h	No change	
	25–50	5 mg/kg q12h		
	10–25	5 mg/kg q24h		
	0–10	2.5 mg/kg q24h		
	HD:	2.5 mg/kg q24h		
Acyclovir (oral)	200 mg q4h	(5 × /d) or 400 mg q12h	No change	
	>10	No change		
	0–10	200 mg q12h		
	800 mg q4h	(5 × /d)		
	>25	No change		
	10–25	800 mg q8h		
	0–10	800 mg q12h		
Alfentanil	No change		Decrease	
Allopurinol	80	250 mg q24h	No change	
	60	200 mg q24h		
	40	150 mg q24h		
	20	100 mg q24h		
	10	100 mg q48h		
	0	100 mg q72h		
Alprazolam	No change		Decrease	

Amantadine	≥80 60–79 40–59 30–39 20–29 10–19	100 mg bid 200 mg/100 mg alternating qod 100 mg qd 200 mg 2 × /week 100 mg 3 × /week 200 mg/100 mg alternating q7d	No change	
Amikacin	>160 100–159 60–99 40–59 <40 HD:	q6–8h q8–12h q12–18h q18–24h q24–48h Monitor serum level 1 h after HD, suppl. dose after HD as needed	No change	Adjust dose based on serum concentrations and patient's clinical response; in critically ill patients, dosing intervals increased secondary to increased fluid accumulation and reduced renal function
Aminophylline	No change		0.3 mg/kg/h	Adjust dose based on serum concentrations and patient's clinical response
Amiodarone	No change		Reduce dosage in severe liver disease	Adjust dose based on serum concentrations and patient's clinical response
Amlodipine	No change		2.5 mg/d to maximum 5 mg/d	
Amoxicillin	10–50 <10 HD:	250–500 mg q6–12h 250–500 mg q12–16h 250–500 mg q16–24h with an additional 250 mg dose after dialysis	No change	

(continued)

TABLE 13.3. *(continued)* **Dosage Adjustments in Renal and Hepatic Failure**

	Adjustment in Renal Failure (CrCl: ml/min/1.73 M^2)			
Agent	**CrCl**	**Dosage**	**Adjustment in Hepatic Failure**	**Comments**
Amoxicillin-clavulanic acid	>30	250–500 mg q8h	No change	
	15–30	250–500 mg q12–18h		
	5–15	250–500 mg q20–36h		
	<5	250–500 mg q48h		
	HD:	Suppl. dose after HD		
Ampicillin (intravenous and oral)	>50	0.25–2 g q4–6h	No change	
	10–50	0.25–2 g q6–12h		
	<10	0.25–2 g q8–16h		
	HD:	Suppl. dose after HD		
Ampicillin-sulbactam	≥30	1.5–3 g q6–8h	No change	
	15–29	1.5–3 g q8–12h		
	5–14	1.5–3 g q24h		
	HD:	Suppl. dose after HD		
Argatroban	No change		Moderate liver disease: 0.5 μg/kg/min	More than 4 h may be required for full reversal of full anticoagulant effects after stopping infusion
Atenolol	15–35	50 mg qd	No change	
	<15	25 mg qd		
	HD:	25–50 mg after dialysis		
Azathioprine	>10	No change	Use with caution; possible decrease in conversion to 6-mercaptopurine	
	<10	May need to decrease		
Aztreonam	>30	0.5–1 g q8–12h	No change	
	10–30	1–2 g initially, then 0.25–1 g q8–12h		
	<10	1–2 g initially, then 0.125–0.5 g q8–12h		
	HD:	same as <10 ml/min with suppl. dose of 0.0625–0.250 g after HD		

Benazepril	<30 or SCr >3 mg/dl: 5 mg qd to maximum 40 mg qd		No change	In patients with a CrCl <30 ml/min, a loop diuretic is preferred to a thiazide diuretic
Betaxolol	Severe renal impairment or HD: 5 mg qd to maximum 20 mg qd		No change	
Bivalirudin	≥60	No change	No change	
	30–60	20% dose reduction		
	10–29	60% dose reduction		
	HD:	90% dose reduction		
Captopril	10–50	75% of usual dose q12–18h	No change	
	<10	50% of usual dose q24h		
Carbamazepine	No change		Decrease	Adjust dose based on serum concentrations and patient's clinical response
Caspofungin	No change		Moderate liver disease: 70 mg loading dose followed by 35 mg q24h	No experience in severe liver disease
Cefadroxil	>50	0.5–1 g q12h	No change	
	25–50	0.5 g q12h		
	10–25	0.5 g q24h		
	<10	0.5 g q36h		
Cefazolin	<55	1 g q6–8h	No change	
	35–54	1 g q8–12h		
	11–34	0.5–1 g q12h		
	<10	0.5–1 g q24h		
	HD:	Suppl. dose after HD		

(continued)

TABLE 13.3. *(continued)* **Dosage Adjustments in Renal and Hepatic Failure**

Agent	Adjustment in Renal Failure (CrCl: ml/min/1.73 M^2)		Adjustment in Hepatic Failure	Comments
	CrCl	Dosage		
Cefepime	>60	0.5–2 g q12h	No change	
	30–60	0.5–2 g q24h		
	11–29	0.5–1 g q24h		
	<10	0.25–0.5 g q24h		
	HD:	Suppl. dose after HD		
Cefixime	21–60	300 mg qd	No change	
	<20	200 mg qd		
	HD:	Suppl. dose not required		
Cefotaxime	>20	1–2 g q4–12h	Possible adjustment in severe disease	Partially metabolized to desacetyl-cefotaxime, which has partial activity
	<20	0.5–1 g q4–12h		
	HD:	0.5–2 g q24h with suppl. dose after HD		
Cefoxitin	>50	1–2 g q6–8h	No change	
	30–50	1–2 g q8–12h		
	10–29	1–2 g q12–24h		
	5–9	0.5–1 g q12–24h		
	<5	0.5–1 g q24–48h		
	HD:	1–2 g after HD		
Cefpodoxime	<30	100–200 mg q24h	No change	
	HD:	100–200 mg 3 × /wk after dialysis		
Cefprozil	<30	250 mg q24h	No change	
	HD:	250 mg after dialysis		
Ceftazidime	>50	1 g q8h	No change	
	31–50	1 g q12h		
	16–30	1 g q24h		
	6–15	0.5 g q24h		
	<5	0.5 g q48h		
	HD:	1 g initially, then 1 g after HD		

Ceftibuten	>50 30–49 5–29 HD:	400 mg qd 200 mg qd 100 mg qd 400 mg after HD		
Cefuroxime	>20 10–20 <10 HD:	0.75–1 g q8h 0.75 g q12h 0.75 g q24h Suppl. dose after HD	No change	
Cephalexin	11–40 5–10 <5	0.5 g q8–12h 0.25 g q12h 0.25 g q12–24h	No change	
Chloramphenicol	See Comments		See Comments	Adjust dose based on serum concentrations and patient's clinical response
Chlorpromazine	No change		Avoid or decrease due to increased cerebral sensitivity	
Cidofovir	Increase in SCr ≥0.3–0.4 mg/dl above baseline: 3 mg/kg Increase in SCr ≥0.5 mg/dl above baseline or urinary protein ≥3+: cidofovir must be discontinued	No change	Contraindicated in patients with preexisting SCr >1.5 mg/dl, CrCl ≤55 ml/min or preexisting urine protein concentration ≥100 mg/dl	
Cimetidine	>30 <30 HD:	300 mg q6–8h 300 mg q12h Suppl. dose after HD and q12h during interdialysis period	No change	Dosage may be based on gastric acid secretory response; further dose reductions when hepatic impairment is also present
Ciprofloxacin (Intravenous)	>30 5–29	200–400 mg q12h 200–400 mg q18–24h	No change	

(continued)

TABLE 13.3. *(continued)* **Dosage Adjustments in Renal and Hepatic Failure**

Agent	Adjustment in Renal Failure (CrCl: ml/min/1.73 M^2)		Adjustment in Hepatic Failure	Comments
	CrCl	Dosage		
Ciprofloxacin (Oral)	30–50 5–29 HD:	250–500 mg q12h 250–500 mg q18h 250–500 mg qd suppl. doses not required	No change	In patients with severe infections and severe renal impairment, 750 mg PO q12–18h with careful monitoring
Clarithromycin	<30	500 mg initially, then 250 mg qd-bid	No change	
Clindamycin	No change		Decrease dose in moderate to severe disease	
Codeine	10–50 <10	Decrease dose by 25% Decrease dose by 50%	Decrease	
Daptomycin	≥30 <30 including HD and CAPD	4 mg/kg q24h 4 mg/kg q48h	No change	
Dexmedetomidine	No change		Reduce	
Desirudin	>60 ≥31–60 <31	15 mg q12h 5 mg q12h 1.7 mg q12h	No change	Moderate renal dysfunction: monitor aPTT and SCr at least daily; if aPTT is >2 × control 1; interrupt therapy until aPTT returns to <2 × control, 2; resume therapy at reduced dose guided by initial degree of aPTT abnormality Severe renal dysfunction: monitor aPTT and SCr at least daily; If aPTT is >2 × control 1; interrupt therapy until aPTT returns to <2 × control, 2; consider additional dose reduction guided by initial degree of aPTT abnormality

Diazepam	No change		Decrease	Active metabolites contribute to effect; use agents without active metabolites
Didanosine	HD:	25% of the usual qd dose	No change	
Digoxin	See Comments		No change	Adjust dosage based on serum concentrations and patient's clinical response
Disopyramide (immediate release capsules)	>40 30–40 15–30 <15	100 mg q6h 100 mg q8h 100 mg q12h 100 mg q24h	No change	Adjust dosage based on serum concentrations and patient's clinical response
Divalproex	No change		Decrease	Adjust dosage based on serum concentrations and patient's clinical response
Dofetilide	>60 40–60 20–<40 <20	500 μg bid 250 μg bid 125 μg bid Contraindicated	No change	
Doxacurium	See Comments		No change	Monitor paralysis with train-of-four nerve stimulation
Doxycycline	No change		Decrease dosage in moderate disease	
Enalaprilat	>30 <30	1.25 mg q6h 0.625 mg q6h	No change	
Enoxaparin	 >30 <30 >30 <30	Prophylactic doses 40 mg q24h 30 mg q24h Treatment doses 1 mg/kg bid 1 mg/kg qd	No change	Anti-Xa levels may be lower in critically ill patients receiving standard doses

(continued)

TABLE 13.3. *(continued)* **Dosage Adjustments in Renal and Hepatic Failure**

Agent	Adjustment in Renal Failure (CrCl: ml/min/1.73 M^2)		Adjustment in Hepatic Failure	Comments
	CrCl	Dosage		
Eptifibatide	ACS: SCr <2 mg/dl: bolus: 180 μg/kg followed by infusion of 2 μg/kg/min SCr 2–4 mg/dl: bolus: 180 μg/kg followed by infusion of 1 μg/kg/min PCI: SCr <2 mg/dl: Bolus: 180 μg/kg followed by infusion of 2 μg/kg/min; a second 180 μg/kg bolus dose is administered 10 minutes after the first; SCr 2–4 mg/dl; bolus: 180 μg/kg followed by infusion of 1 μg/kg/min; a second 180 μg/kg bolus dose is administered 10 min after the first		No change	
Ertapenem	>30 ≤10–30 HD: <6h before HD session HD: ≥6h before HD session	1 g q24h 500 mg q24h 150 mg after HD No supplemental dose	No change	
Erythromycin	No change		Decrease dosage in moderate to severe disease	Increased incidence of reversible hearing loss in patients with renal insufficiency
Esomeprazole	No change		Do not exceed 20 mg in patients with severe liver impairment	
Eszopiclone	No change		1 mg at bedtime in patients with severe liver disease	

Ethambutol	70–100	15 mg/kg q24h	No change	
	10–50	15 mg/kg q24–36h		
	<10	15 mg/kg q48h		
Famciclovir	Herpes zoster (immunocompetent)		No change	
	>60	500 mg q8h		
	40–59	500 mg q12h		
	20–39	500 mg q24h		
	<20	500 mg q48h		
	HD:	250 mg after dialysis		
Famotidine	>10	20 mg q12h	No change	
	<10	20 mg q24h		
Flecainide	<20	Decrease usual dose by 25–50%	Decrease	Initial dose in patients with renal impairment is 100 mg q12h Dose adjustment should be made no faster than every 4 d Adjust dose based on serum concentrations and patient's clinical response
Fluconazole	>50	200–400 mg q24h	No change	Patients with impaired renal function should receive an initial loading dose of 50–400 mg followed by daily maintenance dose based on CrCl
	21–50	50% q24h		
	11–20	25% q24h		
	HD:	Usual dose after HD		
Foscarnet	**Induction Doses**		No change	
		Equal to 60 mg/kg/dose		
	ml/min/kg	q8h		
	≥1.6	60		
	1.5	57		
	1.4	53		
	1.3	49		

(continued)

TABLE 13.3. *(continued)* **Dosage Adjustments in Renal and Hepatic Failure**

Agent	Adjustment in Renal Failure (CrCl: ml/min/1.73 M^2)		Adjustment in Hepatic Failure	Comments
	CrCl	Dosage		
Foscarnet (*continued*)	Induction Doses (*continued*)			
	1.2	46		
	1.1	42		
	1.0	39		
	0.9	35		
	0.8	32		
	0.7	28		
	0.6	25		
	0.5	21		
	0.4	18		
	Maintenance Doses			
		Equal to 90 mg/kg/dose		
	ml/min/kg	q24h		
	≥1.4	90		
	1.2–1.4	78		
	1.0–1.2	75		
	0.8–1.0	71		
	0.6–0.8	63		
	0.4–0.6	57		
		Equal to 120 mg/kg/dose		
	ml/min/kg	q24h		
	≥1.4	120		
	1.2–1.4	104		
	1.0–1.2	100		
	0.8–1.0	94		
	0.6–0.8	84		
	0.4–0.6	76		

Fosphenytoin	No change		Decrease dosage in severe disease	Adjust dosage based on unbound "free" phenytoin serum concentrations and patient's clinical response
Gabapentin	>60	400 mg tid	No change	
	30–60	300 mg bid		
	15–30	300 mg qd		
	<15	300 mg qod		
	HD:	300–400 mg loading dose then 200–300 mg after dialysis		
Ganciclovir (Intravenous)	Induction Dosage		No change	
	≥70	5 mg/kg q12h		
	50–69	2.5 mg/kg q12h		
	25–49	2.5 mg/kg q24h		
	10–24	1.25 mg/kg q24h		
	HD:	1.25 mg/kg 3 × weekly after dialysis		
	Maintenance Dosage			
	≥70	5 mg/kg q24h		
	50–69	2.5 mg/kg q24h		
	25–49	1.25 mg/kg q24h		
	10–24	0.625 mg/kg q24h		
	HD:	0.625 mg/kg 3 × weekly after dialysis		
Gatifloxacin	≥40	400 mg qd	No change	
	<40	200 mg qd		
	HD:	200 mg qd		
Gemifloxacin	>40	320 mg q24h	No change	
	≤40	160 mg q24h		
	HD or CAPD	160 mg q24h		

(continued)

TABLE 13.3. *(continued)* **Dosage Adjustments in Renal and Hepatic Failure**

Agent	Adjustment in Renal Failure (CrCl: ml/min/1.73 M^2)		Adjustment in Hepatic Failure	Comments
	CrCl	Dosage		
Gentamicin	>160	q6–8h	No change	Adjust dosage based on serum concentrations and patient's clinical response; in critically ill patients dosing intervals are increased secondary to increased fluid accumulation and reduced renal function
	100–159	q8–12h		
	60–99	q12–18h		
	40–59	q18–24h		
	<40	q24–48h		
	HD:	Monitor serum level 1 h after HD; supplemental dose after HD as needed		
Imipenem	>71	125–500 mg q6–12h	No change	See manufacturer's recommendations for dose adjustments based on severity of infection, weight, and renal function
	41–70	125–500 mg q6–8h		
	21–40	125–250 mg q6–12h		
	6–20	125–250 mg q12h		
	HD:	Suppl. dose after HD and at 12 h intervals; patients with CrCl <5 ml/min/1.73M^2 should not receive imipenem if HD not instituted within 48 h		
Isoniazid	No change		Decrease	
Labetalol	No change		Decrease	
Lamivudine	>50	150 mg bid	No change	
	30–49	150 mg qd		
	15–29	150 mg once, then 100 mg qd		
	5–14	150 mg once, then 50 mg qd		
	<5	50 mg once, then 25 mg qd		
Lansoprazole	No change		Consider dosage in patients with severe liver disease	

Lepirudin	>60	0.15 mg/kg/h	No change	Maintain aPTT 1.5–2.5 times control
	45–60	0.075 mg/kg/h		
	30–44	0.045 mg/kg/h		
	15–29	0.0225 mg/kg/h		
	<15	Avoid or stop infusion		
Levofloxacin	>50	0.5–1 g q24h	No change	
	20–49	0.5 g initially, then 0.25 g q24h		
	10–19	0.5 g initially, then 0.25 g q48h		
	HD	0.5 g initially, then 0.25 g q48h		
Lidocaine	No change		Maintenance dose 2 mg/min or less	Adjust dosage based on serum concentrations and patient's clinical response
Linezolid	HD	Reduce	No change	
Lisinopril	10–30	5 mg qd	No change	
	<10	2.5 mg qd		
Lorazepam	No change		No change	
Meperidine	>50	q3–4h	Decrease	Should avoid in patients with CrCl <10 ml/min
	10–50	q6h (25% decrease)		Metabolite accumulates in renal failure and may produce seizures
Meropenem	>50	1 g q8h	No change	
	26–50	1 g q12h		
	10–25	0.5 g q12h		
	<10	0.5 g q24h		
	HD:	Unknown		
Methadone	>50	q6h	Decrease	Significant accumulation with repetitive dosing
	10–50	q8h		
	<10	q8–12h		
Methyldopa	>10	0.25–1 g q6h	Avoid	
	<10	Decrease		
Metoclopramide	<40	50% of recommended dose	No change	
Metoprolol	No change		Decrease	

(continued)

TABLE 13.3. *(continued)* **Dosage Adjustments in Renal and Hepatic Failure**

Agent	Adjustment in Renal Failure (CrCl: ml/min/1.73 M^2)		Adjustment in Hepatic Failure	Comments
	CrCl	Dosage		
Metronidazole	<10	500 mg q12h	Decrease dosage in severe disease	
Midazolam	Decrease		Decrease	Active metabolites contribute to effect
Milrinone	50	0.43 μg/kg/min	No change	
	40	0.38 μg/kg/min		
	30	0.33 μg/kg/min		
	20	0.28 μg/kg/min		
	10	0.23 μg/kg/min		
	5	0.2 μg/kg/min		
Minoxidil	See Comments		No change	Patients with renal failure or those receiving dialysis may require approximately 1/3 less drug than in patients who are not receiving dialysis; in patients receiving dialysis, the dose should be administered after dialysis
Moexipril	>40	7.5–30 mg qd		
	<40	3.75–15 mg qd		
Mycophenolate	<25	Avoid doses >1 g bid		
Nadolol	>50	q24h	No change	
	31–50	q24–36h		
	10–30	q24–48h		
	<10	q40–60h		
Nafcillin	No change		Decrease dosage in severe disease	

Nicardipine	20 mg PO tid with conventional capsules or 30 mg PO bid with sustained release capsules		Severe liver failure: 20 mg PO bid with conventional release capsules	In liver failure, oral bioavailability may increase by four-fold Severe hepatic failure dosing should be reduced from tid to bid Use with caution in patients with portal hypertension Sustained-release capsules should be avoided in patients with hepatic failure
Nimodipine	No change		30 mg PO q4h	Blood pressure and heart rate should be monitored
Nitroprusside	See Comments		No change	Maintain thiocyanate concentration <10 mg/dL
Oxacillin	No change		Decrease in severe disease	
Pancuronium	See Comments		See Comments	Active metabolite accumulates in renal failure Monitor paralysis with train-of-four nerve stimulation
Penicillin	>50 10–50 <10 HD:	2–4 MU q2–6h 1–2 MU q4–6h 0.5–1 MU q8–12h or 1–2 MU q12–18h Suppl. dosage after HD	No change	Maximum recommended dose in renal failure is 4–10 MU/24h Patients with combined renal and liver disease may need further dosage reductions
Pentamidine	>50 10–50 <10	4 mg/kg q24h 4 mg/kg q36h 4 mg/kg q48h	No change	
Pentobarbital	No change		See Comments	Adjust dosage based on serum concentrations and patient's clinical response
Phenobarbital	No change		See Comments	Adjust dosage based on serum concentrations and patient's clinical response

(continued)

TABLE 13.3. *(continued)* **Dosage Adjustments in Renal and Hepatic Failure**

Agent	Adjustment in Renal Failure (CrCl: ml/min/1.73 M^2)		Adjustment in Hepatic Failure	Comments
	CrCl	Dosage		
Phenytoin	No change		Decrease dose in severe disease	Adjust dosage based on unbound "free" phenytoin serum concentrations and patient's clinical response
Pindolol	No change		Decrease	
Piperacillin	>40 20–40 <20 HD:	2–4 g q4–6h 3–4 g q8h 3–4 g q12h 2 g q8h and 1 g after HD	No change	
Piperacillin-tazobactam	>40 20–40 <20 HD:	3.375 g q6h 2.25 g q6h 2.25 g q8h 2.25 g q8h and 0.75 g after HD	No change	
Prazosin	1 mg bid		No change	Patients with chronic renal failure may require only small doses of the drug
Primidone	No change		Decrease	Avoid in severe liver disease Adjust dosage based on serum concentrations and patient's clinical response
Procainamide	Normal: Mild: Moderate: Severe:	2.7 mg/kg/h 2.0 mg/kg/h 1.5 mg/kg/h 1.0 mg/kg/h	No change	Adjust dosage based on serum concentrations and patient's clinical response
Propoxyphene	Decrease		Decrease	
Propranolol	No change		Decrease	
Quinidine	No change		Decrease	Adjust dosage based on serum concentrations and patient's clinical response

Quinapril	>60	10 mg qd	No change	
	30–60	5 mg qd		
	10–30	2.5 mg qd		
	<10	Insufficient data for recommendations		
Ramipril	<40	25% of normal dose	No change	
Ranitidine	>50	50 mg IV q6–8h	No change	
	10–50	75% of normal dose q24h		
	<10	50% of normal dose q24h		
Rifampin	No change		Decrease	Dosage should be decreased in patients with hepatic/biliary obstruction
Rimantadine	<10	100 mg qd	Severe liver failure: 100 mg qd	
Rocuronium	No change		See Comments	Hepatic disease extends clinical duration Monitor paralysis with train-of-four nerve stimulation
Sotalol	>60	80 mg q12h	No change	Each incremental dosage increase should be made only after a given dosage has been repeated at least 5 or 6 times at the dosing interval appropriate for the degree of renal impairment
	30–59	80 mg q24h		
	10–30	80 mg q36–48h		
	<10	Individualize		
Stavudine	Weight >60 kg			
	>50	40 mg q12h		
	26–50	20 mg q12h		
	10–25	20 mg q24h		
	<10 or HD:	Unknown		
	Weight <60 kg			
	>50	30 mg q12h		
	26–50	15 mg q12h		
	10–25	15 mg q24h		
	<10 or HD:	Unknown		

(continued)

TABLE 13.3. *(continued)* **Dosage Adjustments in Renal and Hepatic Failure**

Agent	Adjustment in Renal Failure (CrCl: ml/min/1.73 M^2)		Adjustment in Hepatic Failure	Comments
	CrCl	Dosage		
Streptomycin	50–80 10–50 <10 HD:	7.5 mg/kg q24h 7.5 mg/kg q24–72h 7.5 mg/kg q72–96h 50% to 75% of the initial loading dosage after dialysis	No change	Therapy may begin with an initial 1 g loading dose Adjust dosage based on serum levels and patient's clinical response
Tacrolimus	See Comments		See Comments	Adjust dosage based on serum levels and patient's clinical response
Tetracycline	Reduce		Use with caution	Doxycycline is the preferred agent in patients with renal failure
Thiopental	No change		Decrease	
Ticarcillin-clavulanic acid	>60 30–60 10–30 <10 HD:	3.1 g q4–6h 2 g q4h 2 g q8h 2 g q12h 3.1 g initially, then 2 g q12h with suppl. dosage after HD	No change	Patients with CrCl <10 ml/min and hepatic dysfunction should receive 3.1 g initially, then 2 g q24h
Tigecycline	No change		Severe liver disease: 100 mg initially, then 25 mg q12h	No adjustment required in mild to moderate liver disease
Timolol	Decrease		Decrease	
Tirofiban	<30	1/2 the usual infusion rate	No change	
Tobramycin	>160 100–159 60–99 40–59 <40 HD:	q6–8h q8–12h q12–18h q18–24h q24–48h Monitor serum level 1 h after HD, suppl. dosage after HD as needed	No change	Adjust dosage based on serum levels and patient's clinical response In critically ill patients, dosing intervals are increased secondary to increased fluid accumulation and reduced renal function

Torsemide	Edema of chronic renal failure 10–20 mg IV/PO qd as a single dosage, doses may be doubled to maximum 200 mg/d		Edema in patients with hepatic cirrhosis: 5–10 mg IV/PO qd as a single dosage, doses may be doubled to maximum 40 mg/d	
Tramadol	>30	50–100 mg q4–6h	50 mg q12h	
	<30	50–100 mg q12h, not to exceed 200 mg/d		
Tranexamic acid	SCr:	IV dose	No change	
	1.36–2.83	10 mg/kg bid		
	2.83–5.66	10 mg/kg qd		
	> 5.66	10 mg/kg q48h or 5 mg/kg qd		
	SCr:	Tablets		
	1.36–2.83	15 mg/kg bid		
	2.83–5.66	15 mg/kg qd		
	>5.66	15 mg/kg q48h or 7.5 mg/kg qd		
Trimethoprim-sulfamethoxazole	>30	Usual dose	Decrease	Patients with CrCl ≤10 ml/min may receive 5 mg/kg TMP qd
	15–30	50%		Monitor serum concentrations; maintain peak sulfa level <150 mg/L
	<15	Avoid		
Valacyclovir	Acute herpes zoster		No change	The rate, but not extent, of conversion of valacyclovir to acyclovir may be reduced in patients with moderate to severe liver disease
	>50	1 g q8h		
	30–49	1 g q12h		
	10–29	1 g q24h		
	<10	0.5 g q24h		
	HD:	Suppl. dose after dialysis		
Valganciclovir	Induction		No change	
	≥60	900 mg bid		
	40–59	450 mg bid		
	25–39	450 mg qd		
	10–24	450 mg qod		

(continued)

TABLE 13.3. *(continued)* **Dosage Adjustments in Renal and Hepatic Failure**

Agent	Adjustment in Renal Failure (CrCl: ml/min/1.73 M^2)		Adjustment in Hepatic Failure	Comments
	CrCl	Dosage		
Valganciclovir (*continued*)	Maintenance/ Prophylaxis ≥60 40–59 25–39 10–24	 900 mg qd 450 mg qd 450 mg qod 450 mg twice weekly	No change	
Valproic acid	No change		Decrease	Adjust dosage based on serum concentrations and patient's clinical response
Vancomycin	>50 30–50 <30	0.5–1g q12h 0.5–1g q24h Per levels	No change	Adjust dosage based on serum concentrations and patient's clinical response
Vecuronium	See Comments		See Comments	Active metabolite accumulates in renal failure Monitor paralysis with train-of-four nerve stimulation
Verapamil	No change		Decrease	
Voriconazole	No change		Decrease maintenance dose by 50% in patients with mild to moderate liver disease	
Warfarin	No change		Decrease	Monitor INR/PT
Zaleplon	No change		Reduce dose to 5 mg hs	Do not use in patients with severe liver disease
Zidovudine	Severe renal impairment: 300–400 mg/d End-stage renal disease on dialysis: 100 mg PO q6–8h or 1 mg/kg IV q6–8h		Unknown	
Zolpidem	No change		5 mg qhs	

aPTT, activated partial thromboplastin time; CAPD; continuous ambulatory peritoneal dialysis; CrCl, creatinine clearance; HD, hemodialysis; INR, international normalized ratio; IV, intravenous; PO, by mouth; PT prothrombin time; TMP, trimethoprim; TMP-SMX, Trimethoprim-sulfamethoxazole.

TABLE 13.4. Peritoneal Dialysis—Local Antibiotic Instillation

Drug	Initial Systemic (IV) Dose	Dialysate Concentration (mg/2L Bag)	Comments
Aminoglycosides			
Amikacin	7.5 mg/kg	12–15 mg	Monitor serum concentrations
Gentamicin	2 mg/kg	8–16 mg	Monitor serum concentrations
Tobramycin	2 mg/kg	8–16 mg	Monitor serum concentrations
Cephalosporins			
Cefazolin	0.5 g	250–500 mg	
Cefotaxime	2 g	500 mg	
Cefoxitin	1 g	200 mg	
Ceftazidime	1 g	250 mg	
Ceftriaxone	1 g	500 mg	
Penicillins			
Ampicillin-Sulbactam	1–2 g	100 mg	
Piperacillin	4 g	500 mg	
Ticarcillin	1–2 g	250 mg	
Quinolones			
Ciprofloxacin	400 mg	50 mg	
Other Antibiotics			
Aztreonam	1 g	500 mg	
Clindamycin	300 mg	300 mg	
Erythromycin	0.5–1 g	150 mg	
Imipenem	0.5–1 g	100–200 mg	
Trimethoprim/ sulfamethoxazole (TMP/SMX)	320/1,600 mg	80/400 mg	
Vancomycin	1 g	30–50 mg	Monitor serum concentrations
Antifungal Agents			
Amphotericin B	0.5 mg/kg (see Table 10.3)	2–8 mg	For serious infections, amphotericin B must be given IV
Fluconazole	—	150 mg IP qod	Administer intraperitoneal dose qod

IP, intraperitoneal; IV, intravenous

TABLE 13.5. Hemofiltration Drug Removal

Drug	CVVH	CVVHD of CVVHDF
Acyclovir	5–7.5 mg/kg q24h	5–7.5 mg/kg q24h
Amikacin	7.5 mg/kg adjust dose based on serum levels	7.5 mg/kg adjust dose based on serum levels
Amphotericin B deoxycholate	0.4–1 mg/kg q24h	0.4–1 mg/kg q24h
Amphotericin B lipid complex	3–5 mg/kg q24h	3–5 mg/kg q24h
Amphotericin B liposomal	3–5 mg/kg q24h	3–5 mg/kg q24h
Ampicillin/sulbactam	3 g q12h	3 g q8h
Aztreonam	1–2 g q12h	2 g q12h
Cefazolin	1–2 g q12h	2 g q12h
Cefepime	1–2 g q12h	2 g q12h
Cefotaxime	1–2 g q12h	2 g q12h
Ceftazidime	1–2 g q12h	2 g q12h
Ceftriaxone	2 g q12–24h	2 g q12–24h
Cefuroxime	1.5 g initially, then 750 mg q24h	NR
Ciprofloxacin	200 mg q12h	200–400 mg q12h
Clindamycin	600–900 mg q8h	600–900 mg q8h
Colistin	2.5 mg/kg q48h	2.5 mg/kg q48h
Daptomycin	4 or 6 mg/kg q48h	4 or 6 mg/kg q48h
Famotidine	10 mg q12h	10 mg q12h
Fluconazole	200–400 mg q24h	400–800 mg q24h
Ganciclovir	NR	5 mg/kg q48h
Gentamicin	2.5–3 mg/kg adjust dose based on serum levels	2.5–3 mg/kg adjust dose based on serum levels
Imipenem-cilastatin	500 mg q8h	500 mg q6–8h
Levofloxacin	250–500 mg q24h	250–500 mg q24h
Linezolid	600 mg q12h	600 mg q12h
Meropenem	0.5–1 g q8–12h	1 g q8–12h
Moxifloxacin	400 mg q24h	400 mg q24h
Nafcillin	2 g q4–6h	2 g q4–6h
Oxacillin	2 g q4–6h	2 g q4–6h
Piperacillin	4 g q12h	NR
Piperacillin/tazobactam	4.5 g q8h	4.5 g q8h
Ranitidine	50 mg q24h	50 mg q24h
Ticarcillin/clavulanate	2 g q6–8h	3.1 g q6h
Tobramycin	2.5–3 mg/kg adjust dose based on serum levels	2.5–3 mg/kg adjust dose based on serum levels
Vancomycin	1 g adjust dose based on serum levels	1 g adjust dose based on serum levels
Voriconazole	4 mg/kg PO q12h	4 mg/kg PO q12h

CVVH, continuous venovenous hemo filtration; CVVHD, continuous venovenous hemodialysis; CVVHDF, continuous veno-venous hemo diafiltration; NR, not recommended; PO, by mouth

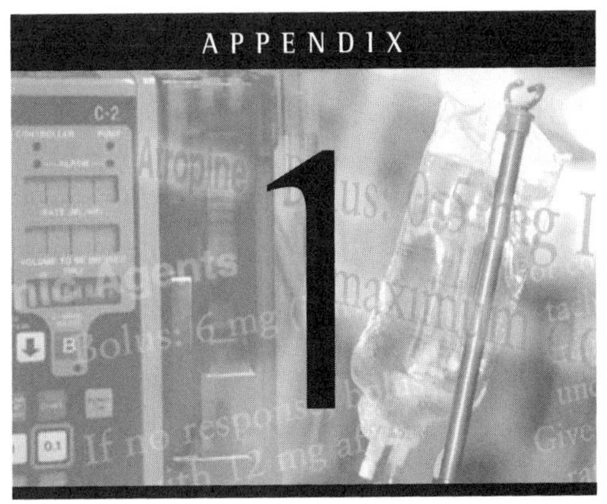

Intravenous Medication Administration Guidelines

Intravenous Medication Administration Guidelines

Drug	Usual Dose Range[a]	Standard Dilution	Maximum Concentration	Adjust for Renal or Hepatic Failure	Infusion Times/Comments/ Drug Interactions
Abciximab					
• Bolus dose:	0.25 mg/kg	Undiluted	2 mg/ml	Renal: no Hepatic: no	Inject over 60 s The dose must be filtered with a 0.22 μm filter prior to injection
• Infusion dose:	10 μg/min for 12 h	9 mg in 250 ml (D5W or 0.9% NaCl)	0.036 mg/ml	Renal: no Hepatic: no	Continuous infusion The dose must be filtered with a 0.22 μm filter prior to dilution
Acetazolamide	5 mg/kg/24h or 250 mg qid-qd	Undiluted	100 mg/ml	Renal: no Hepatic: no	Infuse at 500 mg/min
Acyclovir	5 mg/kg q8h	100 ml (D5W)	7 mg/ml	Renal: yes Hepatic: no	Infuse over at least 60 min
Adenosine	6 mg initially, then 9 mg, then 12 mg	Undiluted	3 mg/ml	Renal: no Hepatic: no	Inject over 1–2 s Drug interactions: theophylline (1), dipyridamole (2)
Alfentanil					
• Bolus dose:	10–25 μg/kg	Undiluted	500 μg/ml	Renal: no Hepatic: yes	Inject over 60 s
• Infusion dose:	0.5–3 μg/kg/min	10,000 μg in 250 ml (D5W)	500 μg/ml	Renal: no Hepatic: yes	Continuous infusion
Amikacin	7.5 mg/kg q12h	50 ml (D5W)	50 mg/ml	Renal: yes Hepatic: no	Infuse over 30 min Drug interaction: neuromuscular blocking agents (3) Therapeutic levels: peak, 20–40 mg/L; trough, <8 mg/L
• High dose extended interval:	20 mg/kg	50 ml (D5W)	50 mg/ml	Renal: yes Hepatic: no	Infuse over 60 min Trough level 0 mg/L before next dose Peak levels unnecessary
Aminocaproic acid	4 g initially, then 1 g/h	20 g in 1000 ml (D5W)	250 mg/ml	Renal: no Hepatic: no	Rapid injection is not recommended, infuse initial dose over 60 min

Drug	Dose	Dilution	Concentration	Dose adjustment	Comments
Aminophylline					
• Loading dose:	6 mg/kg	50 ml (D5W)	25 mg/ml	Renal: no Hepatic: no	Infuse loading dose over 30 min Maximum loading infusion rate 25 mg/min Theophylline dose = 80% of aminophylline dose Drug interactions: cimetidine, ciprofloxacin, erythromycin, clarithromycin (4); see Table 4.6
• Infusion dose: CHF: normal: smoker:	 0.3 mg/kg/h 0.6 mg/kg/h 0.9 mg/kg/h	500 mg in 500 ml (D5W)	10 mg/ml	Renal: no Hepatic: yes	Continuous infusion Therapeutic levels: 10–20 mg/L
Amiodarone					
• First rapid loading infusion:	15 mg/min over first 10 min	150 mg in 100 ml (D5W)	6 mg/ml	Renal: no Hepatic: no	Infuse over 10 min
• Followed by slow loading infusion:	1 mg/min over next 6 h	900 mg in 500 ml (D5W)	6 mg/ml	Renal: no Hepatic: no	Infuse at 33.3 ml/h
• Maintenance infusion:	0.5 mg/min over next 18 h	900 mg in 500 ml (D5W)	6 mg/ml	Renal: no Hepatic: no	Infuse at 16.6 ml/h
• Supplemental infusion:	15 mg/min over 10 min	150 mg in 100 ml (D5W)	6 mg/ml	Renal: no Hepatic: no	Infuse over 10 min
Ammonium chloride	mEq of $H^+ = 0.5 \times$ body weight (kg) $\times$ (103 − serum Cl^-)	100 mEq in 500 ml (0.9% NaCl)	0.2 mEq/ml	Renal: no Hepatic: avoid	Maximum infusion rate is 5 ml/min of a 0.2 mEq/ml solution Correct 1/3 to 1/2 of H^+ deficit while monitoring pH
Amphotericin B	0.5–1.5 mg/kg q24h	250 ml (D5W)	1.4 mg/ml	Renal: no Hepatic: no	Infuse over 2–6 h Do not mix in electrolyte solutions (e.g., 0.9% NaCl, Ringer's lactate)
Amphotericin B Lipid Complex (ABLC)	5 mg/kg/d	D5W to a final concentration of 1 mg/ml	D5W to a final concentration of 2 mg/ml	Renal: no Hepatic: no	Infuse at 2.5 mg/kg/h If the infusion time exceeds 2 h, mix the contents by shaking the bag every 2 h
Ampicillin	0.5–3 g q4–6h	100 ml (0.9% NaCl)	50 mg/ml	Renal: yes Hepatic: no	Infuse over 15–30 min

(continued)

Intravenous Medication Administration Guidelines *(continued)*

Drug	Usual Dose Range[a]	Standard Dilution	Maximum Concentration	Adjust for Renal or Hepatic Failure	Infusion Times/Comments/ Drug Interactions
Ampicillin-sulbactam	1.5–3 g q6h	100 ml (0.9% NaCl)	50 mg/ml	Renal: yes Hepatic: no	Infuse over 15–30 min
Anidulafungin					
• Candidemia and candida infections	200 mg IV on day 1, followed by 100 mg qd	D5W or 0.9% NaCl to a final concentration of 0.5 mg/ml	0.5 mg/ml	Renal: no Hepatic: no	Maximum infusion rate 1.1 mg/min
• Esophageal candidasis	100 mg IV on day 1, followed by 50 mg qd	D5W or 0.9% NaCl to a final concentration of 0.5 mg/ml	0.5 mg/ml	Renal: no Hepatic: no	Maximum infusion rate 1.1 mg/min
Argatroban					Discontinue all parenteral anticoagulants before administering argatroban
• HIT/HITTS	2 μg/kg/min	250 mg in 250 ml (D5W)	1 mg/ml	Renal: no	Continuous infusion
• PCI in HIT/HITTS				Hepatic: yes	Maintain aPTT 1.5–3 times baseline values, not to exceed 100 s
• Bolus dose:	350 μg/kg	250 mg in 250 ml (D5W)	1 mg/ml	Renal: no Hepatic: no	Infuse over 3 to 5 min Check ACT 5–10 min after bolus dose is completed Proceed with procedure if ACT is >300 s
• Infusion:	25 μg/kg/min	250 mg in 250 ml (D5W)	1 mg/ml	Renal: no Hepatic: yes	Continuous infusion
Atenolol	5 mg IV over 5 min, 5 mg IV 10 min later	Undiluted	0.5 mg/ml	Renal: no Hepatic: no	Inject 1 mg/min
Atracurium					
• Intubating dose:	0.4–0.5 mg/kg	Undiluted	10 mg/ml	Renal: no Hepatic: no	Inject over 60 s to prevent histamine release
• Maintenance dose:	0.08–0.1 mg/kg	Undiluted	10 mg/ml	Renal: no Hepatic: no	Drug interactions: aminoglycosides (3), anticonvulsants (5) Monitor train-of-four stimulation
• Infusion dose:	5–9 μg/kg/min	1000 mg in 150 ml (D5W)	10 mg/ml	Renal: no Hepatic: no	Continuous infusion Final volume = 250 ml Concentration = 4 mg/ml Monitor train-of-four stimulation

Azithromycin	500 mg qd for 1–2 d, then convert to oral therapy	1 mg/ml	2 mg/ml	Renal: no Hepatic: no	Infuse the 1 mg/ml final concentration over 3 h and the 2 mg/ml final concentration over 1 h 250 PO = 100 mg IV
Aztreonam	0.5–2 g q6–12h	100 ml (D5W)	200 mg/ml	Renal: yes Hepatic: no	Infuse over 15–30 min
Bivalirudin					
• Bolus dose:	0.75 mg/kg	50 ml (D5W)	5 mg/ml	Renal: yes Hepatic: no	
• Initial infusion:	1.75 mg/kg/h for the duration of the PCI procedure	50 ml (D5W)	5 mg/ml	Renal: yes Hepatic: no	Continuous infusion The ACT should be determined 5 min after the bolus dose; an additional 0.3 mg/kg should be given if needed
• Optional post procedure infusion (up to 4 h):	0.2 mg/kg/h	500 ml (D5W)	0.5 mg/ml	Renal: yes Hepatic: no	Continuous infusion After 4 h the infusion may be continued for up to 20 h post procedure
Bumetanide					
• Bolus dose:	0.5–1 mg	Undiluted	0.5 mg/ml	Renal: no Hepatic: no	Infusion over 3–5 min Maximum rate of injection is 1 mg/min
• Infusion dose:	0.08–0.3 mg/h	2.4 mg in 100 ml (0.9% NaCl)	0.5 mg/ml	Renal: no Hepatic: no	Continuous infusion Monitor electrolytes
Calcium (elemental)	100–200 mg of elemental calcium IV over 15 min followed by 100 mg/h	1,000 mg in 1,000 ml (0.9% NaCl)	1.5 mg/ml	Renal: no Hepatic: no	Ca chloride 1 g = 272 mg (13.6 mEq) of elemental calcium Ca gluconate 1 g = 90 mg (4.65 mEq) of elemental calcium
Caspofungin					
• Day 1 loading dose:	70 mg	250 ml (0.9% NaCl)	0.5 mg/ml	Renal: no Hepatic: yes	Infuse over 60 min
• Maintenance dose:	50 mg qd	250 ml (0.9% NaCl)	0.5 mg/ml	Renal: no Hepatic: yes	Infuse over 60 min
Cefazolin	0.5–1 g q6–8h	50 ml (D5W)	1 g in 10 ml sterile water IVP	Renal: yes Hepatic: no	Infuse over 15–30 min

(continued)

Intravenous Medication Administration Guidelines *(continued)*

Drug	Usual Dose Range[a]	Standard Dilution	Maximum Concentration	Adjust for Renal or Hepatic Failure	Infusion Times/Comments/ Drug Interactions
Cefepime	0.5–2 g q12h	50 ml (D5W)	40 mg/ml	Renal: yes Hepatic: no	Infuse over 30 min
Cefotaxime	1–2 g q4–6h	50 ml (D5W)	1–2 g in 10 ml sterile water IVP	Renal: yes Hepatic: no	Infuse over 15–30 min
Cefoxitin	1–2 g q4–6h	50 ml (D5W)	1–2 g in 10 ml sterile water IVP	Renal: yes Hepatic: no	Infuse over 15–30 min
Ceftazidime	0.5–2 g q8–12h	50 ml (D5W)	1–2 g in 10 ml sterile water IVP	Renal: yes Hepatic: no	Infuse over 15–30 min
Ceftriaxone	0.5–2 g q12–24h	50 ml (D5W)	40 mg/ml	Renal: no Hepatic: no	Infuse over 15–30 min
Cefuroxime	0.75–1.5 g q8h	50 ml (D5W)	0.75 g in 10 ml sterile water IVP	Renal: yes Hepatic: no	Infuse over 15–30 min
Chloramphenicol	0.5–1 g q6h	50 ml (D5W)	100 mg/ml	Renal: yes Hepatic: yes	Infuse over 30 min Therapeutic levels: peak, 10–25 mg/L; trough, 5–10 mg/L
Chlorothiazide	0.5–1 g bid-qid	1 g in 18 ml (sterile water)	1 g in 18 ml	Renal: no Hepatic: no	Inject over 3–5 min
Chlorpromazine	10–50 mg q4–6h	Dilute with 0.9% NaCl to a final concentration of 1 mg/ml	1 mg/ml	Renal: no Hepatic: yes	Infuse at 1 mg/min
Cidofovir	Induction: 5mg/kg q wk × 2 wk Maintenance: 5 mg/kg q2wk	100 ml (0.9% NaCl)	Unknown	Renal: yes Hepatic: no	Infuse over 60 min Cidofovir is contraindicated in patients with a SCr >1.5 mg/dl or CrCl <55 ml/min or urine protein >100 mg/dl

Cimetidine					Drug interactions: theophylline, warfarin, phenytoin, lidocaine, benzodiazepines (6)
• IVPB:	300 mg q6–8h	50 ml (D5W)	15 mg/ml IVP	Renal: yes Hepatic: no	Infuse over 15–30 min
• Infusion dose:	37.5 mg/h	900 mg in 250 ml (D5W)	9 mg/ml	Renal no Hepatic: no	Continuous infusion
Ciprofloxacin	200–400 mg q12h	Premixed solution 2 mg/ml	2 mg/ml	Renal: yes Hepatic: no	Infuse over 60 min Drug interactions: theophylline, warfarin (7)
Cisatracurium					
• Intubating dose:	0.15–0.2 mg/kg	Undiluted	2 mg/ml	Renal: no Hepatic: no	Inject over 60 s
• Maintenance dose:	0.03 mg/kg	Undiluted	2 mg/ml	Renal: no Hepatic: no	Inject over 60 s Monitor train-of-four stimulation
• Infusion dose:	3 μg/kg/min	Add 200 mg (20 ml) to D5W 180 ml	10 mg/ml	Renal: no Hepatic: no	Continuous infusion Final concentrations is 1 mg/ml Monitor train-of-four stimulation
Clindamycin	150–900 mg q8h	100 ml (D5W)	12 mg/ml	Renal: no Hepatic: yes	Infuse over 30–60 min
Conjugated estrogens	0.6 mg/kg/d × 5 d	50 ml (0.9% NaCl)	5 mg/ml	Renal: no Hepatic: no	Infuse over 30 min
Cosyntropin	0.25 mg	Undiluted	0.25 mg/ml	Renal: no Hepatic: no	Inject over 60 s
Cyclosporine	5–6 mg/kg q24h	100 ml (D5W)	2.5 mg/ml	Renal: no Hepatic: no	Infuse over 2–6 h Drug interactions: digoxin (8), erythromycin (9), amphotericin B, nonsteroidal anti-inflammatory drugs (10) IV dose = 1/3 PO dose Therapeutic levels: See Table 13.1
Dantrolene					
• Bolus dose:	1–2 mg/kg (maximum dose 10 mg/kg)	60 ml sterile water (*not* dextrose or electrolyte solutions)	0.33 mg/ml	Renal: no Hepatic: no	Administer as rapidly as possible

(continued)

Intravenous Medication Administration Guidelines *(continued)*

Drug	Usual Dose Range[a]	Standard Dilution	Maximum Concentration	Adjust for Renal or Hepatic Failure	Infusion Times/Comments/ Drug Interactions
Dantrolene (*continued*)					
• Maintenance dose:	2.5 mg/kg q4h × 24 h	60 ml sterile water	0.33 mg/ml	Renal: no Hepatic: no	Infuse over 60 min
Daptomycin	4 mg/kg q24h	100 ml (0.9% NaCl)	5 mg/ml	Renal: yes Hepatic: no	Infuse over 30 min Do not mix with dextrose-containing solutions
Desmopressin	0.3 μg/kg	50 ml (0.9% NaCl)	4 μg/ml	Renal: no Hepatic: no	Infuse over 15–30 min
Dexamethasone	0.5–20 mg q6–24h	50 ml (0.9% NaCl)	4 mg/ml	Renal: no Hepatic: no	May give doses ≤10 mg undiluted IV over 60 s
Dexmedetomidine					
• Loading dose:	1 μg/kg over 10 min	100 μg in 48 ml (0.9% NaCl)	2 μg/ml	Renal: no Hepatic: yes	Infuse over 10 min
• Maintenance dose:	0.2–0.7 μg/kg/h	100 μg in 48 ml (0.9% NaCl)	2 μg/ml	Renal: no Hepatic: yes	Continuous infusion Continuous infusion not to exceed 24 h
Diazepam	2.5–10 mg q2–4h	Undiluted	5 mg/ml	Renal: no Hepatic: yes	Inject at 2–5 mg/m
Diazoxide	50–150 mg q5–15 min	Undiluted	15 mg/ml	Renal: no Hepatic: no	Inject over 30 s Maximum 150 mg/dose
Digoxin					
• Loading dose:	1–1.25 mg over 8–24 h	Undiluted	0.25 mg/ml	Renal: no Hepatic: no	Inject over 3–5 min
• Maintenance dose:	0.125–0.375 mg q24h	Undiluted	0.25 mg/ml	Renal: yes Hepatic: no	Inject over 3–5 min Drug interactions: amiodarone, cyclosporine, quinidine, verapamil (8) Therapeutic levels: 0.5–2 ng/ml
Diltiazem					
• Bolus dose:	0.25–0.35 mg/kg	Undiluted	5 mg/ml	Renal: no Hepatic: no	Inject over 2 min
• Infusion dose:	5–15 mg/h	125 mg in 100 ml (D5W)	1 mg/ml	Renal: no Hepatic: no	Continuous infusion

Diphenhydramine	25–100 mg q2–4h	Undiluted	50 mg/ml	Renal: no Hepatic: no	Inject over 3–5 min Competitive histamine antagonist, doses >1,000 mg/24h may be required
Dobutamine	2.5–20 μg/kg/min	500 mg in 250 ml (D5W)	8 mg/ml	Renal: no Hepatic: no	Continuous infusion
Dolasetron					May prolong QT interval Administer with caution in patients with conduction system abnormalities or electrolyte abnormalities
• Post-op nausea and vomiting:	12.5 mg 15 min before cessation of surgery or as soon as nausea and vomiting present	12.5 mg IVP	12.5 mg	Renal: no Hepatic: no	Inject over 30 seconds
• Chemotherapy induced nausea and vomiting:	100 mg 30 min before chemotherapy	100 mg IVP	100 mg	Renal: no Hepatic: no	Inject over 30 s
Dopamine	2.5–20μg/kg/min	400 mg in 250 ml (D5W)	8 mg/ml	Renal: no Hepatic: no	Continuous infusion
Doxacurium					
• Intubating dose:	0.025–0.08 mg/kg	Undiluted	1 mg/ml	Renal: no Hepatic: no	Inject over 5–10 s
• Maintenance dose:	0.005–0.01 mg/kg	Undiluted	1 mg/ml	Renal: yes Hepatic: no	Inject over 5–10 s Dose based on lean body weight Drug interactions: aminoglycosides (3), anticonvulsants (5) Monitor train-of-four stimulation
• Infusion dose:	0.25 μg/kg/min	10 mg in 100 ml (D5W)	1 mg/ml	Renal: yes Hepatic: no	Continuous infusion Dose based on lean body weight Drug interactions: aminoglycosides (3), anticonvulsants (5) Monitor train-of-four stimulation The 1:10 dilution is only stable for 8 h after preparation

(continued)

Intravenous Medication Administration Guidelines *(continued)*

Drug	Usual Dose Range[a]	Standard Dilution	Maximum Concentration	Adjust for Renal or Hepatic Failure	Infusion Times/Comments/ Drug Interactions
Doxycycline	100–200 mg q12–24h	250 ml (D5W)	1 mg/ml	Renal: no Hepatic: yes	Infuse over 60 min
Droperidol					
• Bolus dose:	0.625–10 mg q1–4h	Undiluted	2.5 mg/ml	Renal: no Hepatic: yes	Inject over 60 s
• Infusion dose:	1–20 mg/h	50 mg in 100 ml (D5W)	2.5 mg/ml (D5W)	Renal: no Hepatic: yes	Continuous infusion Monitor QT interval and electrolytes
Drotrecogin alfa	24 μg/kg/h × 96 h	50–250 ml (0.9% NaCL)	0.2 mg/ml	Renal: no Hepatic: no	Continuous infusion Avoid in patients with single organ dysfunction and recent surgery
Edrophonium	500–1,000 μg/kg	Undiluted	10 mg/ml	Renal: no Hepatic: no	Inject over 60 s Rapid onset, not useful for deep blocks
Enalaprilat	0.625–5 mg q6h	Undiluted	1.25 mg/ml	Renal: yes Hepatic: no	Inject over 5 min Initial dose for patients on diuretics is 0.625 mg
Epinephrine	1–4 μg/min	1 mg in 250 ml (D5W)	0.05 mg/ml	Renal: no Hepatic: no	Continuous infusion
Epoetin α	50–100 U/kg 3 × /wk	Undiluted	20,000 U/ml	Renal: no Hepatic: no	Inject over 3–5 min Maintenance doses range between 12.5–252 U/kg 3 × /wk
Eptifibatide					
• Acute coronary syndrome:	180 μg/kg bolus, then 2 μg/kg/min	Undiluted bolus dose 2 mg/ml Infusion 0.75 mg/ml	Undiluted bolus dose 2 mg/ml Infusion 0.75 mg/ml	Renal: yes Hepatic: no	Withdraw bolus dose from 2 mg/ml, 10 ml vial Continuous infusion
• PCI without ACS:	180 μg/kg bolus × 2, then 2 μg/kg/min				2nd bolus dose administered 10 min after 1st bolus dose
Ertapenem	1 g q24h	1 g in 50 ml (0.9% NaCl)	20 mg/ml	Renal: yes Hepatic: no	Infuse over 30 min

Erythromycin	0.5–1 g q6h	250 ml (0.9% NaCl)	20 mg/ml	Renal: no Hepatic: yes	Infuse over 60 min Drug interactions: theophylline (4), cyclosporine (9)
Esmolol					
• Bolus dose:	500 μg/kg	Undiluted	10 mg/ml	Renal: no Hepatic: no	Inject over 60 s Use 100 mg vial for bolus dose
• Infusion dose:	50–300 μg/kg/min	5g in 500 ml (D5W)	10 mg/ml	Renal: no Hepatic: yes	Continuous infusion
Esomeprazole	20–40 mg q24h	50 ml (0.9% NaCl)	8 mg/ml (IV Bolus)	Renal: no Hepatic: yes	Infuse over 10–30 min Inject IV bolus over at least 3 min
Etomidate	0.3–0.4 mg/kg	Undiluted	2 mg/ml	Renal: no Hepatic: no	Inject over 60 s
Famotidine	20 mg q12h	100 ml (D5W)	20 mg/5ml 0.9% NaCl IVP	Renal: yes Hepatic: no	Infuse over 15–30 min Inject IVP dose over 3–5 min
Fenoldopam	0.01–1.6 μg/kg/min	10 mg in 500 ml (D5W)	40 μg/ml	Renal: no Hepatic: no	Do not use a bolus dose Continuous infusion Titrate infusion no more frequently than every 15 min Recommended increments for titration are 0.05–0.1 μg/kg/min
Fentanyl					
• Bolus dose:	25–75 μg q1–2h	Undiluted	50 μg/ml	Renal: no Hepatic: no	Inject over 5–10 s
• Infusion dose:	50–100 μg/h	50 μg/ml	50 μg/ml	Renal: no Hepatic: no	Continuous infusion
Filgastrim (GCSF)	5–10 μg/kg × 2–4 wk	Dilute in D5W to a final concentration of 5–15 μg/ml	15 μg/ml	Renal: no Hepatic: no	Infuse over 15–30 min Preferred route of administration is SC To protect against adsorption to plastic materials, albumin must be added to a final concentration of 2 mg/ml Do not dilute with saline at any time; product may precipitate

(continued)

Intravenous Medication Administration Guidelines *(continued)*

Drug	Usual Dose Range[a]	Standard Dilution	Maximum Concentration	Adjust for Renal or Hepatic Failure	Infusion Times/Comments/ Drug Interactions
Fluconazole	100–800 mg q24h	Premixed solution 2 mg/ml	2 mg/ml	Renal: yes Hepatic: no	Maximum infusion rate 200 mg/h
Flumazenil					
• Reversal of conscious sedation:	0.2 mg initially, then 0.2 mg q1min to a total of 1 mg	Undiluted	0.1 mg/ml	Renal: no Hepatic: no	Inject over 15 s Maximum dose of 3 mg in any 1 h period
• Benzodiazepine overdose:	0.2 mg initially, then 0.3 mg × 1 dose, then 0.5 mg q30s up to a total of 3 mg	Undiluted	0.1 mg/ml	Renal: no Hepatic: no	Maximum dose of 3 mg in any 1 h period
• Infusion dose:	0.1–0.5 mg/h	5 mg in 1,000 ml (D5W)	0.1 mg/ml	Renal: no Hepatic: no	Continuous infusion
Foscarnet					
• Induction dose:	60 mg/kg q8h	Undiluted	24 mg/ml	Renal: yes Hepatic: no	Infuse over 1 h
• Maintenance dose:	90–120 mg/kg q24h	Undiluted	24 mg/ml	Renal: yes Hepatic: no	Infuse over 2 h
Fosphenytoin					
• Status epilepticus loading dose:	15–20 mg PE/kg	Dilute to a final concentration from 1.5 to 25 mg PE/ml with D5W or 0.9% NaCl	25 mg PE/ml	Renal: no Hepatic: no	Fosphenytoin 75 mg/ml = phenytoin 50 mg/ml Infusion rate 100–150 mg PE/min Continuous monitoring of ECG, BP, respiration Peak phenytoin levels occur approximately 2 h after end of infusion
• Nonemergent loading and maintenance dose:	10–20 mg PE/kg	Dilute to a final concentration from 1.5 to 25 mg PE/ml with D5W or 0.9% NaCl	25 mg PE/ml	Renal: no Hepatic: yes	Should not be administered IM for the treatment of status epilepticus
• Initial daily maintenance dose:	4–6 mg PE/kg/d	Dilute to a final concentration from 1.5 to 25 mg PE/ml with D5W or 0.9% NaCl	25 mg PE/ml	Renal: no Hepatic: yes	Phenytoin therapeutic levels: 10–20 mg/L

• IM/IV substitution for oral phenytoin therapy:	Substitute with same total daily dose	Dilute to a final concentration from 1.5 to 25 mg PE/ml with D5W or 0.9% NaCl	25 mg PE/ml	Renal: no Hepatic: yes	
Furosemide					
• Bolus dose:	20–40 mg q1–2h	Undiluted	10 mg/ml	Renal: no Hepatic: no	Maximum injection rate 40 mg/min Up to 400–800 mg/dose may be required in some patients
• Infusion dose:	2–20 mg/h	100 mg in 100 ml (0.9% NaCl)	10 mg/ml	Renal: no Hepatic: no	Continuous infusion Monitor electrolytes
Ganciclovir	2.5 mg/kg q12h	100 ml (D5W)	10 mg/ml	Renal: yes Hepatic: no	Infuse over 1 h
Gatifloxacin	400 mg qd	250 ml (D5W)	2 mg /ml	Renal: yes Hepatic: no	Infuse over 60 min
Gentamicin					
• Loading dose:	2–3 mg/kg	50 ml (D5W)	40 mg/ml	Renal: no Hepatic: no	Infuse over 30 min
• Maintenance dose:	1.5–2.5 mg/kg q8–24h	50 ml (D5W)	40 mg/ml	Renal: yes Hepatic: no	Infuse over 30 min Critically ill patients have an increased volume of distribution requiring increased doses Drug interaction: neuromuscular blocking agents (3) Therapeutic levels: peak, 4–10 mg/L, trough <2 mg/L
• High dose extended interval:	5–8 mg/kg	50 ml (D5W)	40 mg/ml	Renal: yes Hepatic: no	Infuse over 60 min Trough level 0 mg/L before next dose Peak levels unnecessary
Glucagon	0.5–3 mg followed by 1–20 mg/h	100 mg in 100 ml (D5W)	10 mg/ml	Renal: no Hepatic: no	Continuous infusion May cause hypokalemia, hyperglycemia, and tachycardia
Glycopyrrolate	5–15 μg/kg	Undiluted	0.2 mg/ml	Renal: no Hepatic: no	Inject over 60 s

(continued)

Intravenous Medication Administration Guidelines *(continued)*

Drug	Usual Dose Range[a]	Standard Dilution	Maximum Concentration	Adjust for Renal or Hepatic Failure	Infusion Times/Comments/ Drug Interactions
Granisetron					
• Chemotherapy-induced nausea and vomiting resistant to standard antiemetic therapy	10 μg/kg IVP starting 30 min before the emetogenic drug	Undiluted	1 mg/ml	Renal: no Hepatic: no	Inject over 60 s
• Postoperative nausea and vomiting	20–40 μg/kg as a single dose	Undiluted	1 mg/ml	Renal: no Hepatic: no	Infuse over 5 min
Haloperidol lactate					
• Bolus dose:	1–10 mg q2–4h	Undiluted	5 mg/ml	Renal: no Hepatic: no	Inject over 3–5 min In urgent situations, the dose may be doubled every 20–30 min until an effect is obtained Decanoate salt is only for IM administration
• Infusion dose:	1–10 mg/h	200 mg in 160 ml (D5W) (1 mg/ml)	Pure drug: 5 mg/ml D5W: 3 mg/ml; 0.9% NaCl: 0.75 mg/ml	Renal: no Hepatic: yes	Continuous infusion Monitor QT interval and electrolytes
Hydralazine	5–20 mg q4–6h	Undiluted	20 mg/ml	Renal: no Hepatic: no	Inject over 60 s
Hydrochloric acid	H^+ deficit in mEq = 0.5 × (body weight in kg) × (103-serum Cl^-)	1 mEq/10 ml (sterile water)	1 mEq/10 ml	Renal: no Hepatic: no	Maximum infusion rate = 0.2 mEq/kg/h

Hydrocortisone	12.5–100 mg q6–12h	Undiluted	50 mg/ml	Renal: no Hepatic: no	Inject over 60 s
Hydromorphone	1–4 mg q4–6h	Undiluted	4 mg/ml	Renal: no Hepatic: no	Inject over 60 s Dilaudid-HP available as 10 mg/ml
Ibutilide	≥60 kg: 1 mg <60 kg: 0.01 mg/kg	50 ml (D5W)	Undiluted 1 mg/10 ml	Renal: no Hepatic: no	Infuse over 10 min If arrhythmia does not terminate within 10 min after initial dose, a second dose may be administered over 10 min, 10 min after the completion of the first dose Continuous ECG monitoring for at least 4 h following infusion or until QTc has returned to baseline
Imipenem	0.5–1 g q6–8h	100 ml (D5W)	5 mg/ml	Renal: yes Hepatic: no	Infuse over 30–60 min
Isoniazid	300 mg qd	50 ml (D5W)	Unknown	Renal: yes Hepatic: yes	Infuse over 15–30 min IM preparation is used for IV administration
Isoproterenol	1–10 μg/min	2 mg in 500 ml (D5W)	0.2 mg/ml	Renal: no Hepatic: no	Continuous infusion
Ketamine					
• Bolus dose:	1–2 mg/kg	Undiluted	100 mg/ml	Renal: no Hepatic: no	Inject over 60 s
• Infusion dose:	9–45 μg/kg/min	200 mg in 500 ml (D5W)	100 mg/ml	Renal: no Hepatic: no	Continuous infusion
Labetalol					
• Bolus dose:	20 mg q15min	Undiluted	5 mg/ml	Renal: no Hepatic: no	Inject over 2 min
• Infusion dose:	1–4 mg/min	200 mg in 160 ml (D5W)	1 mg/ml	Renal: no Hepatic: yes	Continuous infusion
Lansoprazole	30 mg qd	30 mg in 50 ml (D5W)	0.6 mg/ml	Renal: no Hepatic: no	Administer over 30 min Must administer through the in-line filter provided

(continued)

Intravenous Medication Administration Guidelines *(continued)*

Drug	Usual Dose Range[a]	Standard Dilution	Maximum Concentration	Adjust for Renal or Hepatic Failure	Infusion Times/Comments/ Drug Interactions
Lepirudin					
• Bolus dose:	0.4 mg/kg	5 mg/ml	5 mg/ml	Renal: yes Hepatic: no	Inject over 15 sec In patients weighing >110 kg, do not exceed the dose for a 110 kg patient
• Infusion dose:	0.15 mg/kg/h	100 mg in 500 ml (D5W)	0.4 mg/ml	Renal: yes Hepatic: no	Continuous infusion Adjust aPTT to 1.5–2.5 times control
Levofloxacin	250–750 mg qd	Premixed solution 5 mg/ml	5 mg/ml	Renal: yes Hepatic: no	Infuse over 60 min
Levorphanol	2 mg q4–6h	Undiluted	2 mg/ml	Renal: no Hepatic: no	Inject over 60 s
Levothyroxine	25–200 μg q24h	Undiluted	100 μg/ml	Renal: no Hepatic: no	Inject over 5–10 s IV dose = 75% of PO dose
Lidocaine					
• Bolus dose:	1 mg/kg	Undiluted	10 mg/ml	Renal: no Hepatic: yes	Inject over 60 s Drug interaction: cimetidine (6)
• Infusion dose:	1–4 mg/min	2 g in 500 ml (D5W)	16 mg/ml	Renal: no Hepatic: yes	Continuous infusion Therapeutic levels: 1.5–5.0 mg/L
Linezolid	600 mg q12h	Undiluted	2 mg/ml	Renal: yes Hepatic: no	Infuse over 30 min
Lorazepam					
• Bolus dose:	0.5–2 mg q1–4h	Undiluted	1 mg/ml	Renal: no Hepatic: no	Inject 2 mg/min Dilute 1:1 with 0.9% NaCl before administration
• Infusion dose:	0.02–0.1 mg/kg/h	20–40 mg in 250 ml (D5W)	2 mg/ml Dilute 1:1 with 0.9% NaCl before administration	Renal: no Hepatic: no	Continuous infusion Lorazepam should be diluted in glass IV containers because it may be adsorbed onto plastic IV containers

Magnesium (elemental)					Magnesium sulfate 1 g = 8 mEq = elemental magnesium 98 mg
• Magnesium deficiency:	25 mEq over 24 h followed by 6 mEq over the next 12 h	25 mEq in 1,000 ml (D5W)	1 mEq/ml	Renal: yes Hepatic: no	
• Ventricular arrhythmias:	16 mEq over 1 h followed by 40 mEq over 6 h	40 mEq in 1,000 ml (D5W)	1 mEq/ml	Renal: yes Hepatic: no	16 mEq (2 g) may be diluted in 100 ml D5W and infused over 1 h
Mannitol					
• Diuretic:	12.5–100 g over 1–2 h	Undiluted	250 mg/ml	Renal: no Hepatic: no	Inject over 3–5 min
• Cerebral edema:	0.25–0.5 g/kg q4h	Undiluted	250 mg/ml	Renal: no Hepatic: no	Inject over 3–5 min
Meperidine	25–100 mg q2–4h	Undiluted	100 mg/ml	Renal: yes Hepatic: yes	Inject over 60 s Avoid in renal failure Neurotoxic metabolite, normeperidine causes seizures
Meropenem	1 g q8h	100 ml (D5W)	1 g/30 ml IVP	Renal: yes Hepatic: no	Infuse over 15–30 min Injection over 3–5 min
Methadone	5–20 mg qd	Undiluted	10 mg/ml	Renal: yes Hepatic: yes	Inject over 3–5 min Accumulation with repetitive dosing
Methyldopa	250–1,000 mg q6h	100 ml (D5W)	10 mg/ml	Renal: yes Hepatic: yes	Infuse over 30–60 min
Methyl-prednisolone	10–250 mg q6h	Undiluted	62.5 mg/ml	Renal: no Hepatic: no	Inject over 60 s
Metoclopramide					
• For intubation of small intestine:	10 mg × 1 dose	Undiluted	5 mg/ml	Renal: no Hepatic: no	Inject over 3–5 min
Metoprolol	5 mg q2min × 3	Undiluted	1 mg/ml	Renal: no Hepatic: yes	Inject over 60 s
Metronidazole	500 mg q6h	Premixed solution 5 mg/ml	5 mg/ml	Renal: yes Hepatic: yes	Infuse over 30 min

(continued)

Intravenous Medication Administration Guidelines *(continued)*

Drug	Usual Dose Range[a]	Standard Dilution	Maximum Concentration	Adjust for Renal or Hepatic Failure	Infusion Times/Comments/ Drug Interactions
Micafungin					
• Treatment:	150 mg qd	100 ml (0.9% NaCl)	1.5 mg/ml	Renal: no Hepatic: no	Infusion over 1 h
• Prophylaxis:	50 mg qd	100 ml (0.9% NaCl)	1.5 mg/ml	Renal: no Hepatic: no	Infusion over 1 h
Midazolam					
• Bolus dose:	0.025–0.35 mg/kg q1–2h	Undiluted	5 mg/ml	Renal: no Hepatic: yes	Inject 0.5 mg/min
• Infusion dose:	0.5–5 μg/kg/min	50 mg in 100 ml (D5W)	5 mg/ml	Renal: yes Hepatic: yes	Continuous infusion Unpredictable clearance in critically ill patients Active metabolites accumulate in renal failure and contribute to pharmacologic effect
Milrinone					
• Loading dose:	50 μg/kg	Undiluted	0.4 mg/ml	Renal: no Hepatic: no	Infuse over 10 min The loading dose may be given undiluted, but diluting to a rounded total volume of 10 or 20 ml may simplify the visualization of the injection rate
• Maintenance dose:	0.375–0.75 μg/kg/min	Premixed solution 0.2 mg/ml	0.4 mg/ml	Renal: yes Hepatic: no	Continuous infusion
Mivacurium					
• Intubating dose:	0.15–0.25 mg/kg	Undiluted	2 mg/ml	Renal: no Hepatic: no	Inject over 60 s Rapid injection associated with histamine release
• Maintenance dose:	0.01–0.1 mg/kg	Undiluted	2 mg/ml	Renal: no Hepatic: no	Inject over 60 s Monitor train-of-four-stimulation Drug interactions: aminoglycosides (3), anticonvulsants (5)
• Infusion dose:	9–10 μg/kg/min	50 mg in 100 ml (D5W)	0.5 mg/ml	Renal: no Hepatic: no	Continuous infusion Monitor train-of-four stimulation

• Bolus dose:	2–10 mg q1–2h	Undiluted	15 mg/ml	Renal: no Hepatic: no	Inject over 60 s
• Infusion dose:	2–5 mg/h	100 mg in 100 ml (D5W)	15 mg/ml	Renal: yes Hepatic: no	Continuous infusion Active metabolites accumulate in renal failure and contribute to pharmacologic effect
Moxifloxacin	400 mg qd	Premixed solution 1.6 mg/ml	1.6 mg/ml	Renal: no Hepatic: no	Infuse over 60 min
Mycophenolate					
• Renal or hepatic transplant:	1 g q12h	D5W final concentration 6 mg/ml	6 mg/ml	Renal: yes Hepatic: no	Infuse over 2 h
• Cardiac transplant:	1.5 g q12h	D5W final concentration 6 mg/ml	6 mg/ml	Renal: yes Hepatic: no	Infuse over 2 h
Nafcillin	0.5–2 g q4–6h	100 ml (D5W)	250 mg/ml	Renal: no Hepatic: yes	Infuse over 30–60 min
Nalmefene	0.25 μg/kg q2-5min up to a max dose of 1 μg/kg	IVP May dilute 1:1 with saline or sterile water	100 μg/ml	Renal: no Hepatic: no	Infuse over 60 s In cases in which the patient is at increased cardiovascular risk, the incremental dose should be 0.1 μg/kg In patients with renal failure, incremental doses should be infused over 60 s to prevent adverse effects, such as hypertension and dizziness
Naloxone					
• Bolus dose:	0.4–2 mg (maximum 10 mg)	Undiluted	1 mg/ml	Renal: no Hepatic: no	Inject over 60 s
• Infusion dose:	4–5 μg/kg/h	2 mg in 250 ml (D5W)	1 mg/ml	Renal: no Hepatic: no	Continuous infusion
Neostigmine	25–75 μg/kg	Undiluted	1 mg/ml	Renal: no Hepatic: no	Inject over 60 s
Nesiritide					Prime IV tubing with an infusion of 25 ml prior to connecting to patient's vascular access port and prior to administering the bolus dose Do not administer through a central heparin-coated catheter

(continued)

Intravenous Medication Administration Guidelines *(continued)*

Drug	Usual Dose Range[a]	Standard Dilution	Maximum Concentration	Adjust for Renal or Hepatic Failure	Infusion Times/Comments/ Drug Interactions
• Bolus dose:	2 μg/kg	IV push	6 μg/ml	Renal: no Hepatic: no	Withdraw from infusion bag administer over 60 seconds through an IV port in the tubing
• Infusion dose:	0.01 μg/kg/min	1.5 mg in 250 ml (D5W)	6 μg/ml	Renal: no Hepatic: no	Continuous infusion
Nicardipine	5–15 mg/h	25 mg in 250 ml (D5W)	0.1 mg/ml	Renal: yes Hepatic: no	Continuous infusion Infusion site should be changed every 12 h if administered by peripheral vein
Nitroglycerin	20–300 μg/min	50 mg in 250 ml (D5W)	1.6 mg/ml	Renal: no Hepatic: no	Drug interaction: heparin (11)
Nitroprusside	0.5–10 μg/kg/min	50 mg in 250 ml (D5W)	0.8 mg/ml	Renal: yes Hepatic: no	Maintain thiocyanate <10 mg/dl
Norepinephrine	4–35 μg/min	4 mg in 250 ml (D5W)	0.08 mg/ml	Renal: no Hepatic: no	Continuous infusion
Octreotide					
• Continuous infusion:	50–100 μg bolus, followed by continuous infusion at 25–100 μg/h for 24–48 h	500 mg in 250 ml (D5W)	1000 μg/ml	Renal: no Hepatic: no	Continuous infusion:
Ondansetron	16–32 mg 30 min before chemotherapy	50 ml (D5W)	1 mg/ml	Renal: no Hepatic: no	Infuse over 15–30 min
• Postoperative nausea and vomiting:	4 mg IV × 1	Undiluted	2 mg/ml	Renal: no Hepatic: no	Infuse over 2–5 min
Oxacillin	0.5–2 g q4–6h	100 ml (D5W)	250 mg/ 1.5 ml	Renal: no Hepatic: yes	Infuse over 30 min
Pamidronate	60–90 mg × 1 dose	1,000 ml (D5W)	Dilute in at least 1,000 ml	Renal: no Hepatic: no	Infuse over 24 h

Pancuronium					
• Intubating dose:	0.06–0.1 mg/kg	Undiluted	2 mg/ml	Renal: no Hepatic: no	Inject over 60 s
• Maintenance dose:	0.01–0.015 mg/kg	Undiluted	2 mg/ml	Renal: no Hepatic: no	Inject over 60 s Active metabolite accumulates in renal failure and contributes to pharmacologic effect Monitor train-of-four stimulation Drug interactions: aminoglycosides (3), anticonvulsants (5)
• Infusion dose:	1 μg/kg/min	25 mg in 250 ml (D5W)	2 mg/ml	Renal: yes Hepatic: yes	Active metabolite accumulates in renal failure and contributes to pharmacologic effect Monitor train-of-four stimulation Drug interactions: aminoglycosides (3), anticonvulsants (5)
Pantoprazole					
• 2 min infusion:	40 mg qd	10 ml (0.9% NaC)	4 mg/ml	Renal: no Hepatic: no	Infuse over 2 min
• 15 min infusion:	40 mg qd	100 ml (D5W)	0.4 mg/ml	Renal: no Hepatic: no	Infuse over 15 min
Penicillin G	8–24M U divided q4h	100 ml (D5W)	100,000 U/ml	Renal: yes Hepatic: no	Infuse over 15–30 min
Pentamidine	4 mg/kg q24h	50 ml (D5W)	100 mg/ml	Renal: yes Hepatic: no	Infuse over 60 min
Pentobarbital					
• Bolus dose:	20 mg/kg	100 ml (0.9% NaCl)	20 mg/ml	Renal: no Hepatic: no	Infuse over 2 h
• Infusion dose:	1 mg/kg/h initially, then 0.5–4 mg/kg/h	250 ml (0.9% NaCl)	10 mg/ml	Renal: no Hepatic: yes	Therapeutic levels: 20–50 mg/L
Phenobarbital	20 mg/kg	Undiluted	130 mg/ml	Renal: no Hepatic: yes	Maximum infusion rate 50 mg/min Therapeutic levels: 15–40 mg/L
Phentolamine					
• Bolus dose:	5–10 mg	Undiluted	5 mg/ml	Renal: no Hepatic: no	Inject over 3–5 min

(continued)

Intravenous Medication Administration Guidelines *(continued)*

Drug	Usual Dose Range[a]	Standard Dilution	Maximum Concentration	Adjust for Renal or Hepatic Failure	Infusion Times/Comments/ Drug Interactions
Phentolamine (*continued*)					
• Infusion dose:	1–5 mg/min	100 ml (D5W)	5 mg/ml	Renal: no Hepatic: no	Continuous infusion
Phenylephrine	20–30 μg/min	15 mg in 250 ml (D5W)	6.4 mg/ml	Renal: no Hepatic: no	Continuous infusion
Phenytoin	15–20 mg/kg	Undiluted	50 mg/ml	Renal: no Hepatic: yes	Maximum infusion rate 25 to 50 mg/min Drug interactions: cimetidine (6), neuromuscular blocking agents (5) Therapeutic levels: 10–20 mg/L
Phosphate (potassium)	0.16–0.64 mmol/kg	Function of K^+ concentration	Function of K^+ concentration	Renal: yes Hepatic: no	Infuse over 6–8 h 1 mmol of PO_4 = 31 mg of phosphorus Maximum infusion rate 10 mmol/h
Piperacillin	2–4 g q4–6h	100 ml (D5W)	200 mg/ml	Renal: yes Hepatic: no	Infuse over 15–30 min
Pipercillin and tazobactam	3.375 g q6h	100 ml (D5W)	60 mg of piperacillin/ml	Renal: yes Hepatic: no	Infuse over 30 min
Potassium chloride	5–40 mEq/h	40–80 mEq in 1000 ml (0.9% NaCl, D5W, etc.)	0.4 mEq/ml	Renal: yes Hepatic: no	Cardiac monitoring should be used with infusion rates >20 mEq/h
Prednisolone	4–60 mg q24h	Undiluted	20 mg/ml	Renal: no Hepatic: no	Inject over 60 s
Procainamide					
• Loading dose:	15 mg/kg	50 ml (D5W)	20 mg/ml	Renal: no Hepatic: no	Maximum infusion rate 25–50 mg/min
• Infusion dose:	1–4 mg/min	2 g in 500 ml (D5W)	8 mg/ml	Renal: yes Hepatic: no	Therapeutic levels: Procainamide, 4–10 mg/L, NAPA, 10–20 mg/L
Propofol					
• Bolus dose:	0.25–2 mg/kg	Undiluted	10 mg/ml	Renal: no Hepatic: no	Infuse over 1–2 min
• Infusion dose:	5–50 μg/kg/min	Undiluted	10 mg/ml	Renal: no Hepatic: no	Dilute only with 0.9% NaCl to no less than 2 mg/ml Avoid infusion rates >80 μg/kg/min

Propranolol	0.5–1 mg q5–15 min	Undiluted	1 mg/ml	Renal: no Hepatic: yes	Inject over 60 s
• Infusion dose:	1–3 mg/h	50 mg in 500 ml (D5W)	1 mg/ml	Renal: no Hepatic: yes	Continuous infusion
Protamine	<30 min: 1–1.5 mg/100 U heparin 30–60 min: 0.5–0.75 mg/100 U heparin >120 min: 0.25–0.375 mg/100 U heparin	50 mg in 5 ml sterile water	10 mg/ml	Renal: no Hepatic: no	Inject over 3–5 min Do not exceed 50 mg in 10 min
Pyridostigmine	100–300 μg/kg	Undiluted	5 mg/ml	Renal: no Hepatic: no	Inject over 60 s Use to reverse long-acting neuromuscular blocking agents
Quinidine gluconate	600 mg initially, then 400 mg q2h Maintenance 200–300 mg q6h	800 mg in 50 ml (D5W)	16 mg/ml	Renal: no Hepatic: yes	Infusion rate 1 mg/min Therapeutic levels: 1.5–5 mg/L
Quinupristin/ dalfopristin	7.5 mg/kg q8–12h	250 ml (D5W) (approx. 2 mg/ml)	100 ml (D5W) (approx. 5 mg/ml)	Renal: no Hepatic: yes	Infuse over 1 h Infusion volume of 100 ml may be used for central line infusions Not compatible with saline containing solutions
Ranitidine					
• IVPB:	50 mg q6–8h	50 ml (D5W)	2.5 mg/ml	Renal: yes Hepatic: no	Infuse over 15–30 min IVP dose should be injected over at least 5 min
• Infusion dose:	6.25 mg/h	150 mg in 150 ml (D5W)	2.5 mg/ml	Renal: no Hepatic: no	Continuous infusion
Rasburicase	0.15–0.2 mg/kg qd × 5 d	Achieve a final total volume of 50 ml (0.9% NaCl)	Achieve a final total volume of 50 ml (0.9% NaCl)	Renal: no Hepatic: no	Infuse over 30 min

(continued)

Intravenous Medication Administration Guidelines *(continued)*

Drug	Usual Dose Range[a]	Standard Dilution	Maximum Concentration	Adjust for Renal or Hepatic Failure	Infusion Times/Comments/Drug Interactions
Remifentanil					
Continuation in the immediate postoperative period	0.0125–0.025 μg/kg/min	2 mg in 80 ml (D5W)	250 μg/ml	Renal: no Hepatic: no	Continuous infusion Bolus doses to treat postoperative pain are not recommended Infusion rates should not exceed 0.025 μg/kg/min Failure to clear IV tubing of residual drug has been associated with respiratory depression, apnea, and muscle rigidity upon administration of additional fluids through the same IV tubing
Reteplase	10 U followed by a second 10 U dose 30 min later	Diluted with sterile water to a final concentration of 1 U/ml	Diluted with sterile water to a final concentration of 1 U/ml	Renal: no Hepatic: no	Inject over 2 min
Rh_OD Immune Globulin Intravenous	20–250 μg/kg	Undiluted	120 μg/ml	Renal: no Hepatic: no	Inject over 3–5 min
Rifampin	300–600 mg q24h	100 ml (D5W)	3 mg/ml	Renal: no Hepatic: yes	Infuse over 30 min
Rocuronium					
• Bolus dose:	0.6–1.2 mg/kg	Undiluted	10 mg/ml	Renal: no Hepatic: no	Inject over 60 s
• Maintenance dose:	0.1–0.2 mg/kg	Undiluted	10 mg/ml	Renal: no Hepatic: yes	Inject over 60 s Monitor train-of-four stimulation Drug interactions: aminoglycosides (3), anticonvulsants (5)
• Infusion dose:	4–16 μg/kg/min	50 mg in 50 ml (D5W)	10 mg/ml	Renal: no Hepatic: yes	Continuous infusion Monitor train-of-four stimulation Drug interactions: aminoglycosides (3), anticonvulsants (5)

RSV Immune Globulin	750 mg/kg q month	50 mg/ml	50 mg/ml	Renal: no Hepatic: no	Infuse 1.5 ml/kg/h 0–15 min Infuse 3 ml/kg/h 15–30 min Infuse 6 ml/kg/h 30 min to end of infusion
Sargramostim (GM-CSF)	250 mg/M^2/d × 21 d	50 ml (NS)	Should be diluted to >10 μg/ml	Renal: no Hepatic: no	Infuse over 2 h If final concentration is <10 μg/ml, albumin should be added to a final concentration of 0.1%
Sodium bicarbonate	HCO_3^- deficit in mEq = 0.4 × (body weight in kg) × (desired HCO_3^- − measured HCO_3^-)	Premixed solution 0.6 mEq/ml	150 mEq in 1,000 ml SW or D5W	Renal: no Hepatic: no	Continuous infusion Sodium bicarbonate syringes contain 1 mEq/ml Many incompatibilities; flush IV line before and after use
Streptomycin	0.5–1 g qd–q12h	100 ml (0.9% NaCl)	100 ml (0.9% NaCl)	Renal: yes Hepatic: no	Infuse over 30 min IM product is used for IV administration
Succinylcholine	1–2 mg/kg	Undiluted	100 mg/ml	Renal: no Hepatic: no	Infuse over 60 s
Sufentanil					
• Bolus dose:	0.2–0.6 μg/kg	Undiluted	50 μg/ml	Renal: no Hepatic: no	Inject over 60 s
• Infusion dose:	0.01–0.05 μg/kg/min	Undiluted	50 μg/ml	Renal: no Hepatic: no	Continuous infusion
Tacrolimus	50–100 μg/kg/day	100 ml (D5W)	0.02 mg/ml	Renal: yes Hepatic: yes	Infuse over 24 h
Thiamine	100 mg qd × 3	50 ml (D5W)	2 mg/ml	Renal: no Hepatic: no	Infuse over 15–30 min
Thiopental	3–4 mg/kg	Undiluted	4 mg/ml	Renal: no Hepatic: yes	Infuse over 3–5 min
Ticarcillin-clavulanic acid	3.1 g q4–6h	100 ml (D5W)	100 mg/ml	Renal: yes Hepatic: no	Infuse over 15–30 min
Tigecycline	100 mg initially, then 50 mg q12h	100 ml (D5W)	1 mg/ml	Renal: no Hepatic: yes	Reconstituted solution should be yellow to orange in color Infuse over 30–60 min

(continued)

Intravenous Medication Administration Guidelines *(continued)*

Drug	Usual Dose Range[a]	Standard Dilution	Maximum Concentration	Adjust for Renal or Hepatic Failure	Infusion Times/Comments/ Drug Interactions
Tirofiban	0.4 μg/kg/min for 30 min, then 0.1 μg/kg/min	25 mg in 500 ml (D5W)	50 μg/ml	Renal: yes Hepatic: no	Continuous infusion Can be administered through the same IV catheter as heparin
Tissue Plasminogen Activator (rtPA)					
• Myocardial infarction:	100 mg	100 mg in 100 ml (sterile water)	1 mg/ml	Renal: no Hepatic: no	Accelerated infusion: 15 mg bolus, followed by 50 mg over 30 min, then 35 mg over the next 60 min 3 hour infusion: 60 mg in the first h, 20 mg over the second h, and 20 mg over the third h
• Acute ischemic stroke:	0.9 mg/kg (to maximum 90 mg)	Appropriate volume of a 1 mg/ml solution	1 mg/ml	Renal: no Hepatic: no	Infuse over 60 min with 10% of total dose administered as an initial bolus over 1 min
• Pulmonary embolism:	100 mg	100 mg in 100 ml (sterile water)	1 mg/ml	Renal: no Hepatic: no	Infuse over 2 h
Tobramycin					
• Loading dose:	2–3 mg/kg	50 ml (D5W)	40 mg/ml	Renal: no Hepatic: no	Infuse over 30 min
• Maintenance dose:	1.5–2.5 mg/kg q8–24h	50 ml (D5W)	40 mg/ml	Renal: yes Hepatic: no	Infuse over 30 min Critically ill patients have an increased volume of distribution requiring increased doses Drug interaction: neuromuscular blocking agents (3) Therapeutic levels: peak, 4–10 mg/L, trough <2 mg/L
Torsemide					
• Bolus dose:	5–40 mg qd	10 mg/ml	10 mg/ml	Renal: no Hepatic: no	Inject over 2 min
• Infusion dose:	25 mg bolus dose followed by 3 mg/h	100 mg in 100 ml (0.9% NaCl)	10 mg/ml	Renal: no Hepatic: no	Continuous infusion Monitor electrolytes

Tranexamic acid					
• Presurgical:	10 mg/kg immediately prior to surgery	100 ml (D5W)	Unknown	Renal: no Hepatic: no	Infuse over 30 min
• Postsurgical:	10 mg/kg q6–8h for 2–8 d	100 ml (D5W)	Unknown	Renal: yes Hepatic: no	Infuse over 30 min
• Bladder irrigation:	1 g in 1,000 ml (0.9% NaCl) at 1 ml/min for 2–5 d	1 g in 1,000 ml (0.9% NaCl)	1 g in 1,000 ml (0.9% NaCl)	Renal: no Hepatic: no	Not for IV use Instill in bladder at 1 ml/min
Trimethoprim-sulfamethoxazole (TMP-SMX)					
• General:	4–5 mg/kg q12h	TMP 16 mg-SMX 80 mg per 25 ml (D5W)	TMP 16 mg-SMX 80 mg per 10 ml (D5W)	Renal: yes Hepatic: yes (SMX)	Infuse over 60 min
• For pneumocystis carinii:	5 mg/kg q6h	TMP 16 mg-SMX 80 mg per 25 ml (D5W)	TMP 16 mg SMX 80 mg per 10 ml (D5W)	Renal: yes Hepatic: yes (SMX)	Infuse over 60 min Therapeutic levels (SMX): <150 mg/L
Trimetrexate	22–45 mg/m^2 q24h	100 ml (D5W)	2 mg/ml	Renal: no Hepatic: no	Infuse over 60–90 min Trimetrexate must be given with leucovorin 20–40 mg/m^2 q6h to avoid serious or life-threatening toxicities
Valproate sodium	IV dose = PO dose	50 ml (D5W)	10 mg/ml	Renal: no Hepatic: yes	Maximum infusion rate = 20 mg/min
Vancomycin	1 g q12h	250 ml (D5W)	20 mg/ml	Renal: yes Hepatic: no	Infuse over at least 1 h to avoid "red-man" syndrome Therapeutic levels: peak, 20–40 mg/L, trough, <10 mg/L

(continued)

Intravenous Medication Administration Guidelines *(continued)*

Drug	Usual Dose Range[a]	Standard Dilution	Maximum Concentration	Adjust for Renal or Hepatic Failure	Infusion Times/Comments/ Drug Interactions
Vasopressin					
Upper GI bleed:	0.2–0.3 U/min	100 U in 250 ml (D5W)	1 U/ml	Renal: no Hepatic: no	Maximum infusion rate 0.9 U/min
Septic shock:	0.01–0.04 U/min	100 U in 100 ml (D5W)	1 U/ml	Renal: no Hepatic: no	Continuous infusion
Vecuronium					
• Bolus dose:	0.1–0.28 mg/kg	Undiluted	1 mg/ml	Renal: no Hepatic: no	Inject over 60 s
• Maintenance dose:	0.01–0.15 mg/kg	Undiluted	1 mg/ml	Renal: yes Hepatic: yes	Inject over 1–2 min Active metabolite accumulates in renal failure and contributes to pharmacologic effect Monitor train-of-four stimulation Drug interactions: aminoglycosides (3), anticonvulsants (5)
• Infusion dose:	1 μg/kg/min	20 mg in 100 ml (D5W)	1 mg/ml	Renal: yes Hepatic: yes	Continuous infusion Active metabolite accumulates in renal failure and contributes to pharmacologic effect Monitor train-of-four stimulation Drug interactions: aminoglycosides (3), anticonvulsants (5)

Verapamil					
• Bolus dose:	5–10 mg	Undiluted	2.5 mg/ml	Renal: no Hepatic: no	Inject over 1–2 min Drug interaction: digoxin (8)
• Infusion dose:	0.1–5 μg/kg/min	40 mg in 250 ml (D5W)	2.5 mg/ml	Renal: no Hepatic: yes	Continuous infusion
Voriconazole					
• Loading dose:	6 mg/kg q12h × 24 h	100 ml (D5W)	≤5 mg/ml	Renal: no Hepatic: no	Infuse over 1–2 h Maximum infusion rate 3 mg/kg/h
• Maintenance dose:	4 mg/kg q12h	100 ml (D5W)	≤5 mg/ml	Renal: no Hepatic: no	Infuse over 1–2 h Maximum infusion rate 3 mg/kg/h
Zidovudine	1 mg/kg q4h	D5W (50 ml)	4 mg/ml	Renal: yes Hepatic: no	Infuse over 1 h 1 mg/kg IV q4h is the equivalent to the oral dose of 100 mg q4h
Zoledronic acid	4 mg IV × 1	D5W (100 ml)	0.04 mg/ml	Renal: yes Hepatic: no	Infuse over 15 min

ACT, activated clotting time; APPT, activated partial thromboplastin time; BP, blood pressure; D5W, dextrose 5% in water; ECG, electrocardiogram; HF, heart failure; IM, intramuscular; INP, intravenous push; IV, intravenous; NAPA, N-acetylprocainamide; PE, phenytoin equivalents; PO, by mouth; SC, subcutaneous; SMX, sulfamethoxazole; TMP, trimethoprim

[a]Usual dose ranges are listed, refer to appropriate disease state for specific dose.

Drug interactions: (1) antagonizes adenosine effect; (2) potentiates adenosine effect; (3) potentiates effect of neuromuscular blocking agents; (4) inhibits theophylline metabolism; (5) antagonizes effect of neuromuscular blocking agents; (6) metabolism inhibited by cimetidine; (7) metabolism inhibited by ciprofloxacin; (8) increased digoxin concentrations; (9) metabolism inhibited by erythromycin; (10) increased nephrotoxicity; (11) increased heparin requirement.

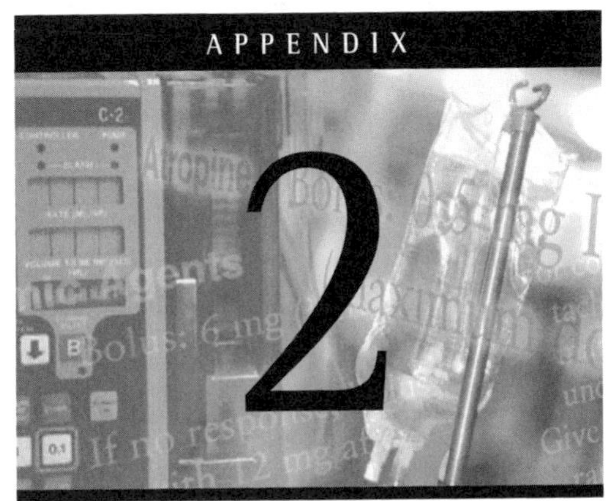

Intravenous to Oral Conversions

Intravenous to Oral Conversions

IV Product	Oral Conversion Product	Comments
Acyclovir	Acyclovir: Herpes simplex: 200 mg PO q4h (5 × /d) Herpes zoster acute treatment: 800 mg PO q4h (5 × /d) Varicella zoster: 800 mg PO qid × 5 d Valacyclovir: Herpes zoster: 1 g PO tid × 7 d	Valacyclovir is rapidly and nearly completely converted to acyclovir
Allopurinol	Allopurinol 100–300 mg PO qd	Oral dose = IV dose
Aminocaproic acid	1–1.25 g/h for 8 h or until bleeding is controlled	
Aminophylline infusion dose	1. Multiply the hourly aminophylline infusion rate (mg/h) by 24 to determine the total daily dose. 2. Multiply the total daily dose by 0.80 to convert aminophylline to theophylline. 3. Divide the total daily theophylline dose by the number of dosing intervals appropriate for the oral theophylline product selected (q24h: 1; q12h: 2; q8h: 3; q6h: 4). 4. Select the closest available dose strength of the product selected. 5. Stop the IV infusion with the first administered oral dose. 6. Monitor theophylline concentration 24–48 h after switching to oral product.	Theophylline = 0.80 × aminophylline Monitor serum concentrations after conversion to oral therapy and adjust oral dose as needed
Amiodarone maintenance infusion	Duration of IV amiodarone infusion — Initial oral daily dose <1 wk — 800–1,600 mg 1–3 wk — 600–800 mg >3 wk — 400 mg	Monitor serum concentrations after conversion to oral therapy and adjust oral dose as needed
Ampicillin	Ampicillin 250–500 mg PO qid or amoxicillin 250–500 mg tid	
Ampicillin-sulbactam	Amoxicillin-Clavulanic acid 250–500 mg PO q8h	
Argatroban	Warfarin Initiate oral anticoagulation only after substantial recovery of platelet counts (i.e., $>100 \times 10^9$/L) Do not use a warfarin loading dose Initiate therapy with expected daily dose of warfarin Overlap argatroban and warfarin therapy for 4–5 d to avoid prothrombotic effect	
Atenolol	Postmyocardial infarction: 50 mg PO after last IV dose, 50 mg PO 12 h later, then 50 mg PO bid for 6–9 days or until discharge from the hospital	
Azithromycin	250 mg PO qd for 5–10 d	

(continued)

Intravenous to Oral Conversions *(continued)*

IV Product	Oral Conversion Product	Comments
Cefazolin	Cefadroxil 500 mg PO q12h, cephalexin 500 mg PO q6h, or cefaclor 500 mg PO q8h	Cefaclor provides gram (−) coverage similar to cefazolin that is not provided by cefadroxil or cephalexin
Cefepime	Ceftibuten 400 mg PO qd	The spectrum of ceftibuten closely approximates the spectrum of cefepime except for *Ps. aeruginosa*
Cefotaxime	Cefpodoxime 100–200 mg PO q12h, cefixime 400 mg PO qd, or ceftibuten 400 mg PO qd	Ceftibuten may provide additional gram (−) coverage not provided by cefpodoxime or cefixime
Cefoxitin	Cefuroxime 250–500 mg PO bid, cefixime 400 mg PO qd, or ceftibuten 400 mg PO qd PLUS metronidazole 250–500 mg PO q6–8h	The spectrum of cefuroxime, cefixime, and ceftibuten closely approximates the gram (+) and gram (−) spectrums of cefoxitin; metronidazole covers the anaerobic organisms not covered by the cephalosporins
Ceftazidime	Ceftibuten 400 mg PO qd	The spectrum of ceftibuten closely approximates the spectrum of ceftazidime except for *Ps. aeruginosa*
Ceftriaxone	Cefpodoxime 100–200 mg PO q12h, cefixime 400 mg PO qd, or ceftibuten 400 mg PO qd	Ceftibuten may provide additional gram (−) coverage not provided by cefpodoxime or cefixime
Cefuroxime	Cefuroxime 250–500 mg PO q12h	
Chloramphenicol	Convert IV dose to equivalent oral dose	The oral formulation has increased bioavailability compared to IV formulation Monitor serum concentrations after conversion to oral therapy and adjust oral dose as needed
Cimetidine	300 mg PO qid, 400 mg PO bid, or 800 mg PO qhs	Oral dose = IV dose
Ciprofloxacin	250–750 mg PO q12h	
Clindamycin	150–450 mg PO q6h	
Cyclosporine	Oral dose equals 3 × IV dose	Monitor serum concentrations after conversion to oral therapy and adjust oral dose as needed
Digoxin maintenance dosage	Convert IV dose to equivalent oral dose	Oral dose approximately equal to IV dose Monitor serum concentrations after conversion to oral therapy and adjust oral dose as needed
Diltiazem continuous infusion	3 mg/h = diltiazem CD 120 mg PO qd 5 mg/h = diltiazem CD 180 mg PO qd 7 mg/h = diltiazem CD 240 mg PO qd 11 mg/h = diltiazem CD 300 mg PO qd	After constant IV infusion, diltiazem exhibits nonlinear pharmacokinetics over the infusion range of 5–13 mg/h The oral conversions are expected to produce approximately equivalent steady-state plasma concentrations to the IV dose
Doxycycline	50–100 mg PO bid	
Enalaprilat	CrCl >30 ml/min: 5 mg PO qd CrCl <30 ml/min: 2.5 mg PO qd	

(continued)

Intravenous to Oral Conversions *(continued)*

IV Product	Oral Conversion Product	Comments
Erythromycin	Tab: 250 mg PO q6h, 333 mg PO q8h, 500 mg PO q12h Susp.: 400 mg PO q6h, 800 mg PO q12h Legionnaire's disease: 250–1,000 mg PO qid	Multiple erythromycin salts and products are available; refer to hospital formulary for available products
Esomeprazole	20–40 mg PO qd	Oral dose = IV dose
Famotidine	10–20 mg PO bid or 40 mg PO qhs	Oral dose = IV dose
Fluconazole	50–400 mg PO qd	Oral dose = IV dose
Fosphenytoin	Switch to Dilantin brand of phenytoin at same total daily dose	Monitor phenytoin serum concentrations after conversion to oral therapy and adjust oral Dilantin dose as needed
Ganciclovir	CMV retinitis maintenance dosing: 1,000 mg PO tid with food or 500 mg PO 6 × /d (q3h while awake) with food	
Gatifloxacin	400 mg PO qd	Oral dose = IV dose
Granisetron	1 mg PO bid, with the first dose given up to 1 h before highly emetogenic chemotherapy, and the second dose given 12 h after the first dose	
Hydralazine	10–50 mg PO qid	
Hydrocortisone	25–100 mg PO q8h	Oral dose equals IV dose
Isoniazid	300 mg PO qd	Oral dose = IV dose
Ketamine	10 mg/kg PO	
Ketorolac	10 mg PO qid	Maximum combined duration of therapy is 5 d
Labetalol	100–400 mg PO bid	
Lansoprazole	15–30 mg PO qd	Oral dose = IV dose
Levofloxacin	250–750 mg PO qd	Oral dose = IV dose
Levothyroxine	Oral dose equals 1.33 times IV dose	
Linezolid	400–600 mg PO bid	Oral dose = IV dose
Methyldopa	250–500 mg PO bid-qid	
Methylprednisolone	4–20 mg qd	Oral dose equals IV dose
Metoclopramide	5–15 mg PO qid	
Metoprolol	Tab: 25–200 mg PO bid SR-tab: 50–100 mg PO qd	
Metronidazole	250–500 mg PO tid	
Midazolam	0.5–1 mg/kg PO	
Moxifloxacin	400 mg PO qd	Oral dose = IV dose
Nafcillin	Dicloxacillin 250–500 mg PO qid	
Nicardipine continuous infusion	0.5 mg/h = 20 mg PO q8h 1.2 mg/h = 30 mg PO q8h 2.2 mg/h = 40 mg PO q8h	
Ondansetron	Administer first dose (4–8 mg) 30 min before start of chemotherapy, with subsequent doses 4 h and 8 h after first dose, then 4–8 mg PO tid for 1–2 d after completion of chemotherapy	
Oxacillin	Oxacillin 250–1,000 mg PO q4–6h or dicloxacillin 250–500 mg PO qid	
Pantoprazole	20–40 mg PO qd	Oral dose = IV dose

(continued)

Intravenous to Oral Conversions *(continued)*

IV Product	Oral Conversion Product	Comments
Penicillin G	Penicillin VK 250–500 mg PO qid	
Phenobarbital	15–60 mg PO qd	Oral dose equals IV dose Monitor serum concentrations after conversion to oral therapy and adjust oral dose as needed
Phenytoin	Convert IV dose to equivalent oral dose	Oral dose approximately equal to IV dose Only Dilantin brand of phenytoin may be given as a single daily dose Monitor serum concentrations after conversion to oral therapy and adjust oral dose as needed
Phosphate	1 g (228 mg or 7.4 mmol) PO qid with meals and at bedtime Must be thoroughly dissolved in 180–240 ml water	
Potassium chloride	Oral dose equals IV dose	Oral powder or elixir must be diluted in at least 120 ml of fluid before administration to prevent osmotic diarrhea
Procainamide continuous infusion	1. Multiply the hourly procainamide infusion rate (mg/h) by 24 to determine the total daily dose. 2. Divide the total daily procainamide dose by the number of dosing intervals appropriate for the oral procainamide product selected (q12h: 2; q6h: 4; q3h: 8). 3. Select the closest available dose strength of the product selected. 4. Stop the IV infusion with the first administered oral dose. 5. Monitor procainamide concentration 24–48 h after switching to oral product.	Monitor serum concentrations after conversion to oral therapy and adjust oral dose as needed
Quinidine gluconate continuous infusion	1. Multiply the hourly quinidine gluconate infusion rate (mg/h) by 24 to determine the total daily dose. 2. Multiply the total daily quinidine gluconate dose by 1.4 to determine the equivalent oral quinidine gluconate dose. 3. Divide the total daily dose by the number of dosing intervals appropriate for the oral quinidine gluconate product selected (q6h: 4; q8h: 3). 4. Select the closest available dose strength of the product selected. 5. Stop the IV infusion with the first administered oral dose. 6. Monitor quinidine concentration 24–48 h after switching to oral product.	The bioavailability of oral quinidine gluconate is approximately 70% Quinidine gluconate delivers 62% quinidine alkaloid Quinidine gluconate is available as a 324 mg sustained release tablet; this formulation may be broken in half for administration Monitor serum concentrations after conversion to oral therapy and adjust oral dose as needed
Ranitidine	150 mg PO bid or 300 mg PO qd	

(continued)

Intravenous to Oral Conversions *(continued)*

IV Product	Oral Conversion Product	Comments
Rifampin	300–600 mg PO qd	Oral dose = IV dose
Tacrolimus	0.15–0.3 mg/kg/d PO in q12h divided doses; administer initial dose no sooner than 6 h after transplantation; if IV therapy was initiated, begin 8–12 h after discontinuing IV therapy	Monitor serum concentrations after conversion to oral therapy and adjust oral dose as needed
Tranexamic acid	25 mg/kg PO tid-qid starting 1 d before surgery and continued for 2–8 d postsurgery	
Trimethoprim-sulfamethoxazole (TMP-SMX)	1 Septra or 1 Septra DS tab (or equivalent susp. volume) PO q12h	
Verapamil	Tab: 40–120 mg PO q8h SR-tab/cap: 120–240 mg PO qd	
Voriconazole	Maintenance dose: 200 mg PO q12h	

IV, intravenous; PO, by mouth

The patient, degree of organ impairment, severity of infection or disease state, and duration of IV therapy at time of switch are important in determining the most appropriate oral dose. Many hospitals with switch programs have predetermined the most appropriate oral dose for the switch.

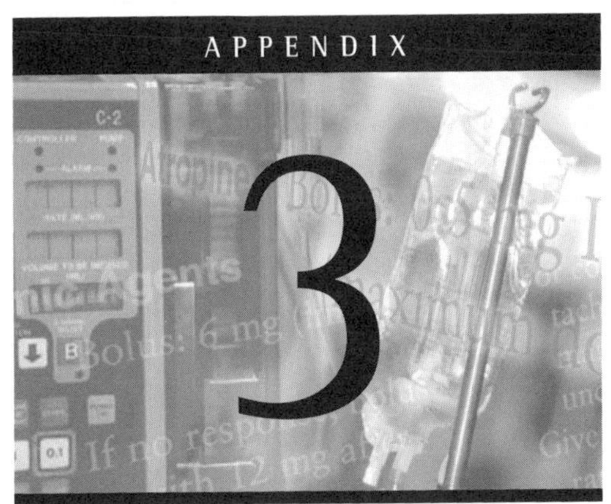

Selected Oral Drug Doses

Selected Oral Drug Doses

Generic Name (Trade Name)	Therapeutic Category	Preparation	Usual Adult Dose/Comments
Abacavir (Ziagen)	Antiretroviral	Tab: 300 mg Soln: 20 mg/ml	300 mg PO bid
Acarbose (Precose)	Hypoglycemic	Tab: 50, 100 mg	Initial: 25 mg PO tid at the start of each main meal Maintenance: Increase dose as needed at 4- to 8-wk intervals Maximum: ≤60 kg: 50 mg PO tid; >60 kg: 100 mg PO tid Not recommended in diabetics with SCr >2 mg/dl
Acebutolol (Sectral)	Antihypertensive, antiarrhythmic	Cap: 200, 400 mg	HTN: 400–800 mg PO qd Arrhythmias: 200 mg PO bid; maximum: 600–1,200 mg/d
Acyclovir (Zovirax)	Antiviral	Cap: 200 mg Tab: 400, 800 mg Susp: 200 mg/5 ml	*Herpes simplex*: Initial treatment genital herpes: 200 mg PO q4h (5 × /d) *Herpes zoster*: Acute treatment: 800 mg PO q4h (5 × /d) *Varicella zoster:* 20 mg/kg (up to 800 mg) PO qid × 5d
Albuterol (Proventil, Ventolin)	Bronchodilator	Tab: 2, 4 mg SR-Tab: 4 mg Syr: 2 mg/5 ml	Tab/Syr: 2–4 mg PO tid-qid, maximum 16 mg/d SR-Tab: 4–8 mg PO q12h
Allopurinol (Zyloprim)	Antigout	Tab: 100, 300 mg	Mild gout: 200–300 mg PO qd Moderate-severe gout: 400–600 mg PO qd
Alprazolam (Xanax)	Antianxiety	Tab: 0.25, 0.5, 1, 2 mg	0.25–0.5 mg PO tid
Amantadine (Symmetrel)	Antiparkinsonian, antiviral	Cap: 100 mg Syr: 50 mg/5 ml	Influenza: 200 mg PO qd or 100 mg PO bid
Amiloride (Midamor)	Potassium-sparing diuretic	Tab: 5 mg	5–10 mg PO qd
Aminocaproic acid (Amicar)	Hemostatic	Tab: 500 mg Syr: 250 mg/ml	5 g PO during the first hour, then by 1–1.25 g/h for 8 h or until bleeding is controlled
Amiodarone (Cordarone)	Antiarrhythmic	Tab: 200 mg	Loading: 800–1,600 mg PO qd for 1–3 wk Maintenance: 600–800 mg PO qd for 1 mo, then 200–400 mg PO qd
Amlodipine (Norvasc)	Antihypertensive, antianginal	Tab: 2.5, 5, 10 mg	HTN: 2.5–5 mg PO qd Angina: 5–10 mg PO qd
Amoxicillin (*multiple*)	Antibiotic	Cap: 250, 500 mg Tab: 125, 250 mg Susp: 125, 250 mg/5 ml	250–500 mg PO tid

(continued)

Selected Oral Drug Doses *(continued)*

Generic Name (Trade Name)	Therapeutic Category	Preparation	Usual Adult Dose/Comments
Ampicillin (*multiple*)	Antibiotic	Cap: 250, 500 mg Susp: 125, 250, 500 mg/5 ml	250–500 mg PO qid
Amprenavir (Agenerase)	Antiretroviral	Cap: 50 mg Soln: 15 mg/ml	1,200 mg PO bid
Atazanavir (Reyataz)	Antiretroviral	Cap: 100, 150, 200 mg	300–400 mg PO qd
Atenolol (Tenormin)	Antihypertensive, antianginal	Tab: 25, 50, 100 mg	HTN, angina: 25–100 mg PO qd Postmyocardial infarction: 50 mg PO after last IV dose, 50 mg PO 12 h later, then 50 mg PO bid for 6–9 d or until discharge from the hospital
Azathioprine (Imuran)	Immunosuppressant	Tab: 50 mg	Organ transplant: maintenance after IV therapy 1–3 mg/kg/d
Azithromycin (Zithromax)	Antibiotic	Tab: 250, 500, 600 mg Susp: 100 mg/5 ml, 200 mg/5 ml 1 g packs	500 mg on day one, then 250 mg PO qd × 4 d MAC: 1,200 mg q wk Oral tablets and suspension may be taken with or without food The 1 g packet should be mixed thoroughly with 60 ml water before administration
Bacitracin	Antibiotic	Inj: 50,000 units	*Clostridium difficile*: 20,000–25,000 units PO q6h for 7–10 d
Benazepril (Lotensin)	Antihypertensive	Tab: 5, 10, 20, 40 mg	10–40 mg PO qd in 1 or 2 doses
Betaxolol (Kerlone)	Antihypertensive	Tab: 10, 20 mg	10–20 mg PO qd
Bisacodyl (*multiple*)	Laxative	Tab: 5 mg Suppos: 10 mg	PO: 5–15 mg qd prn PR: 10 mg qd prn
Bumetanide (Bumex)	Loop diuretic	Tab: 0.5, 1, 2 mg	0.5–2 mg PO qd
Candesartan (Atacand)	Antihypertensive	4, 8, 16, 32 mg	2–32 mg PO qd
Captopril (Capoten)	Antihypertensive, heart failure, postmyocardial infarction	Tab: 6.25, 12.5, 25, 50, 100 mg	HTN, CHF: 6.25–100 mg PO bid-tid Postmyocardial infarction: 6.25 mg initially increasing up to 50 mg PO tid
Carbamazepine (Tegretol)	Anticonvulsant	Tab: 100, 200 mg Susp: 100 mg/5 ml	200 mg PO qid up to 1,200 mg/d Adjust dose monitoring serum concentrations
Carvedilol (Coreg)	Antihypertensive, HF	Tab: 3.125, 6.25, 12.5, 25 mg	3.125–25 mg PO bid

(continued)

Selected Oral Drug Doses *(continued)*

Generic Name (Trade Name)	Therapeutic Category	Preparation	Usual Adult Dose/Comments
Cefaclor (Ceclor)	Antibiotic	Cap: 250, 500 mg Susp: 125, 250, 375 mg/5 ml	125–500 mg PO q8h
Cefadroxil (Duricef)	Antibiotic	Cap: 500, 1000 mg Susp: 125, 250, 500 mg/5 ml	500–1000 mg PO bid
Cefixime (Suprax)	Antibiotic	Tab: 200, 400 mg Susp: 100 mg/5 ml	400 mg PO qd or 200 mg PO bid
Cefpodoxime (Vantin)	Antibiotic	Tab: 100, 200 mg Susp: 50, 100 mg/5 ml	100–200 mg PO q12h
Cefprozil (Cefzil)	Antibiotic	Tab: 250, 500 mg Susp: 125, 250 mg/5 ml	500 mg PO q24h to 250–500 mg PO q12h
Ceftibuten (Cedax)	Antibiotic	Cap: 400 mg Susp: 90, 180 mg/5 ml	400 mg PO qd for 10 d The bioavailability of ceftibuten is decreased with food, therefore it should be administered at least 2 h before or 1 h after meals
Cefuroxime (Ceftin)	Antibiotic	Tab: 125, 250, 500 mg Susp: 125 mg/5 ml	125–500 mg PO bid
Cephalexin (Keflex)	Antibiotic	Cap: 250, 500 mg Tab: 250, 500, 1,000 mg Susp: 125, 250 mg/5 ml	250–1,000 mg PO qid
Chloral Hydrate (*multiple*)	Sedative-hypnotic	Cap: 250, 500 mg Syr: 250, 500 mg/5 ml Suppos: 324, 500, 648 mg	Sedative: 250 mg PO tid Hypnotic: 500–1,000 mg PO hs
Chloramphenicol (Chloromycetin)	Antibiotic	Cap: 250 mg Susp: 150 mg/5 ml	50 mg/kg/day divided q6h The oral preparations have a bioavailability greater than the intravenous preparation
Chlorpromazine (Thorazine)	Antipsychotic	Tab: 10, 25, 50, 100, 200 mg Syr: 2 mg/ml Liquid conc.: 30, 100 mg/ml SR-Cap: 30, 75, 150, 200, 300 mg Suppos: 25, 100 mg	Psychosis: 10–25 mg PO tid up to 1–2 g/d Hiccups: 25–50 mg PO tid-qid
Chlorthalidone (Hygroton)	Thiazide diuretic	Tab: 15, 25, 50, 100 mg	15–100 mg PO qd
Cimetidine (Tagamet)	H_2-antagonist	Tab: 100, 200, 300, 400, 800 mg Liq: 300 mg/5 ml	300 mg PO qid, 400 mg PO bid, or 800 mg PO qhs

(continued)

Selected Oral Drug Doses *(continued)*

Generic Name (Trade Name)	Therapeutic Category	Preparation	Usual Adult Dose/Comments
Ciprofloxacin (Cipro)	Antibiotic	Tab: 100, 250, 500, 750 mg XR Tab: 500, 1,000 mg Susp: 250, 500 mg/5 ml	250–750 mg PO q12h XR: 500–1,000 mg PO qd (urinary tract infections only) Oral doses should be at least 2 h before or after antacids containing magnesium or aluminum, as well as sucralfate, metal cations such as iron, and multivitamins containing zinc
Clarithromycin (Biaxin)	Antibiotic	Tab: 250, 500 mg SR-Tab: 500 mg Susp: 125, 250 mg/5 ml	250–500 mg PO q12h SR-Tab: 1,000 mg PO qd
Clindamycin (Cleocin)	Antibiotic	Cap: 75, 150, 300 mg Susp: 75 mg/5 ml	150–450 mg PO q6h
Clonidine (Catapres)	Antihypertensive	Tab: 0.1, 0.2, 0.3 mg	0.1–1.2 mg PO bid
Clopidogrel (Plavix)	Antiplatelet agent	Tab: 75 mg	Recent MI, stroke, peripheral vascular disease: 75 mg qd Acute coronary syndrome: 300 mg PO loading dose followed by 75 mg PO qd
Codeine (*multiple*)	Opiate analgesic	Tab: 15, 30, 60 mg	15–60 mg PO q3–6h prn
Cyclosporine (Sandimmune, Neoral)	Immunosuppressant	Sandimmune Cap: 25, 50 100 mg Liq: 100 mg/ml Neorol Cap: 25, 100 mg Liq: 100 mg/ml	15 mg/kg PO 4–12 h before transplant, then taper to maintenance of 5–10 mg/kg/d monitoring cyclosporine concentrations
Delavirdine (Rescriptor)	Antiviral	Tab: 100, 200 mg	400 mg PO tid on empty stomach
Dexamethasone (*multiple*)	Corticosteroid	Tab: 0.25, 0.5, 0.75, 1.5, 2, 4, 6 mg Elixir: 0.1 mg/ml, 0.5 mg/0.5 ml	0.75–10 mg PO qd-qid depending on condition being treated
Diazepam (Valium)	Sedative-hypnotic	Tab: 2, 5, 10 mg SR-Cap: 15 mg Liq: 5 mg/5 ml, 5 mg/ml	2–10 mg PO bid-qid SR-Cap: 15 mg PO qd
Dicloxacillin (*multiple*)	Antibiotic	Cap: 250, 500 mg Susp: 62.5 mg/5 ml	250–500 mg PO qid

(continued)

Generic Name (Trade Name)	Therapeutic Category	Preparation	Usual Adult Dose/Comments
Didanosine (Videx)	Antiviral	Tab: 25, 50, 100, 150 mg Pwd: 100, 167, 250, 375 mg	Tab: <60 kg: 125 mg PO q12h; ≥60 kg: 200 mg PO q12h Take 2 tablets at each dose for adequate buffering to prevent degradation by gastric acid; chew or crush and disperse 2 tablets in ≥1 oz water prior to consumption; take on empty stomach Pwd: <60 kg: 167 mg PO q12h; >60 kg: 250 mg PO q12h Dissolve contents of packet in 4 oz water and drink on empty stomach
Digoxin (Lanoxin, Lanoxicaps)	Heart failure, antiarrhythmic	Tab: 0.125, 0.25, 0.5 mg Cap: 0.05, 0.1, 0.2 mg Elixir: 0.05 mg/ml	0.125–0.5 mg PO qd Adjust dose monitoring serum concentrations
Diltiazem (Cardizem, Dilacor)	Antihypertensive, antianginal	Tab: 30, 60, 90, 120 mg SR-Cap: Cardizem SR 60, 90, 120 mg Cardizem CD 120, 180, 240, 300 mg Dilacor XR 120, 180, 240 mg	Tab: 30–90 mg PO qid Cardizem SR: 60–120 mg PO bid up to 360 mg/d Cardizem CD: 120–480 mg PO qd Dilacor XR: 120–480 mg PO qd
Diphenhydramine (Benadryl)	Antihistamine, hypnotic	Tab/Cap: 25, 50 mg Liq: 12.5 mg/5 ml	25–50 mg PO q4–6h prn Hypnotic: 25–50 mg PO hs
Dipyridamole (Persantine)	Antiplatelet	Tab: 25, 50, 75 mg	25–100 mg PO qid
Disopyramide (Norpace, Norpace CR)	Antiarrhythmic	Cap: 100, 150 mg SR-Cap: 100, 150 mg	Cap: 100–150 mg PO q6h SR-Cap: 100–300 mg PO q12h Adjust dose monitoring serum concentrations
Divalproex (Depakote)	Anticonvulsant	SR-Tab: 125, 250, 500 mg SR-Cap: 125 mg sprinkle caps	125–500 mg PO qid Adjust dose monitoring serum concentrations
Dofetilide (Tikosyn)	Antiarrhythmic	Cap: 125, 250, 500 μg	Starting dose: 125–500 μg bid based on renal function; maintenance dose: 125 μg qd to 250 μg bid based on renal function

(continued)

Generic Name (Trade Name)	Therapeutic Category	Preparation	Usual Adult Dose/Comments
Dolasetron (Anzemet)	Antiemetic	Tab: 50 mg, 100 mg	Chemotherapy induced nausea and vomiting (CINV): 100 mg 1 h PO before chemotherapy Post-operative nausea and vomiting (PONV): 100 mg 2 h PO before surgery
Doxazosin (Cardura)	Antihypertensive, BPH	Tab: 1, 2, 4, 8 mg	1–16 mg PO qd
Doxycycline (Vibramycin)	Antibiotic	Tab: 100 mg Cap: 50, 100 mg Syr: 50 mg/5 ml	50–100 mg PO bid
Efavirenz (Sustiva)	Antiretroviral	Cap: 50, 100, 200 mg Tab: 600 mg	600 mg PO qd
Emtricitabine (Emtriva)	Antiretroviral	Cap: 200 mg	200 mg PO qd
Enalapril (Vasotec)	Antihypertensive, heart failure	Tab: 2.5, 5, 10, 20 mg	2.5 mg PO qd to 20 mg PO bid
Eplerenone (Inspra)	Antihypertensive, heart failure	Tab: 25, 50 mg	HTN: 50 mg PO qd CHF: 25–50 mg PO qd
Eprosartan (Teveten)	Antihypertensive	Tab: 400, 600 mg	400–600 mg PO qd
Erythromycin (*multiple*)	Antibiotic	Tab: 250, 500 mg SR-Tab: 250, 333, 500 mg SR-Cap: 250 mg Susp: 200, 400 mg/5 ml	Tab: 250 mg PO q6h, 333 mg PO q8h, 500 mg PO q12h Susp: 400 mg PO q6h, 800 mg PO q12h Legionnaire's Disease: 250–1000 mg PO qid
Esomeprazole	Proton pump inhibitor	SR-Cap: 20, 40 mg	20–40 mg PO qd
Eszopiclone (Lunesta)	Hypnotic	Tab: 1, 2, 3 mg	Nonelderly adults: 2 mg PO hs Elderly: 1 mg PO hs
Ethambutol (Myambutol)	Antituberculous	Tab: 100, 400 mg	Initial: 15 mg/kg PO qd Retreatment: 25 mg/kg PO qd, after 60 d, decrease to 15 mg/kg PO qd
Famciclovir (Famvir)	Antiviral	Tab: 125, 250, 500 mg	500 mg PO q8h for 7 d
Famotidine (Pepcid)	H_2-antagonist	Tab: 10, 20, 40 mg Pwd: 40 mg/5 ml	10–20 mg PO bid or 40 mg PO qhs
Felodipine (Plendil)	Antihypertensive	SR-Tab: 2.5, 5, 10 mg	2.5–10 mg PO qd
Flecainide (Tambocor)	Antiarrhythmic	Tab: 50, 100, 150 mg	Initially 100–150 mg PO bid, increasing by 50 mg PO bid increments every 4 d Adjust dose monitoring serum concentrations

(continued)

Selected Oral Drug Doses *(continued)*

Generic Name (Trade Name)	Therapeutic Category	Preparation	Usual Adult Dose/Comments
Fluconazole (Diflucan)	Antifungal	Tab: 50, 100, 150, 200 mg Susp: 10, 40 mg/ml	200 mg initially, then 100 mg PO qd
Fosamprenavir (Lexiva)	Antiretroviral	Tab: 700 mg	700–1,400 mg PO qd with or without ritonavir
Fosinopril (Monopril)	Antihypertensive, HF	Tab: 10, 20, 40 mg	HTN/HF: 10–40 mg/d in 1 or 2 doses
Furosemide (Lasix)	Loop diuretic	Tab: 20, 40, 80 mg Liq: 10 mg/ml, 40 mg/5 ml	10–80 mg PO bid
Gabapentin (Neurontin)	Anticonvulsant	Cap: 100, 300, 400 mg	300 mg PO on day 1; 300 mg PO bid on day 2; 300 mg PO tid on day 3; up to 1,800 mg/d divided tid
Ganciclovir (Cytovene)	Antiviral	Cap: 250 mg	Cytomegalovirus retinitis maintenance dosing: 1,000 mg PO tid with food or 500 mg PO 6 × /d (q3h while awake) with food
Gatifloxacin (Tequin)	Antibiotic	Tab: 200, 400 mg	200–400 mg PO qd Oral doses should be at least 2 h before or after antacids containing magnesium or aluminum, as well as sucralfate, metal cations such as iron, and multivitamins containing zinc
Gemifloxacin (Factive)	Antibiotic	Tab: 320 mg	320 mg PO qd
Glimepiride (Amaryl)	Hypoglycemic	Tab: 1, 2, 4 mg	1–4 mg PO qd
Glipizide (Glucotrol, Glucotrol XL)	Hypoglycemic	Tab: 5, 10 mg SR-Tab: 5, 10 mg	Tab: 5 mg PO q AM before breakfast, increasing to 15 mg/d divided bid prn SR-Tab: 5 mg PO q AM with breakfast, increasing to 10 mg PO q AM prn
Glyburide (Diabeta, Micronase)	Hypoglycemic	Tab: 1.25, 2.5, 5 mg	Tab: Initial: 1.25–5 mg PO q AM with breakfast
Glyburide micronized (Glynase PresTab)		PresTab: 1.5, 3, 6 mg	Maintenance: 1.25 to 20 mg/d in single or divided doses PresTab: Initial: 0.75 to 3 mg PO q AM with breakfast. Maintenance: 0.75 to 12 mg PO in single or divided doses

(continued)

Selected Oral Drug Doses *(continued)*

Generic Name (Trade Name)	Therapeutic Category	Preparation	Usual Adult Dose/Comments
Granisetron (Kytril)	Antiemetic	Tab: 1.12 mg (1 mg as the base)	1 mg PO bid, with the first dose given up to 1 h before highly emetogenic chemotherapy, and the 2nd dose given 12 h after the first dose
Haloperidol (Haldol)	Antipsychotic	Tab: 0.5, 1, 2, 5, 10, 20 mg Liq: 2, 5 mg/ml	0.5–5 mg PO bid-tid
Hydralazine (Apresoline)	Antihypertensive	Tab: 10, 25, 50, 100 mg	10–50 mg PO qid
Hydrochlorothiazide (*multiple*)	Thiazide diuretic	Tab: 25, 50, 100 mg Liq: 50 mg/5 ml, 100 mg/ml	25–100 mg PO qd
Hydrocortisone (*multiple*)	Corticosteroid	Tab: 5, 10, 20 mg	10–240 mg/d depending on disease being treated
Hydromorphone (Dilaudid)	Opioid analgesic	Tab: 1, 2, 3, 4, mg Liq: 1 mg/ml	1–2 mg PO q4–6h prn titrating dose to severity of pain
Hydroxyzine (Atarax, Vistaril)	Antihistamine, sedative, antianxiety	Tab/Cap: 10, 25, 50, 100 mg Syr: 10 mg/5 ml Susp: 25 mg/5 ml	Pruritis: 25 mg PO tid-qid Sedation/antianxiety: 10–100 mg PO qid
Ibuprofen (Motrin, Advil)	NSAID	Tab: 200, 300, 400, 600, 800 mg Susp: 100 mg/5 ml	Analgesia: 200–600 mg PO qid Arthritis: 300–800 mg PO tid-qid
Indapamide (Lozol)	Thiazide-like diuretic	Tab: 1.25, 2.5 mg	1.25–5 mg PO qd
Indinavir (Crixivan)	Antiviral	Cap: 100, 200, 333, 400 mg	800 mg PO tid on empty stomach or with light low fat meals; drink plenty of water
Indomethacin (Indocin)	NSAID	Cap: 25, 50 mg Susp: 25 mg/5 ml Suppos: 50 mg	25–50 mg PO bid-qid
Irbesartan (Avapro)	Antihypertensive	Tab: 75, 150, 300 mg	150–300 mg PO qd
Isoniazid (*multiple*)	Antituberculous	Tab: 50, 100, 300 mg Liq: 50 mg/5 ml	300 mg PO qd
Isosorbide dinitrate (Isordil, Sorbitrate, Dilatrate SR)	Antianginal	Tab: 5, 10, 20, 30, 40 mg SL-Tab: 2.5, 5, 10 mg SR-Tab: 40 mg	Tab: 5–40 mg PO q6h SL-Tab: 2.5–10 mg SL q2–3h SR-Tab: 20–80 mg PO q8–12h (40 mg tablets are scored and may be broken in half) SR-Cap: 40–80 mg PO q8–12h
Isosorbide mononitrate (Ismo, Monoket, Imdur)	Antianginal	Tab: 10, 20 mg SR-Tab: 60 mg	Tab: 20 mg PO bid with the two doses given 7 h apart SR-Tab: 30–120 mg PO qd
Isradipine (Dynacirc)	Antihypertensive	Cap: 2.5, 5 mg	2.5–10 mg PO bid

(continued)

Generic Name (Trade Name)	Therapeutic Category	Preparation	Usual Adult Dose/Comments
Itraconazole (Sporanox)	Antifungal	Cap: 200 mg Liq: 50 mg/5 ml	Cap: 200–400 mg PO qd with meals Liq: 200–400 mg PO qd on empty stomach
Ketoconazole (Nizoral)	Antifungal	Tab: 200 mg	200–400 mg PO qd
Ketorolac (Toradol)	NSAID	Tab: 10 mg	Indicated only as continuation therapy to parenteral ketorolac; maximum combined duration of use (parenteral and oral) 5 d 10 mg PO q6h not to exceed 40 mg/d
Labetalol (Normodyne, Trandate)	Antihypertensive	Tab; 100, 200, 300 mg	100–400 mg PO bid
Lactulose (Cephulac, Chronulac)	Laxative	Syr: 10 g/15 ml	15–60 ml/dose qd-tid
Lamivudine (Epivir)	Antiviral	Tab: 100, 150, 300 mg Liq: 5, 10 mg/ml	≥50 kg; 150 mg PO bid in combination with zidovudine <50 kg; 2 mg/kg PO bid in combination with zidovudine
Lamotrigine (Lamictal)	Anticonvulsant	Tab: 25, 50, 150, 200 mg	Patients on enzyme-inducing agents but not valproate: 50 mg PO qd for 2 wk, then 50 mg PO bid for 2 wk, then 300–500 mg/d divided bid Patients on enzyme-inducing agents including valproate: 25 mg PO qod for 2 wk, then 25 mg PO qd for 2 wk, then 100–150 mg/d divided bid
Lansoprazole (Prevacid)	Proton pump inhibitor	SR-Cap; 15, 30 mg SR-Tab, orally disintegrating: 15, 30 mg SR-granules for oral suspension: 15, 30 mg	15–60 mg PO qd
Levofloxacin (Levaquin)	Antibiotic	Tab: 250, 500, 750 mg Oral soln: 25 mg/ml	250–750 mg PO qd Oral doses should be at least 2 h before or after antacids containing magnesium or aluminum, as well as sucralfate, metal cations such as iron, and multivitamins containing zinc

(continued)

Selected Oral Drug Doses *(continued)*

Generic Name (Trade Name)	Therapeutic Category	Preparation	Usual Adult Dose/Comments
Levothyroxine (Synthroid, Levothroid)	Thyroid hormone	Tab: 25, 50, 75, 88, 100, 112, 125, 137, 150, 175, 200, 300 μg	Initial dose: 25–50 μg/d increasing to 100–200 μg/d with monitoring of T_4 and TSH levels
Linezolid (Zyvox)	Antibiotic	Tab: 400, 600 mg PWD for Susp: 100 mg/5 ml	400–600 mg PO bid
Liothyronine (Cytomel)	Thyroid hormone	Tab: 5, 25, 50 μg	25 μg initially, increase up to 25–75 μg qd
Lisinopril (Prinivil, Zestril)	Antihypertensive, heart failure	Tab: 2.5, 5, 10, 20, 40 mg	2.5–40 mg PO qd
Loperamide (Imodium)	Antidiarrheal	Cap/Tab: 2 mg Liq: 1 mg/5 ml	4 mg PO initially, then 2 mg PO after each loose stool to a maximum of 8 mg/d
Lorazepam (Ativan)	Sedative-hypnotic	Tab: 0.5, 1, 2 mg Liq: 2 mg/ml	Antianxiety: 0.5–3 mg PO bid-tid Hypnotic: 0.5–4 mg PO hs
Losartan (Cozaar)	Antihypertensive	Tab: 25, 50, 100 mg	25–100 mg PO qd Initial dose for patients on diuretics 25 mg PO qd
Meperidine (Demerol)	Opioid analgesic	Tab: 50, 100 mg Syr: 50 mg/5 ml	50–150 mg PO q3–4h prn
Metformin (Glucophage)	Hypoglycemic	Tab: 500, 850 mg	500 mg: PO bid with morning and evening meals up to 2,500 mg/d divided bid 850 mg: PO q AM with morning meal up to 2,550 mg/d divided bid Should not be used in patients with renal disease or dysfunction and should be avoided in patients with clinical or laboratory evidence of hepatic disease
Methadone (Dolophine)	Opioid analgesic	Tab: 5, 10 mg Liq: 5, 10 mg/5 ml, 10 mg/ml, 10 mg/10 ml	2.5–10 mg PO q3–4h prn
Methyldopa (Aldomet)	Antihypertensive	Tab: 125, 250, 500 mg Susp: 250 mg/5 ml	250–500 mg PO bid-qid
Methylprednisolone (Medrol)	Corticosteroid	Tab: 2, 4, 8, 16, 24, 32 mg	4–48 mg/d depending on disease being treated
Metoclopramide (Reglan)	GI motility, antiemetic	Tab: 5, 10 mg Syr: 5 mg/5 ml	5–15 mg PO qid
Metolazone (Zaroxolyn)	Thiazide-like diuretic	Tab: 0.5, 2.5, 5, 10 mg	2.5–20 mg PO qd

(continued)

Generic Name (Trade Name)	Therapeutic Category	Preparation	Usual Adult Dose/Comments
Metoprolol (Lopressor, Toprol XL)	Antihypertensive antianginal	Tab: 50, 100 mg SR-Tab: 50, 100, 200 mg (equal to 47.5, 95, 190 mg of metoprolol)	Tab: 25–200 mg PO bid SR-Tab: 50–200 mg PO qd
Metronidazole (Flagyl)	Antibiotic	Tab: 250, 500 mg	250–500 mg PO tid
Mexiletine (Mexitil)	Antiarrhythmic	Cap: 150, 200, 250 mg	200 mg PO q8h with food Adjust dose monitoring serum concentrations
Minoxidil (Loniten)	Antihypertensive	Tab: 2.5, 10 mg	5–40 mg PO qd in single or divided doses bid
Moexipril (Univasc)	Antihypertensive	Tab: 7.5, 15 mg	7.5–30 mg/d in 1 or 2 doses 1h before meals
Montelukast (Singulair)	Leukotriene receptor antagonist	Tab: 10 mg Chew tab: 4, 5 mg Granules: 4 mg	10 mg PO qd
Moricizine (Ethmozine)	Antiarrhythmic	Tab: 200, 250, 300 mg	200–300 mg PO q8h
Morphine **Morphine sustained-release (MS-Contin, Kadian, Oramorph-SR)**	Opiate analgesic	Tab: 15, 30 mg Liq: 2, 4, 20 mg/ml, 10, 20 mg/5 ml SR-Tab: 15, 30, 60, 100, 200 mg SR-Cap: 20, 50, 100 mg Suppos: 5, 10, 20, 30 mg	Tab/Liq/Suppos: 10–30 mg PO/PR q4h prn SR-Tab: 15–30 mg PO q12h initially, then adjust dose and interval according to the requirements of individual patient SR-Cap: 20 mg PO qd initially, then adjust dose and interval according to the requirements of individual patient
Moxifloxacin (Avelox)	Antibiotic	Tab: 400 mg	400 mg PO qd
Mycophenolate (CellCept, Myfortic)	Immunosuppressive	Cap: 250 mg Tab: 500 mg SR-Tab: 180 mg Pwd for susp: 200 mg	1,000–1,500 mg PO bid SR-Tab: 720 mg PO bid
Nadolol (Corgard)	Antihypertensive, antianginal	Tab; 20, 40, 80, 120, 160 mg	20–160 mg PO qd
Nelfinavir (Viracept)	Antiviral	Tab: 250, 625 mg Pwd: 50 mg/g	750 mg PO tid with food or 1250 mg PO bid
Nevirapine (Viramune)	Antiviral	Tab: 200 mg Susp: 10 mg/ml	200 mg PO qd × 14 d, then 200 mg PO bid
Nicardipine (Cardene)	Antihypertensive, antianginal	Cap: 20, 30 mg SR-Cap: 30, 45, 60 mg	Cap: 20–40 mg PO tid SR-Cap: 30–60 mg PO bid
Nifedipine (Adalat Procardia)	Antihypertensive, antianginal	Cap: 10, 20 mg SR-Tab: 30, 60, 90 mg	Cap: 10–30 mg PO tid SR-Tab: 30–90 mg PO qd

(continued)

Selected Oral Drug Doses *(continued)*

Generic Name (Trade Name)	Therapeutic Category	Preparation	Usual Adult Dose/Comments
Nifedipine sustained release (Adalat CC, Procardia XL)			
Nimodipine (Nimotop)	Subarachnoid hemorrhage	Cap: 30 mg	60 mg PO q4h, beginning within 96 h after a subarachnoid hemorrhage and continuing for 21 d
Nitroglycerin (*Multiple*)	Antianginal	SL-Tab: 0.15, 0.3, 0.4, 0.6 mg SL-spray: 0.4 mg/dose SR-Cap: 2.5, 6.5, 9, 13 mg SR-Tab: 2.6, 6.5, 9 mg SR-buccal Tab: 1, 2, 3 mg Top: 2% ointment (NTG 15 mg/in) Patch: 0.1, 0.2, 0.3, 0.4, 0.6, 0.8 mg/h	SL-Tab: 0.15–0.6 mg under tongue q5min as needed for relief of chest pain SL-spray: 0.4–0.8 mg on or under tongue q5min as needed for relief of chest pain SR-Cap: 2.5–9 mg PO q8–12h SR-Tab: 1.3–6.5 mg PO q8–12h SR-buccal Tab: 1–3 mg dissolved in place on oral mucosa q5h while awake Top: 0.5–2 in q6–8h Patch: 0.1–0.8 mg/h patch q24h, removing the patch for a 10–12 h nitrate free period before applying the next patch
Olmesartan (Benicar)	Antihypertensive	Tab: 5, 20, 40 mg	20–40 mg PO qd
Omeprazole (Prilosec)	Proton pump inhibitor	SR-Tab: 20 mg SR-Cap: 10, 20, 40 mg Powder for oral susp: 20, 40 mg	20 mg PO qd up to 80 mg/d divided bid
Ondansetron (Zofran)	Antiemetic	Tab: 4, 8 mg	Administer first dose (4–8 mg) 30 min before start of chemotherapy, with subsequent doses 4 h and 8 h after first dose, then 4–8 mg PO tid for 1–2 d after completion of chemotherapy
Opium, tincture, deodorized	Antidiarrheal	Liq: 10% (morphine 6 mg/0.6 ml)	0.2–0.6 ml qd-qid
Oseltamivir (Tamiflu)	Antiviral	Cap: 75 mg Powder for Susp: 12 mg/ml	75 mg PO bid for 5 d
Oxacillin (*multiple*)	Antibiotic	Cap: 250, 500 mg Susp: 250 mg/5 ml	500–1,000 mg PO q4–6h
Oxazepam (Serax)	Sedative-hypnotic	Cap: 10, 15, 30 mg Tab: 15 mg	Sedative: 10–30 mg PO tid-qid Hypnotic: 10–30 mg PO hs

(continued)

Selected Oral Drug Doses *(continued)*

Generic Name (Trade Name)	Therapeutic Category	Preparation	Usual Adult Dose/Comments
Oxybutynin (Ditropan)	Urinary antispasmodic	Tab: 5 mg Syr: 5 mg/5 ml	5 mg PO tid
Oxycodone (*multiple*)	Opioid analgesic	Tab: 5 mg Liq: 5 mg/5 ml, 20 mg/ml	10–30 mg PO q4h prn
Pantoprazole (Protonix)	Proton pump inhibitor	SR-Tab: 20, 40 mg	20–40 mg PO qd
Paregoric	Antidiarrheal	Liq: morphine 2 mg/5 ml	5–10 ml PO qd-qid
Penicillin VK (*Multiple*)	Antibiotic	Tab: 125, 250, 500 mg Susp: 125, 250 mg/5 ml	250–500 mg PO qid
Pentobarbital (Nembutal)	Hypnotic	Cap: 50, 100 mg Elixir: 20 mg/5 ml Suppos: 30, 60, 120, 200 mg	Cap/elixir: Hypnotic: 100 mg PO qhs Pre-op: 100 mg PO 1–2 h preprocedure Suppos: 120–200 mg PR qhs
Perindopril (Aceon)	Antihypertensive	Tab: 2, 4, 8 mg	2–16 mg PO qd
Phenazopyridine (Pyridium)	Urinary analgesic	Tab: 100, 200 mg	100–200 mg PO tid
Phenobarbital (*multiple*)	Anticonvulsant, sedative	Tab: 15, 30, 60, 100 mg Elixir: 15, 20 mg/5 ml	Sedative: 30–100 mg/d divided in 3 doses Hypnotic: 30–200 mg PO hs Anticonvulsant: 30–200 mg/d in single or divided doses Adjust dose monitoring serum concentrations
Phenoxybenzamine (Dibenzyline)	Antihypertensive	Cap: 10 mg	10 mg PO bid up to 40 mg bid-tid
Phenytoin (Dilantin)	Anticonvulsant	Cap: 30, 100 mg Tab: 50 mg Susp: 25 mg/ml	100 mg PO tid Only the Dilantin brand of phenytoin sodium may be given in a single daily dose Adjust dose monitoring serum concentrations
Phosphate, potassium phosphate (K-Phos Original, Neutra-Phos-K), potassium and sodium phosphate (K-Phos M.F., Neutra-Phos)	Electrolyte replacement	*Potassium phosphate*: Tab: K-Phos Original: PO_4 114 mg (3.7 mmol), K 3.7 mEq Cap: Neutra-Phos-K: PO_4 250 mg (8 mmol), K 14.25 mEq *Potassium and sodium phosphate*: Cap: Neutra-Phos: PO_4 250 mg (8 mmol), K 7.125 mEq, Na 7.125 mEq Tab: K-Phos M.F.: PO_4 125.6 mg (4 mmol), K 1.14 mEq, Na 2.9 mEq	1 g (228 mg or 7.4 mmol) PO qid with meals and at bedtime Must be thoroughly dissolved in 180–240 ml water

(continued)

Selected Oral Drug Doses *(continued)*

Generic Name (Trade Name)	Therapeutic Category	Preparation	Usual Adult Dose/Comments
Pindolol (Visken)	Antihypertensive	Tab: 5, 10 mg	5 mg PO bid up 60 mg/d divided bid
Potassium chloride (*multiple*)	Electrolyte replacement	SR-Tab: 6, 8, 10, 20 mEq SR-Cap: 8, 10 mEq Liq: 10, 20, 30, 40 mEq/15 ml Packets: 10, 15, 20, 25 mEq	Hypokalemia (treatment or prophylaxis): 10–40 mEq PO qd-qid, with titration as needed Oral solution and powder must be diluted and stirred in 60–180 ml water before swallowing; these dosage forms may also be added to orange, tomato, or apple juice Sustained-release tablets without a wax matrix may be swallowed whole or broken Sustained-release capsules may be opened and sprinkled on food Some sustained-release products utilize a wax matrix from which the drug is slowly leached out as it passes through the GI tract; the expended wax matrix may appear intact in the stool
Prazosin (Minipress)	Antihypertensive	Cap: 1, 2, 5 mg	1 mg PO bid-tid up to 20 mg/d divided tid
Prednisolone (*multiple*)	Corticosteroid	Tab: 5 mg Syr: 15 mg/5 ml	5–60 mg/day depending on disease being treated
Prednisone (*Multiple*)	Corticosteroid	Tab: 1, 2.5, 5, 10, 20, 50 mg Liq: 5 mg/5 ml, 5 mg/ml	5–60 mg/day depending on disease being treated
Primidone (Mysoline)	Anticonvulsant	Tab: 50, 250 mg Susp: 250 mg/5 ml	250 mg PO tid Adjust those monitoring serum concentrations
Procainamide (Pronestyl), Procainamide sustained-release (Procan-SR, Pronestyl-SR)	Antiarrhythmic	Tab/cap: 250, 375, 500 mg SR-Tab: 250, 500, 750, 1,000 mg	Cap: up to 50 mg/kg/d in divided doses q3h SR-Tab: 50 mg/kg/day in divided doses q6–12h Some sustained-release products utilize a wax matrix from which the drug is slowly leached out as it passes through the GI tract; the expended wax matrix may appear intact in the stool Adjust dose monitoring serum concentrations

(continued)

Selected Oral Drug Doses *(continued)*

Generic Name (Trade Name)	Therapeutic Category	Preparation	Usual Adult Dose/Comments
Prochlorperazine (Compazine)	Antiemetic	Tab: 5, 10, 25 mg Syr: 5 mg/5 ml SR-Cap: 10, 15, 30 mg Suppos: 2.5, 5, 25 mg	Tab/Syr: 5–10 mg PO tid-qid SR-Cap: 10–30 mg PO q12h Suppos: 25 mg PR q12h
Promethazine (Phenergan)	Antiemetic	Tab: 12.5, 25, 50 mg Syr: 6.25, 25 mg/5 ml Suppos: 12.5, 25, 50 mg	Tab/Syr/Suppos: 12.5–50 mg PO/PR q4–6h prn
Propafenone (Rythmol)	Antiarrhythmic	Tab: 150, 225, 300 mg SR-Cap: 225, 325, 425 mg	150–300 mg PO q8h SR: 225–425 mg q12h
Propoxyphene HCl (Darvon)	Opioid analgesic	Cap: 32, 65 mg	32–65 mg PO q4h prn
Propranolol (Inderal, Inderal LA)	Antihypertensive, antianginal	Tab: 10, 20, 30, 40, 80, 90 mg SR-Cap: 60, 80, 120, 160 mg Liq: 4, 8, 80 mg/ml	Tab/Liq: 10–40 mg PO tid-qid up to 240 mg/d divided tid-qid Postmyocardial infarction: 180–240 mg/d divided tid-qid SR-Cap: 60–240 mg PO qd
Pyrazinamide (*Multiple*)	Antituberculous	Tab: 500 mg	15–30 mg/kg up to 2 g PO qd
Pyrimethamine (Daraprim)	Antiparasitic	Tab: 25 mg	Toxoplasmosis: 50–75 mg PO qd with 1–4 g of sulfadiazine, continued for 1–3 wk, decrease by 50% and continued for an additional 4–5 wk
Quinidine gluconate (Quinaglute)	Antiarrhythmic	SR-Tab: 324 mg	324–648 mg PO q6–12h Adjust dose monitoring serum concentrations Contains 62% quinidine alkaloid
Quinidine polygalacturonate (Cardioquin)	Antiarrhythmic	Tab: 275 mg	275 mg PO bid-tid Adjust dose monitoring serum concentrations Contains 60% quinidine alkaloid
Quinidine sulfate (*multiple*), Quinidine sulfate sustained-release (Quinidex)	Antiarrhythmic	Tab: 200, 300 mg SR-Tab: 300 mg	Tab/SR-Tab: 200–600 mg PO q6–8h Adjust dose monitoring serum concentrations Contains 83% quinidine alkaloid
Quinapril (Accupril)	Antihypertensive, heart failure	Tab: 5, 10, 20, 40 mg	HTN: 10–80 mg/d in 1 or 2 doses HF: 5 mg PO bid to 40 mg/d in 1 or 2 doses

(continued)

Selected Oral Drug Doses *(continued)*

Generic Name (Trade Name)	Therapeutic Category	Preparation	Usual Adult Dose/Comments
Rabeprazole (Aciphex)	Proton pump inhibitor	SR-Tab: 20 mg	20 mg PO qd
Ramipril (Altace)	Antihypertensive, HF, MI	Cap: 1.25, 2.5, 5, 10 mg	HTN: 2.5–20 mg/d in 1 or 2 doses HF: 2.5 mg PO bid to 5 mg PO bid MI: 1.25 mg PO qd to 2.5 mg PO bid
Ranitidine (Zantac)	H_2-antagonist	Tab: 75, 150, 300 mg Cap: 150, 300 mg Syr: 75 mg/5 ml Effervescent tab: 150 mg Effervescent granules: 150 mg/packet	150 mg PO bid or 300 mg PO qd
Rifabutin (Mycobutin)	Antituberculous	Cap: 150 mg	300 mg PO qd
Rifampin (Rifadin)	Antituberculous	Cap: 150, 300 mg	300–600 mg PO qd
Rifapentine (Priftin)	Antituberculous	Tab: 150 mg	Intensive phase: 600 mg PO twice weekly for 2 mo Continuation phase: 600 mg PO once weekly for 4 mo
Rimantadine (Flumadine)	Antiviral	Tab: 100 mg Syr: 50 mg/5 ml	Influenza: Prophylaxis: 100 mg PO bid Treatment: 100 mg PO bid starting within 48 h of symptoms and continuing for 7 d
Ritonavir (Norvir)	Antiviral	Cap: 100 mg Liq: 80 mg/ml	600 mg PO bid
Salsalate (Disalcid)	NSAID	Tab: 500, 750 mg Cap: 500 mg	1,500 mg PO bid or 1,000 mg PO tid
Saquinavir (Invirase)	Antiviral	Cap: 200 mg	600 mg PO tid within 2 h of food and in combination with zidovudine or zalcitabine
Simethicone (Mylicon, Phazyme, Mylanta Gas)	Antiflatulent	Tab: 60, 95 mg Chewable tab: 40, 80, 125 mg Gelcap: 62.5, 125 mg Liq: 40 mg/0.6 ml	40–125 mg PO qd after meals
Sirolimus (Rapamune)	Immunosuppressive	Tab: 1, 2 mg Soln: 1 mg/ml	6 mg loading dose followed by 2 mg PO qd
Sodium polystyrene sulfonate (Kayexalate)	Potassium removing resin	Pwd: 10–12 g/heaping teaspoon Susp: 15 gm/60 ml	15–60 g PO, repeat as necessary to lower serum potassium level
Sotalol (Betapace)	Antiarrhythmic	Tab: 80, 160, 240 mg	80–160 mg PO bid
Spironolactone (Aldactone)	Potassium sparing diuretic	Tab: 25, 50, 100 mg	25–100 mg PO qd or in divided doses

(continued)

Selected Oral Drug Doses *(continued)*

Generic Name (Trade Name)	Therapeutic Category	Preparation	Usual Adult Dose/Comments
Stavudine (Zerit)	Antiviral	Cap: 15, 20, 30, 40 mg Pwd for soln: 1 mg/ml SR-Cap: 37.5, 50, 75, 100 mg	40 mg PO q12h 50 mg PO qd
Sucralfate (Carafate)	Antiulcer	Tab: 1 g Susp: 1 g/10 ml	1 g PO qid on empty stomach
Tacrolimus (Prograf)	Immunosuppressant	Cap: 0.5, 1, 5 mg	0.15–0.3 mg/kd/d PO in q12h divided doses; administer initial dose no sooner than 6 h after transplantation; if IV therapy was initiated, begin 8–12 h after discontinuing IV therapy
Telithromycin (Ketek)	Antibiotic	Tab: 400 mg	800 mg PO qd
Telmisartan (Micardis)	Antihypertensive	Tab: 20, 40, 80 mg	20–80 mg PO qd
Temazepam (Restoril)	Hypnotic	Cap: 7.5, 15, 30 mg	7.5–30 mg PO hs
Terazosin (Hytrin)	Antihypertensive	Cap: 1, 2, 5, 10 mg	1–10 mg PO qhs
Terbutaline (Brethine, Bricanyl)	Bronchodilator	Tab 2.5, 5 mg	2.5–5 mg PO tid
Tetracycline (*multiple*)	Antibiotic	Cap: 250, 500 mg Syr: 125 mg/5 ml	250–500 mg PO qid
Theophylline (Elixophyllin, Slo-phyllin, Theolair), sustained-release (Slo-Bid, Theo-Dur, Theo-24, Uni-Dur)	Bronchodilator	Theophylline Cap: 100, 200, 300 mg Tab: 100, 125, 200, 250, 300 mg Liq: 27 mg/5 ml SR-Tab: 100, 200, 250, 300, 400, 450, 500, 600 mg SR-Cap: 50, 75, 100, 125, 200, 250, 260, 300, 400 mg	Initially 300 mg/d; if tolerated, the dose may be increased after 3 d to 400 mg/d; and then if necessary after 3 d to 600 mg/d; depending on product selected, dosing interval may be 6, 8, or 12 h; dose and interval should be adjusted using serum levels
Ticlopidine (Ticlid)	Antiplatelet	Tab: 250 mg	250 mg PO bid with meals Contraindicated in patients with liver disease
Timolol (Blocadren)	Antihypertensive myocardial	Tab: 5, 10, 20 mg	10–20 mg PO bid Postmyocardial infarction: 100 mg PO bid
Topiramate (Topamax)	Anticonvulsant	Tab: 25, 100, 200 mg	200 mg PO bid
Torsemide (Demadex)	Loop diuretic	Tab: 5, 10, 20, 100 mg	5–20 mg PO qd to maximum 200 mg/d
Tramadol (Ultram)	Analgesic	Tab: 50 mg	50–100 mg PO q4–6h up to 400 mg/d
Trandolapril (Mavik)	Antihypertensive	Tab: 1, 2, 4 mg	1–8 mg PO qd

(continued)

Selected Oral Drug Doses *(continued)*

Generic Name (Trade Name)	Therapeutic Category	Preparation	Usual Adult Dose/Comments
Tranexamic acid (Cyklokapron)	Hemostatic	Tab: 500 mg	25 mg/kg PO tid-qid starting 1 d before surgery and continued for 2–8 d postsurgery
Triamterene (Dyrenium)	Potassium sparing diuretic	Cap: 50, 100 mg	50–100 mg PO bid
Trimethobenzamide (Tigan)	Antiemetic	Cap: 100, 250 mg Suppos: 200 mg	100–250 mg PO tid-qid Suppos: 200 mg PR tid-qid
Troglitazone (Rezulin)	Hypoglycemic	Tab: 200, 400 mg	400–600 mg PO qd
Valacyclovir (Valtrex)	Antiviral	Tab: 500 mg	1000 mg PO tid for 7 d
Valganciclovir (Valcyte)	Antiviral	Tab: 450 mg	900 mg PO qd-bid
Valproic acid (Depakene)	Anticonvulsant	Cap: 250 mg Syr: 250 mg/5 ml	15 mg/kg/day divided bid-tid to maximum 60 mg/kg/d Adjust dose monitoring serum concentrations
Valsartan (Diovan)	Antihypertensive	Cap: 40, 80, 160, 320 mg	80–320 mg PO qd
Vancomycin (Vancocin)	Antibiotic	Cap: 125, 250 mg Liq: 125, 250 mg/5 ml	*Clostridium difficile*: 125 mg PO q6h for 7–10 d Oral solution may be prepared using the injection dose form
Verapamil (Calan, Isoptin), Verapamil sustained release (Calan-SR, Isoptin-SR)	Antihypertensive, antianginal	Tab: 40, 80, 120 mg SR-Tab/Cap: 120, 180, 240 mg	Tab: 20–120 mg PO qid SR-Tab: 120 mg PO qd up to 240 mg PO q12h
Voriconazole (Vfend)	Antifungal	Tab: 50, 200 mg Oral Susp: 40 mg/ml	100–300 mg PO q12h
Warfarin (Coumadin)	Anticoagulant	Tab: 1, 2, 2.5, 4, 5, 7.5, 10 mg	5 mg PO qd × 3, then individualize dose based on PT or INR results
Zaleplon (Sonata)	Hypnotic	Cap: 5, 10 mg	5–10 mg PO hs Avoid doses >5 mg in the elderly
Zanamivir (Relenza)	Antiviral	Pwd for inhalation: 5 mg	10 mg inhaled bid × 5 days
Zidovudine (Retrovir)	Antiviral	Cap: 100, 300 mg Syr: 50 mg/5 ml	100 mg PO q4h (5–6 × /d)
Zafirlukast (Accolate)	Leukotriene receptor antagonist	Tab: 10, 20 mg	20 mg PO bid
Zolpidem (Ambien)	Hypnotic	Tab: 5, 10 mg	2.5–10 mg PO hs

Selected Combination Oral Drug Products

Brand Name (Ingredients)	Therapeutic Category	Preparation	Usual Adult Dose
Aggrenox (extended-release dipyridamole, aspirin)	Antiplatelet	Cap: Extended-release dipyridamole 200 mg, aspirin 25 mg	Stroke: 1 tablet bid
Augmentin (amoxicillin, clavulanic acid)	Antibiotic	Tab: Amoxicillin 250 mg, clavulanic acid 125 mg Amoxicillin 500 mg, clavulanic acid 125 mg Amoxicillin 875 mg, clavulanic acid 125 mg SR-Tab: Amoxicillin 1,000 mg, clavulanic acid 62.5 mg Chew Tab: Amoxicillin 125 mg, clavulanic acid 32.5 mg Amoxicillin 200 mg, clavulanic acid 28.5 mg Amoxicillin 250 mg, clavulanic acid 62.5 mg Amoxicillin 400 mg, clavulanic acid 57 mg Susp (per 5 ml): Amoxicillin 250 mg, clavulanic acid 62.5 mg Amoxicillin 400 mg, clavulanic acid 57 mg Amoxicillin 600 mg, clavulanic acid 42.9 mg	Augmentin 250–500 PO q8–12h Augmentin-XR 2 tablets q12h
Avandamet (rosiglitazone, metformin)	Antidiabetic agent	Tab: Rosiglitazone 1 mg, metformin 500 mg Rosiglitazone 2 mg, metformin 500 mg Rosiglitazone 2 mg, metformin 1,000 mg Rosiglitazone 4 mg, metformin 500 mg Rosiglitazone 4 mg, metformin 1,000 mg	1 mg/500 mg PO qd up to 8 mg/2,000 mg qd
Bactrim, Septra (sulfamethoxazole, trimethoprim)	Antibiotic	Tab: Sulfamethoxazole 400 mg, trimethoprim 80 mg DS Tab: Sulfamethoxazole 800 mg, trimethoprim 160 mg Susp (per 5 ml): Sulfamethoxazole 200 mg, trimethoprim 40 mg	1 Bactrim to 1 Bactrim DS tab (or equivalent susp volume) PO q12h *P. carinii* pneumonia treatment: 20 mg/kg/d trimethoprim divided q6h *P. carinii* pneumonia prophylaxis: 1 DS tablet or 20 ml of susp PO q24h

(continued)

Selected Combination Oral Drug Products *(continued)*

Brand Name (Ingredients)	Therapeutic Category	Preparation	Usual Adult Dose
Bicitra (sodium citrate, citric acid)	Electrolyte replacement, systemic alkalinizer	Liq (per 5 ml): Sodium citrate 500 mg, citric acid 334 mg (Each 1 ml delivers 1 mEq of Na and the equivalent of 1 mEq of bicarbonate)	Systemic alkalinizer: 10–30 ml diluted in 30–90 ml water qid, after meal and at bedtime, the dose being titrated as needed Neutralizing buffer; 15–30 ml as a single dose; may be diluted in 15–30 ml water
Darvocet-N (propoxyphene napsylate, acetaminophen)	Analgesic	Tab: Darvocet-N 50: Propoxyphene napsylate 50 mg, acetaminophen 325 mg Darvocet-N 100: Propoxyphene napsylate 100 mg, acetaminophen 650 mg	1–2 tabs PO q4–6h prn pain
Dyazide (triamterene, hydrochlorothiazide)	Diuretic, antihypertensive	Cap: Triamterene 37.5 mg, hydrochlorothiazide 25 mg	1–2 cap PO qd
Fansidar (pyrimethamine, sulfadoxine)	Antimalarial	Tab: Sulfadoxine 500 mg, pyrimethamine 25 mg	Treatment of acute attack of malaria: 2–3 tablets with or without quinine Malaria prophylaxis: 1 tablet PO weekly or 2 tablets once every 2 wk
Glucovance (glyburide, metformin)	Antidiabetic agent	Tab: Glyburide 1.25 mg, metformin 250 mg Glyburide 2.5 mg, metformin 500 mg Glyburide 5 mg, metformin 500 mg	1.25/250 mg PO qd-bid up to 20 mg/2,000 mg/d
Lomotil (diphenoxylate, atropine)	Antidiarrheal	Tab: Diphenoxylate 2.5 mg, atropine 0.025 mg Liq (per 5 ml): Diphenoxylate 2.5 mg, atropine 0.025 mg	Tab: 2 tabs PO qid until control of diarrhea is achieved Liq: 10 ml PO qid until control of diarrhea is achieved
Maxzide (triamterene, hydrochlorothiazide)	Diuretic, antihypertensive	Tab: Maxzide-25: Triamterene 37.5 mg, hydrochlorothiazide 25 mg Maxzide: Triamterene 75 mg, hydrochlorothiazide 50 mg	Maxzide-25: 1–2 tabs PO qd Maxzide: 1 tab PO qd

(continued)

Selected Combination Oral Drug Products *(continued)*

Brand Name (Ingredients)	Therapeutic Category	Preparation	Usual Adult Dose
Metaglip (glipizide, metformin)	Antidiabetic agent	Tab: Glipizide 2.5 mg, metformin 250 mg Glipizide 2.5 mg, metformin 500 mg Glipizide 5 mg, metformin 500 mg	2.5 mg/250 mg PO once daily with a meal up 20 mg/ 2,000 mg/d
Percocet (oxycodone HCl, acetaminophen)	Analgesic	Tab: Oxycodone HCl 5 mg, acetaminophen 325 mg	1 tab PO q6h prn pain
Percodan (oxycodone HCl, oxycodone terephthalate, aspirin)	Analgesic	Tab: Oxycodone HCl 4.5 mg, oxycodone terephthalate 0.038 mg, aspirin 325 mg	1 tab PO q6h prn pain
Polycitra (sodium citrate, potassium citrate, citric acid)	Electrolyte replacement, systemic alkalinizer	Liq (per 5 ml): Sodium citrate 500 mg, potassium citrate 500 mg, citric acid 334 mg (Each 1 ml delivers 1 mEq of Na, 1 mEq of K, and the equivalent of 2 mEq of bicarbonate)	Systemic alkalinizer: 10–30 ml diluted in 30–90 ml water qid, after meals and at bedtime, the dose being titrated as needed Neutralizing buffer: 15–30 ml as a single dose; may be diluted in 15–30 ml water
Trilisate (choline magnesium salicylate, magnesium salicylate)	NSAID	Tab: 500 mg tablet: Choline salicylate 293 mg, magnesium salicylate 362 mg 750 mg tablet: Choline salicylate 400 mg, magnesium salicylate 544 mg 1,000 mg tablet: Choline salicylate 587 mg, magnesium salicylate 725 mg Liq: 500 mg/5 ml: Choline salicylate 293 mg, magnesium salicylate 362 mg	1,000–1,500 mg PO bid or 3,000 mg PO qhs
Tylenol with codeine (acetaminophen, codeine)	Analgesic	Tab: Tylenol #2: Acetaminophen 300 mg, codeine 15 mg Tylenol #3: Acetaminophen 300 mg, codeine 30 mg Tylenol #4: Acetaminophen 300 mg, codeine 60 mg Elixir (per 5 ml): Acetaminophen 120 mg, codeine 12 mg	Tylenol #2: 2–3 tabs PO q4h prn pain Tylenol #3: 1–2 tabs PO q4h prn pain Tylenol #4: 1 tab PO q4h prn pain Elixir: 15 ml PO q4h prn pain

(continued)

Selected Combination Oral Drug Products *(continued)*

Brand Name (Ingredients)	Therapeutic Category	Preparation	Usual Adult Dose
Vicodin, Vicodin ES (hydrocodone, acetaminophen)	Analgesic	Tab: Hydrocodone 5 mg, acetaminophen 500 mg ES tab: Hydrocodone 7.5 mg, acetaminophen 750 mg	Vicodin: 1–2 tabs PO q4h prn pain Vicodin ES: 1 tab PO q4h prn pain

BPH, benign prostatic hypertrophy; Cap, capsule; HF, heart failure; HTN, hypertension; Inj, injection; INR, international normalized ratio; Liq, liquid; MI, myocardial infarction; PO, by mouth; PR, per rectum; PT, prothrombin time; Pwd, powder; NSAID, nonsteroidal anti-inflammatory drug; NTG, nitroglycerin; SCr, serum creatinine; SL, sublingual; soln, solution; SR, sustained-release; Suppos, suppository; Susp, suspension; Syr, syrup; Tab, tablet; Top, topical

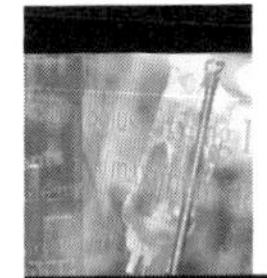

Index

B

C

F

H

I

K

N

O

S

T

U

V

W